Lecture Notes in Computer Science   11167

Commenced Publication in 1973
Founding and Former Series Editors:
Gerhard Goos, Juris Hartmanis, and Jan van Leeuwen

Editorial Board

David Hutchison
  Lancaster University, Lancaster, UK
Takeo Kanade
  Carnegie Mellon University, Pittsburgh, PA, USA
Josef Kittler
  University of Surrey, Guildford, UK
Jon M. Kleinberg
  Cornell University, Ithaca, NY, USA
Friedemann Mattern
  ETH Zurich, Zurich, Switzerland
John C. Mitchell
  Stanford University, Stanford, CA, USA
Moni Naor
  Weizmann Institute of Science, Rehovot, Israel
C. Pandu Rangan
  Indian Institute of Technology Madras, Chennai, India
Bernhard Steffen
  TU Dortmund University, Dortmund, Germany
Demetri Terzopoulos
  University of California, Los Angeles, CA, USA
Doug Tygar
  University of California, Berkeley, CA, USA
Gerhard Weikum
  Max Planck Institute for Informatics, Saarbrücken, Germany

More information about this series at http://www.springer.com/series/7412

Martin Reuter · Christian Wachinger
Hervé Lombaert · Beatriz Paniagua
Marcel Lüthi · Bernhard Egger (Eds.)

Shape in Medical Imaging

International Workshop, ShapeMI 2018
Held in Conjunction with MICCAI 2018
Granada, Spain, September 20, 2018
Proceedings

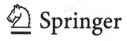
Springer

Editors
Martin Reuter (iD)
German Center for
Neurodegenerative Diseases
Bonn, Germany

and

Harvard Medical School
Boston, USA

Christian Wachinger (iD)
Ludwig Maximilian University of Munich
Munich, Germany

Hervé Lombaert (iD)
École de Technologie Supérieure
Montreal, QC, Canada

Beatriz Paniagua
Kitware Inc.
Carrboro, NC, USA

and

University of North Carolina at Chapel Hill
Chapel Hill, USA

Marcel Lüthi (iD)
University of Basel
Basel, Switzerland

Bernhard Egger (iD)
Massachusetts Institute of Technology
Cambridge, MA, USA

ISSN 0302-9743   ISSN 1611-3349   (electronic)
Lecture Notes in Computer Science
ISBN 978-3-030-04746-7   ISBN 978-3-030-04747-4   (eBook)
https://doi.org/10.1007/978-3-030-04747-4

Library of Congress Control Number: 2018962145

LNCS Sublibrary: SL6 – Image Processing, Computer Vision, Pattern Recognition, and Graphics

© Springer Nature Switzerland AG 2018
This work is subject to copyright. All rights are reserved by the Publisher, whether the whole or part of the material is concerned, specifically the rights of translation, reprinting, reuse of illustrations, recitation, broadcasting, reproduction on microfilms or in any other physical way, and transmission or information storage and retrieval, electronic adaptation, computer software, or by similar or dissimilar methodology now known or hereafter developed.
The use of general descriptive names, registered names, trademarks, service marks, etc. in this publication does not imply, even in the absence of a specific statement, that such names are exempt from the relevant protective laws and regulations and therefore free for general use.
The publisher, the authors, and the editors are safe to assume that the advice and information in this book are believed to be true and accurate at the date of publication. Neither the publisher nor the authors or the editors give a warranty, express or implied, with respect to the material contained herein or for any errors or omissions that may have been made. The publisher remains neutral with regard to jurisdictional claims in published maps and institutional affiliations.

This Springer imprint is published by the registered company Springer Nature Switzerland AG
The registered company address is: Gewerbestrasse 11, 6330 Cham, Switzerland

Preface

This volume contains the proceedings of the International Workshop on **Shape** in Medical Imaging (ShapeMI 2018) held in conjunction with the 21st International Conference on Medical Image Computing and Computer Assisted Intervention (MICCAI 2018) on September 20, 2018, in Granada, Spain. This workshop is a continuation of the previous MICCAI SeSAMI 2016 and SAMI 2015 Workshops as well as the Shape Symposium 2015 and 2014.

This workshop presented original methods and applications related to shape analysis and processing. It provided a venue for researchers working in shape modeling, analysis, statistics, classification, geometric learning, and their applications to share novel ideas, to present recent research results, and to interact with each other.

Today's image data usually represents 3D geometric structures, often describing continuous and time-varying phenomena. Therefore, shape and geometry processing methods have been receiving increased attention, for example, thanks to their higher sensitivity to local variations relative to traditional markers, such as the volume of a structure. Shape and spectral analysis, geometric learning and modeling algorithms, as well as application-driven research were the focus of this workshop. Shape analysis methods are broadly applicable to many different fields from medical image computing to paleontology, anthropology and beyond.

This workshop brought together medical imaging scientists to discuss novel approaches and applications in shape and geometry processing and their use in research and clinical studies and applications. Another aim was to explore novel, cutting-edge theoretical methods and their usefulness for medical applications, such as from the fields of geometric learning or spectral shape analysis. As a single-track workshop, ShapeMI featured excellent keynote speakers, technical paper presentations, and demonstrations of state-of-the-art software for shape processing in medical research.

We thank all the contributors to this workshop for making it such a huge success, with an audience of around 80 people throughout the day. We thank all authors who shared their latest findings, as well as the Program Committee members who contributed quality reviews in a very short time. We especially thank our keynote speakers, who kindly accepted our invitation and enriched the workshop with their excellent presentations: Stanley Durrleman (Co-Director of the Inria/ICM Aramis Lab at the Brain and Spine Institute within the Pitié-Salpêtrière Hospital in Paris), Michael Bronstein (Professor at USI Lugano, Italy, and at Imperial College London, UK), and Daniel Rueckert (Professor and Head of the Department of Computing at Imperial

College London, UK). We congratulate Kris M. Campbell and Thomas Fletcher, who received the best paper award, kindly sponsored by Kitware.

September 2018

Martin Reuter
Christian Wachinger
Hervé Lombaert
Beatriz Paniagua
Marcel Lüthi
Bernhard Egger

Organization

Advisory Board/Program Committee

Diana Mateus	École Centrale de Nantes, France
Ender Konukoglu	ETH Zürich, Switzerland
Guido Gerig	New York University, USA
James Fishbaugh	New York University, USA
Julien Lefèvre	Aix-Marseille University, France
Kilian Pohl	SRI International, USA
Marc Niethammer	University of North Carolina at Chapel Hill, USA
Martin Styner	University of North Carolina at Chapel Hill, USA
Marius Linguraru	Children's National Medical Center, USA
Miaomiao Zhang	Lehigh University, USA
Orcun Goksel	ETH Zürich, Switzerland
Philippe Buechler	University of Bern, Switzerland
Sailesh Cojeti	DZNE Bonn, Germany
Stefan Sommer	University Copenhagen, Denmark
Steve Pizer	University of North Carolina at Chapel Hill, USA
Tim Cootes	University of Manchester, UK
Tinashe Mutsvangwa	University of Cape Town, South Africa
Thomas Vetter	University of Basel, Switzerland
Umberto Castellani	University of Verona, Italy
Washington Mio	Florida State University, USA
Xavier Pennec	Inria Sophia Antipolis, France
Yonggang Shi	University of Southern California, USA
Yoshinobu Sato	NARA Institute of Science and Technology, Japan

Contents

Shape Applications/Validation/Software

Shape Methods

Shape Classification and Deep Learning

Shape Applications/Validation/Software

Deformetrica 4: An Open-Source Software for Statistical Shape Analysis

Alexandre Bône[1,2,3,4,5](✉), Maxime Louis[1,2,3,4,5], Benoît Martin[1,2,3,4,5], and Stanley Durrleman[1,2,3,4,5]

[1] Institut du Cerveau et de la Moelle épinière, ICM, 75013 Paris, France
{alexandre.bone,stanley.durrleman}@icm-institute.org
[2] Inserm, U 1127, 75013 Paris, France
[3] CNRS, UMR 7225, 75013 Paris, France
[4] Sorbonne Université, 75013 Paris, France
[5] Inria, Aramis project-team, 75013 Paris, France

Abstract. Deformetrica is an open-source software for the statistical analysis of images and meshes. It relies on a specific instance of the large deformation diffeomorphic metric mapping (LDDMM) framework, based on control points: local momenta vectors offer a low-dimensional and interpretable parametrization of global diffeomorphims of the 2/3D ambient space, which in turn can warp any single or collection of shapes embedded in this physical space. Deformetrica has very few requirements about the data of interest: in the particular case of meshes, the absence of point correspondence can be handled thanks to the current or varifold representations. In addition to standard computational anatomy functionalities such as shape registration or atlas estimation, a bayesian version of atlas model as well as temporal methods (geodesic regression and parallel transport) are readily available. Installation instructions, tutorials and examples can be found at http://www.deformetrica.org.

Keywords: Statistical shape analysis · Computational anatomy
Large deformation diffeomorphic metric mapping
Open-source software

1 Introduction

D'Arcy Thomson first proposed the idea to compare two distinct shapes through the ambient-space deformations that transform one into the other [17]. Many years later, this insight still proves relevant, and one of its state-of-the-art avatar is the large deformation diffeomorphic metric mapping (LDDMM) [7,15], which offers a modern and principled framework for the construction of such transformations. Deformetrica relies on a specific instance of this framework, based on control points [7]. Section 2 details this theoretical backbone of our software, along with the current and varifold representations, which allow to handle mesh

---

A. Bône and M. Louis—Equal contributions.

© Springer Nature Switzerland AG 2018
M. Reuter et al. (Eds.): ShapeMI 2018, LNCS 11167, pp. 3–13, 2018.
https://doi.org/10.1007/978-3-030-04747-4_1

without point correspondence. Section 3 reports the competitive execution times of those core operations. Section 4 describes how this computation core is leveraged to offer ready-to-use higher level models to study shape dataset.

2   Theoretical Background

2.1   Control-Points-Based LDDMM: Constructing Diffeomorphisms

Deformetrica offers a low-dimensional and interpretable parametrization of diffeomorphisms of the ambient space $\mathbb{R}^d$, $d \in \{2, 3\}$. Let $(q_k)_{k=1,...,p}$ a set of p "control" points in $\mathbb{R}^d$ and $(\mu_k)_{k=1,...,p}$ be a set of p "momentum" vectors of $\mathbb{R}^d$. Those paired sets define a vector "velocity" field v of the ambient space through a convolution filter:

$$v : x \in \mathbb{R}^d \rightarrow v(x) = \sum_{k=1}^{p} K(x, q_k) \cdot \mu_k \tag{1}$$

where K is typically a gaussian kernel $K(x, y) = \exp\left(-\|x - y\|^2 / \sigma^2\right)$ of kernel width $\sigma > 0$. The kernel width σ will control the typical width of the generated deformation patterns. The set of vector fields v of the form (1) is a reproducible kernel Hilbert space (RKHS) V, with norm:

$$\|v\|_V^2 = \sum_{k,l=1,...,n} K(q_k, q_l) \cdot \mu_k^\top \mu_l. \tag{2}$$

Evolution equations are prescribed for the control point and momentum sets, called the "Hamiltonian" equations:

$$\begin{cases} \dot{q}(t) = K(q(t), q(t)) \cdot \mu(t) \\ \dot{\mu}(t) = -\frac{1}{2} \nabla_q \left\{ K\left(q(t), q(t)\right) \cdot \mu(t)^\top \mu(t) \right\} \end{cases} \tag{3}$$

These equations are integrated using an Euler or a Runge-Kutta of order 2 scheme. Is therefore obtained a time-varying velocity field $v(x, t)$ that can be computed at any time t using Eq. (1) with the corresponding control points $q(t)$ and momenta $\mu(t)$.

Let $x \in \mathbb{R}^d$ be any point of the ambient space. We define the transformed point $\Phi(x)$ as the value at time 1 of the function $l : [0, 1] \mapsto \mathbb{R}^d$ with initial condition $l(0) = x$ and which obeys the ordinary differential equation:

$$l'(t) = v(l(t), t). \tag{4}$$

The obtained mapping $\Phi : \mathbb{R}^d \mapsto \mathbb{R}^d$ is a diffeomorphism of the ambient space $\mathbb{R}^d$. Mathematical details are available in [19].

Overall, the obtained diffeomorphism Φ is fully parametrized by initial sets of control points q and momenta μ: we will note $\Phi = \Phi_{q,\mu}$. This simple parametrization of a large family of diffeomorphisms paves the way to the optimization of the initial control points q and momenta μ to estimate a desired transformation of the ambient space.

On a more theoretical note, for a fixed number of control points p the obtained set of diffeomorphisms has the structure of a finite-dimensional manifold, its geodesics are defined by the Hamiltonian equations (3), its tangent space at any point is the set of velocity fields obtained by the convolution of any momenta on the corresponding control points, and its cometric is given by the kernel matrix $[K(q_k, q_l)]_{k,l=1,\ldots,p}$.

2.2   Diffeomorphic Action on Shapes: Deforming Meshes or Images

Once a diffeormorphism of the ambient space is constructed, the way it deforms a shape must be specified. We distinguish the cases of mesh data and image data. A diffeormophism acts on a mesh by direct and independent application onto its vertices. On an image $I : \mathbb{R}^d \mapsto \mathbb{R}$, a diffeomorphism acts according to:

$$\Phi_{q,\mu}(I) = I \circ \Phi_{q,\mu}^{-1}.$$

This computation is done the following way:

1. A initial regular grid of points $(s_k)_{k=1,\ldots,r}$ corresponding to the voxel positions of the original image I is determined.
2. The positions $\Phi^{-1}(s_k)$ are computed. This is achieved using Eq. (4) for $k \in \{1,\ldots,r\}$, integrated from 1 to 0, with initial position $l(s_k) = s_k$ and using the opposite of the momenta $\mu(t)$ describing the diffeomorphism. This operation is exactly as expensive as the computation of the deformation of a mesh with r vertices.
3. The intensities at the positions $\Phi^{-1}(s_k)$ are computed by bi/tri-linear interpolation from the original image intensities, and assigned as being the intensity of the deformed image on the grid at position s_k. Zero padding is applied outside the original image. This operation is massively parellelizable.

In the rest of the paper, we will note $\Phi_{q,\mu} \star S$ the result of the action of a diffeomorphism $\Phi_{q,\mu}$ on a shape S.

2.3   Shape Attachments: Evaluting Deformation Residuals

To evaluate if the deformed shape is close to its target, a metric is needed. For images, the Euclidian ℓ^2 distance is trivially available. For meshes, the same ℓ^2 metric can be used if there is a point-to-point correspondence. In the general case of meshes without point correspondence, the "current" or "varifold" distances are available, and described in the rest of this section.

Whether the connectivity of the mesh is made of segments or triangles, it is possible to compute the centers $(c_k)_{k=1,\ldots,r}$ and the normals $(n_k)_{k=1,\ldots,r}$ of the edges. Equipped with those, one can compute either the current distance [18]:

$$d\left((n_k^\alpha, c_k^\alpha)_{p=1,\ldots,r^\alpha}, (n_l^\beta, c_l^\beta)_{l=1,\ldots,r^\beta}\right)^2 = \sum_k \sum_l K_W(c_k^\alpha, c_l^\beta) \cdot (n_k^\alpha)^\top n_l^\beta$$

or rather the varifold distance [5], which ignores the orientation of the normals:

$$d\left((n_k^\alpha, c_k^\alpha)_{k=1,\ldots,r^\alpha}, (n_l^\beta, c_l^\beta)_{l=1,\ldots,r^\beta}\right)^2 = \sum_k \sum_l K_W(c_k^\alpha, c_l^\beta) \cdot \frac{\left((n_k^\alpha)^\top n_l^\beta\right)^2}{\|n_k^\alpha\|\|n_l^\beta\|}$$

where K_W is a Gaussian kernel with width σ_W.

Deformetrica offers the possibility to compute simultaneous deformations of several shapes all embedded in the same ambient space $\mathbb{R}^d$. If $O^\alpha = (S_1^\alpha, \ldots, S_{n_s}^\alpha)$ and $O^\beta = (S_1^\beta, \ldots, S_{n_s}^\beta)$ are two objects constituted of n_s homologous shapes, Deformetrica computes the squared distance via:

$$d(O^\alpha, O^\beta)^2 = \sum_{k=1}^{n_s} \frac{d(S_k^\alpha, S_k^\beta)^2}{\sigma_k^2} \tag{5}$$

which is a weighted average of the squared distances of the corresponding objects. The parameters σ_k can be used to tune the relative importances of each part of the composite "multi-object" of study.

2.4   A Glimpse at Optimization

Each Deformetrica model leverages those deformation and attachment mechanics to define a specific cost function, that will then be optimized either by steepest gradient descent or with the limited-memory Broyden-Fletcher-Goldfarb-Shanno (L-BFGS) method [12]. Deformetrica 4 exploits the automatic differentiation functionalities offered by the PyTorch project [16] to compute the required gradients, as suggested in [11].

3   Performances

The deformation mechanics heavily rely on convolution operations, as well as computing current or varifold attachments. Computing a convolution has a quadratic numerical complexity with the number of considered points, and is therefore a very critical operator in Deformetrica. A second constraint arise with automatic differentiation memory requirements, which are also quadratic with the input data sizes in the case of a naive implementation. Deformetrica features two ways to perform convolution, both either on CPU or GPU:

- using a naive PyTorch-based code [16], typically faster for small data sizes but unreasonably memory-greedy with larger data;
- using the dedicated PyKeops library [4] which offers a PyTorch-compatible python wrapper for memory-efficient kernel operations with their derivatives. This library is typically required to deal with real-size data.

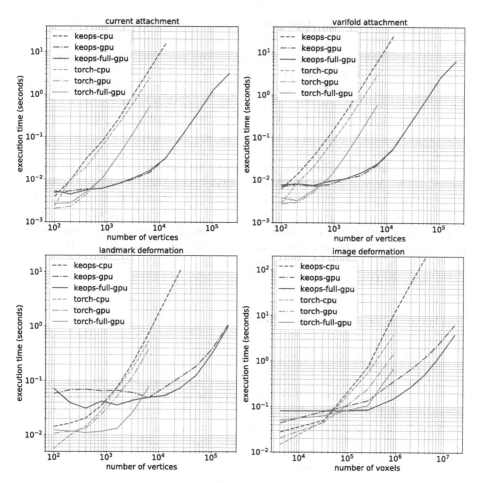

Fig. 1. Top: needed time to compute either the current or varifold attachment and the associated gradient, versus the number of vertices in each mesh. Bottom: needed time to compute either a landmark or image deformation and the associated gradient, versus the number of vertices and voxels respectively. The reported times are averages over 100 evaluations.

An additional performance switch is offered by the PyTorch library: all linear algebra operations can be ported directly on GPU with a single flag. Obviously, this come at the cost of an increased GPU memory usage.

Figure 1 reports typical execution times against the data size, respectively for the attachment and deformation atomic operations. The reported times include the (automatic) computation of the gradient. This benchmark has been made on an Ubuntu 14.04 machine, equipped with an Intel Xeon E5-1630 v3 CPU and Nvidia Quadro M4000 GPU with Nvidia driver version 384.130. Note that both the PyTorch and PyKeops libraries are quite recent, and can be expected to improve their performances in the near future.

In all cases, the "torch"-based convolutions are faster for small data sizes, but are overtaken by the "keops"-based ones at some point. The CPU-only operations can prove efficient to compute the deformation of small shapes, but quickly become order of magnitudes slower than their GPU equivalents for larger data. The "full-gpu" option does not lower the execution times for attachments, when it consistently does so for deformations. Note that the torch-based curves are interrupted earlier than their keops-based counterparts, because the memory requirements due to automatic differentiation becomes unreasonable for too large data sizes.

We can finally underline the satisfyingly fast image deformation performances, allowing to register two full-resolution ($181 \times 217 \times 181$) T1-weighted magnetic resonance images (MRIs) in 1 min and 42 s (after 50 iterations of the L-BFGS estimator), with a GPU memory footprint around 2 gigabytes. Choosing the slower but much less memory-intensive "keops-gpu" mode instead of "keops-full-gpu", the same registration takes 3 min and 22 s with a GPU memory footprint of 60 megabytes. In absence of gpu, the "keops-cpu" option allows to still estimate the registration, but requires around 10 h.

4   Deformetrica Applications

4.1   Atlas and Registration

Cost Function. We consider here a cross-sectional collection of shapes $(S_i)_{i=1,\ldots,n}$. The atlas model offers to compute a mean T of the shapes and a collection of diffeomorphisms $(\Phi_i)_{i=1,\ldots,n}$ such that for all $i \in \{1, \ldots, n\}$, we have $\Phi_i \star T \simeq S_i$. This is achieved by minimization of the cost function:

$$C(T, q, \mu_{i=1,\ldots,n}) = \sum_i d(\Phi_{q,\mu_i} \star T, S_i)^2 / \sigma_\epsilon^2 + R(q, (\mu_i)_{i=1,\ldots,n}), \qquad (6)$$

$$\text{with} \quad R(q, (\mu_i)_{i=1,\ldots,n}) = \sum_i \mu_i^\top K(q, q) \mu_i \qquad (7)$$

noting $K(q,q)$ the p-by-p "kernel" matrix $[K(q_k, q_l)]_{k,l=1,\ldots,p}$. The first term in Eq. (6) controls the data attachment i.e. how well the collection of objects is fitted by the deformation of the template, while the second term acts as a regularizer by penalizing the kinetic energy of the deformations. The relative importance of those two terms is specified by the user through the parameter σ_ϵ. The resulting atlas obtained from images of digits is displayed by Fig. 2.

Smoothing the Gradient. When working with meshes with boundaries, the gradient of the cost function (6) with respect to the mesh vertices positions T can be very large near the boundary, inducing the estimated template T to have a non-natural shape. A workaround consists in convolving the analytic gradient with a Gaussian kernel. It provides a different descent direction which results in a smoother estimated template.

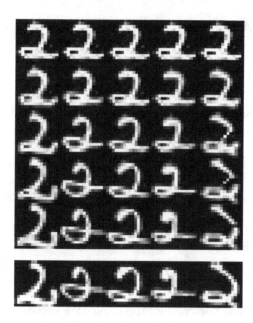

Fig. 2. Illustration of an estimated "deterministic" atlas model on the five images represented at the bottom row. The top row represents five repetitions of the estimated template shape, when the following rows represent the progressive deformations of this template that eventually match well the input dataset shown on the last row. The somehow unnatural rightmost deformation indicates that the σ_ϵ parameter might advantageously be chosen slightly greater, since less energetic deformations would be estimated.

Registration. The registration problem is a particular instantiation of the atlas cost function with a single target S and a fixed template T:

$$C(q, \mu) = d(\Phi_{q,\mu} \star T, S)^2 / \sigma_\epsilon^2 + R(q, \mu) \tag{8}$$

It has numerous applications in medical imaging. For instance, registering MRIs from two different patients allows to perform relevant voxel-wise intensity comparisons, after removal of their natural anatomical differences. Alternatively, it can be leveraged to transfer some standard brain segmentation towards a new particular subject.

4.2 Bayesian Atlas

The atlas cost function (6) can be seen as an approximation of the negative complete log-likelihood of a generative, hierarchical, mixed-effects statistical model, that we call the Bayesian atlas one [10].

Statistical Model. From a common template T and control points q, the individual shapes S_i are considered as random deformations of T plus noise:

$$S_i = \Phi_{q,\mu_i} \star T + \epsilon_i, \quad \text{with} \quad \mu_i \overset{\text{iid}}{\sim} \mathcal{N}(0, \Sigma_\mu) \quad \text{and} \quad \epsilon_i \overset{\text{iid}}{\sim} \mathcal{N}(0, \sigma_\epsilon). \tag{9}$$

To fit the framework of mixed-effects models, we distinguish the model fixed effects $\theta = (T, q, \Sigma_\mu, \sigma_\epsilon)$ and the model random effects $z = (\mu_i)_i$. Inverse-Wishart bayesian priors are chosen for the variance parameters: $\Sigma_\mu \sim \mathcal{IW}(\Gamma_\mu, m_\mu)$ and $\sigma_\epsilon \sim \mathcal{IW}(\gamma_\epsilon, m_\epsilon)$. The introduced additional hyper-parameters are by default automatically set following the heuristics given in [10].

Log-Likelihood. Noting $S = (S_i)$ the collection of all the observations, the complete log-likelihood is given by:

$$-2\log p(S, \theta, z) = \sum_i \left\{ d(\Phi_{q,\mu_i} \star T, S_i)^2/\sigma_\epsilon^2 + \mu_i^\perp \Sigma_\mu^{-1} \mu_i \right\} \qquad (10)$$
$$+ m_\mu \left\{ \log\left(\det \Sigma_\mu\right) + \text{Tr}\left(\Sigma_\mu^\perp \Gamma_\mu^{-1}\right) \right\} + m_\epsilon \left\{ \log \sigma_\epsilon^2 + \gamma_\epsilon^2/\sigma_\epsilon^2 \right\}.$$

The maximum a posteriori (MAP) estimate of the model parameters can be approximated as follow:

$$\theta_{map} = \text{argmax}_\theta \int p(S, \theta, z)\mathrm{d}z \approx \text{argmax}_{\theta,z}\, p(S, \theta, z). \qquad (11)$$

This classical "max-max" or "mode" approximation becomes an equality in the limit case where $p(z)$ is a Dirac distribution, i.e. $\Sigma_\mu = 0$.

Note that computing this approximate MAP amounts to finding the minimum of the negative log-likelihood (10), which echoes the previously introduced atlas cost function (6). The introduced modeling provides a statistical interpretation to the regularization term, which arises from assumed underlying random structures on the momenta μ_i and the residuals ϵ_i. Those assumptions are weaker, more intrinsic than arbitrarily prescribing the regularization term (7): the estimated atlas can therefore be expected to be more data-driven, or in other words more representative of the input data.

Estimation. The Bayesian atlas is estimated in Deformetrica with gradient-based methods following the iterative procedure described in [10], which alternates gradient steps over the current estimates of $T, q, (\mu_i)$ and closed-form updates of the variance parameters $\Sigma_\mu, \sigma_\epsilon$.

A second class of estimation methods, based on a stochastic approximation of the classical expectation-maximization algorithm (see [1,6]) will be released in Deformetrica 4.1. This so-called SAEM estimator will compute the exact θ_{map}, integrating out the full distribution of the momenta random effects.

4.3   Geodesic Regression

Geodesic regression generalizes linear regression to manifold-valued data [8,9]. We consider here a time-series dataset $(S_i)_{i=1,\ldots,n}$ observed at times $(t_i)_{i=1,\ldots,n}$. Practical examples could be repeated MRIs of the same individual, or repeated observations of the growth of a plant. The cost function for geodesic regression is:

$$C(T, q, \mu) = \sum_i d(\Phi_{q,t_i\mu} \star T, S_i)^2/\sigma_\epsilon^2 + R(q, \mu). \qquad (12)$$

where $R(q, \mu)$ is given by Eq. (7). The first term in (12) controls the attachment of the data while the second penalizes the "kinetic" energy of the deformation. The data-attachment versus regularity tradeoff is addressed by the user-specified parameter σ_ϵ. Note that the trajectory $t \mapsto \Phi_{q,t\mu} \star T$ is the action of a geodesic on the q-manifold of diffeomorphisms onto the template shape T.

Optimization of this cost yields an estimated template shape T as well as sets of control points and associated initial momenta, so that the induced time-continuous flow of diffeomorphisms applied to the template shape $t \mapsto \Phi_{q,t\mu} \star T$ is as close as possible to the input observations. Figure 3 shows an example of geodesic regression on 3D meshes of human faces (data courtesy of Paolo Piras, Sapienza Universitá di Roma, Italy).

4.4 Parallel Transport in Shape Analysis

Deformetrica implements the parallel transport method for shape analysis described in [13]. Given two sets of control points and momenta q^α, q^β and μ^α, μ^β, the parallel transport is a differential geometry notion which allows to consider the translation of the deformation described by q^β, μ^β along the deformation defined by q^α, μ^α. The computation of this transport can be done following a procedure whose convergence is proven in [14].

An interesting example occurs when q^α, μ^α describes a known progression, for example a geodesic regression learned from repeated observation of a reference subject and when q^β, μ^β describes a registration between an observation of the reference subject and a new subject. In that case, the flow of the parallel-transported deformation can be used to obtain a prediction of the future state of the subject [3]. It is in some sense a transfer learning operation.

Figure 4 shows an example of parallel translation of the geodesic progression obtained on Fig. 3 onto a face with a different form.

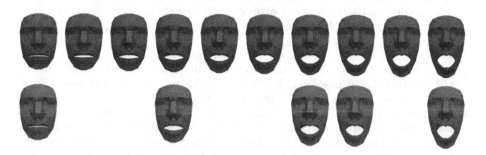

Fig. 3. Estimated geodesic regression. Top row: the estimated trajectory. Bottom row: observations from which the top trajectory is learned.

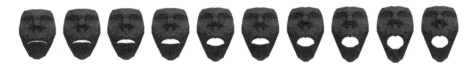

Fig. 4. Parallel transport of the human face trajectory shown on Fig. 3 onto a different face.

5   Conclusion

Deformetrica implements common computational anatomy methods both on meshes and images. Future releases of the software will include probabilistic principal geodesic analysis [20] as well as the longitudinal atlas statistical model [2].

One of the main limitation of the software for a wider range of applications lies in the purely geometrical modeling of the shapes. Mainly, a deformation model cannot change the topology of the deformed image, thus restricting the range of applications. Using the metamorphosis framework or including functional shapes could increase the impact of the software.

Acknowledgments. This work has been partly funded by the European Research Council (ERC) under grant agreement No 678304, European Union's Horizon 2020 research and innovation program under grant agreement No. 666992, and the program Investissements d'avenir ANR-10-IAIHU-06.

References

1. Allassonnière, S., Kuhn, E., Trouvé, A.: Construction of bayesian deformable models via a stochastic approximation algorithm: a convergence study. Bernoulli **16**(3), 641–678 (2010)
2. Bône, A., Colliot, O., Durrleman, S.: Learning distributions of shape trajectories from longitudinal datasets: a hierarchical model on a manifold of diffeomorphisms. In: Proceedings of the IEEE Conference on Computer Vision and Pattern Recognition, pp. 9271–9280 (2018)
3. Bône, A., et al.: Prediction of the progression of subcortical brain structures in Alzheimer's disease from baseline. In: Cardoso, M.J., et al. (eds.) GRAIL/MFCA/MICGen-2017. LNCS, vol. 10551, pp. 101–113. Springer, Cham (2017). https://doi.org/10.1007/978-3-319-67675-3_10
4. Charlier, B., Feydy, J., Glaunès, J.A., Trouvé, A.: An efficient kernel product for automatic differentiation libraries, with applications to measure transport (2017)
5. Charon, N., Trouvé, A.: The varifold representation of nonoriented shapes for diffeomorphic registration. SIAM J. Imaging Sci. **6**(4), 2547–2580 (2013)
6. Delyon, B., Lavielle, M., Moulines, E.: Convergence of a stochastic approximation version of the EM algorithm. Ann. Stat. **27**, 94–128 (1999)
7. Durrleman, S., et al.: Morphometry of anatomical shape complexes with dense deformations and sparse parameters. NeuroImage **101**, 35–49 (2014)
8. Fishbaugh, J., Prastawa, M., Gerig, G., Durrleman, S.: Geodesic regression of image and shape data for improved modeling of 4D trajectories. In: ISBI 2014–11th International Symposium on Biomedical Imaging, pp. 385–388, April 2014

9. Fletcher, T.: Geodesic regression on Riemannian manifolds. In: Proceedings of the Third International Workshop on Mathematical Foundations of Computational Anatomy-Geometrical and Statistical Methods for Modelling Biological Shape Variability, pp. 75–86 (2011)

10. Gori, P., et al.: A Bayesian framework for joint morphometry of surface and curve meshes in multi-object complexes. Med. Image Anal. **35**, 458–474 (2017)

11. Kühnel, L., Sommer, S.: Computational anatomy in Theano. In: Cardoso, M.J., et al. (eds.) GRAIL/MFCA/MICGen-2017. LNCS, vol. 10551, pp. 164–176. Springer, Cham (2017). https://doi.org/10.1007/978-3-319-67675-3_15

12. Liu, D.C., Nocedal, J.: On the limited memory BFGS method for large scale optimization. Math. Program. **45**(1–3), 503–528 (1989)

13. Louis, Maxime, Bône, Alexandre, Charlier, Benjamin, Durrleman, Stanley: Parallel transport in shape analysis: a scalable numerical scheme. In: Nielsen, Frank, Barbaresco, Frédéric (eds.) GSI 2017. LNCS, vol. 10589, pp. 29–37. Springer, Cham (2017). https://doi.org/10.1007/978-3-319-68445-1_4

14. Louis, M., Charlier, B., Jusselin, P., Susovan, P., Durrleman, S.: A fanning scheme for the parallel transport along geodesics on Riemannian manifolds. SIAM J. Numer. Anal. **56**, 2563–2584 (2018)

15. Miller, M.I., Trouvé, A., Younes, L.: Geodesic shooting for computational anatomy. J. Math. Imaging Vis. **24**(2), 209–228 (2006)

16. Paszke, A., et al.: Pytorch: tensors and dynamic neural networks in python with strong GPU acceleration, May 2017

17. Thompson, D.W., et al.: On growth and form (1942)

18. Vaillant, M., Glaunès, J.: Surface matching via currents. In: Christensen, G.E., Sonka, M. (eds.) IPMI 2005. LNCS, vol. 3565, pp. 381–392. Springer, Heidelberg (2005). https://doi.org/10.1007/11505730_32

19. Younes, L.: Shapes and Diffeomorphisms, vol. 171. Springer, Heidelberg (2010). https://doi.org/10.1007/978-3-642-12055-8

20. Zhang, M., Singh, N., Fletcher, P.T.: Bayesian estimation of regularization and atlas building in diffeomorphic image registration. IPMI **23**, 37–48 (2013)

On the Evaluation and Validation of Off-the-Shelf Statistical Shape Modeling Tools: A Clinical Application

Anupama Goparaju[1]($\boxtimes$), Ibolya Csecs[2], Alan Morris[2], Evgueni Kholmovski[2,3], Nassir Marrouche[2], Ross Whitaker[1], and Shireen Elhabian[1]

[1] Scientific Computing and Imaging Institute, University of Utah, Salt Lake City, UT, USA
anupama.goparaju@utah.edu, {whitaker,shireen}@sci.utah.edu
[2] Comprehensive Arrhythmia Research and Management Center, Division of Cardiovascular Medicine, School of Medicine, University of Utah, Salt Lake City, UT, USA
{alan.morris,nassir.marrouche}@carma.utah.edu
[3] Department of Radiology and Imaging Sciences, School of Medicine, University of Utah, Salt Lake City, UT, USA
evgueni.kholmovski@hsc.utah.edu

Abstract. Statistical shape modeling (SSM) has proven useful in many areas of biology and medicine as a new generation of morphometric approaches for the quantitative analysis of anatomical shapes. Recently, the increased availability of high-resolution in vivo images of anatomy has led to the development and distribution of open-source computational tools to model anatomical shapes and their variability within populations with unprecedented detail and statistical power. Nonetheless, there is little work on the evaluation and validation of such tools as related to clinical applications that rely on morphometric quantifications for treatment planning. To address this lack of validation, we systematically assess the outcome of widely used off-the-shelf SSM tools, namely ShapeWorks, SPHARM-PDM, and Deformetrica, in the context of designing closure devices for left atrium appendage (LAA) in atrial fibrillation (AF) patients to prevent stroke, where an incomplete LAA closure may be worse than no closure. This study is motivated by the potential role of SSM in the geometric design of closure devices, which could be informed by population-level statistics, and patient-specific device selection, which is driven by anatomical measurements that could be automated by relating patient-level anatomy to population-level morphometrics. Hence, understanding the consequences of different SSM tools for the final analysis is critical for the careful choice of the tool to be deployed in real clinical scenarios. Results demonstrate that estimated measurements from ShapeWorks model are more consistent compared to models from Deformetrica and SPHARM-PDM. Furthermore, ShapeWorks and Deformetrica shape models capture clinically relevant population-level variability compared to SPHARM-PDM models.

© Springer Nature Switzerland AG 2018
M. Reuter et al. (Eds.): ShapeMI 2018, LNCS 11167, pp. 14–27, 2018.
https://doi.org/10.1007/978-3-030-04747-4_2

Keywords: Statistical shape models · Surface parameterization
Correspondence optimization · Evaluation

1   Introduction

Morphometric techniques for the quantitative analysis of anatomical shapes have been important for the study of biology and medicine for more than 100 years. Statistical shape modeling (SSM) is the computational extension of classical morphometric techniques to more detailed representations of complex anatomy and their variability within populations with high levels of geometric detail and statistical power. SSM is beginning to impact a wide spectrum of clinical applications, e.g., implants design [26], anatomy reconstruction from less-expensive 2D images [4], surgical planning [18], and reconstructive surgery [25].

Learning Population-Level Metric: Developing computational tools for shape modeling is contingent upon defining a *metric* in the space of shapes to enable comparing shapes and performing shape statistics (e.g., averaging). That is, two shapes that differ in a manner that is typical of the variability in the population should be considered *similar* relative to two shapes that differ in atypical ways. For instance, size is such a typical mode of anatomical variation that most shape-based analyses factor it out, thereby treating two anatomical objects that differ only in size as the *same*. Populations of anatomic objects typically show other common variations. There is a growing consensus in the field that such a metric should be adapted to the specific population under investigation, which entails finding correspondences across an ensemble of shapes. The scientific premise of existing correspondence techniques falls in two broad categories: a *groupwise* approach to estimating correspondences (e.g., ShapeWorks [5], Minimum Description Length - MDL [9], Deformetrica [11]) that considers the variability in the entire cohort and a *pairwise* approach (e.g., SPHARM-PDM [23]) that considers mapping to a predefined surface parameterization. Pairwise methods lead to biased and suboptimal models [7,8,19]. On the other hand, groupwise methods learn a population-specific metric in a way that does not penalize natural variability and therefore can capture the underlying parameters in an anatomical shape space. Other publicly available tools, e.g., FreeSurfer [12], BrainVoyager [14], FSL [16], and SPM [1], provide shape modeling capabilities, but they tend to be tailored to specific anatomies or limited topologies. SPHARM-PDM [23], for example, is a parameterization-based correspondence scheme that relies on a smooth one-to-one mapping from each surface instance to the unit sphere. Here, we consider a representative set of open-source SSM tools (see Table 1) that can be used for general anatomy; ShapeWorks, Deformetrica, and SPHARM-PDM.

Proof-of-Concept: Consider the simple example of an ensemble of 3D boxes with a bump at a varying location. Ideally, one would want the correspondences to reflect the fact that the *bump* is a single feature whose position on the main box shape varies across the population. When comparing the shape of different

Table 1. Open-source SSM tools considered for evaluation and validation

SSM tools	Groupwise	Topology-independent	Parameterization-free	General anatomy
ShapeWorks [5]	✓	✓	✓	✓
SPHARM-PDM [23]	X	X	X(sphere)	✓ (spherical topology)
Deformetrica [11]	✓	✓	✓	✓

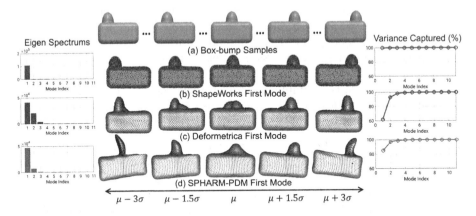

Fig. 1. Proof-of-concept: (a) Box-bump samples. The mean ±3 stds of the 1st mode of (b) ShapeWorks [5], (c) Deformetrica [11], and (d) SPHARM-PDM [23].

boxes, one would want to downplay the impact of the bump location on the comparing metric to respect the natural population variability that is not captured by simple affine transformations. Figure 1 illustrates how the groupwise aspect of the corresponence optimization of ShapeWorks is able to discover the underlying mode of variation in the box-bump ensemble in comparison to a pairwise diffeomorphism-based shape modeling approach (Fig. 1(c)) in which shapes are embedded in the image intensity values at voxels, and nonlinear registration is used to map all sample images to a reference image, which is estimated based on the Frechet mean of all samples [11]. As illustrated in Fig. 1(a), shapes from ShapeWorks remain more faithful to those described by the original training set, even out to three standard deviations, at which the diffeomorphic description breaks down. In particular, diffeomorphic warps recovered an incorrect shape model in which the mean shape showed a box with two bumps rather than a single bump. Furthermore, SPHARM-PDM does not guarantee an efficient solution in the parameter space of the resulting shape model (Fig. 1(d)), with an inherent limitation of only modeling anatomies with spherical topology.

Lack of Validation in a Clinical Scenario: Computer-assisted diagnosis and surgical planning can help clinicans making objective decisions [17,21]. In particular, shape modeling has played an important role in clinical applications that benefit from both qualitative and quantitative insights of population-level variability, e.g., diagnosis of liver cirrhosis [17] and finding associations between surgical parameters and head shapes following cranioplasty [21]. Recent advances in vivo imaging of anatomy and the wide spectrum of shape modeling applications have led to the development and distribution of open-source SSM tools, further enabling their use in an *off-the-shelf* manner. Evaluation of SSM tools has been performed using non-clinical applications such as image segmentation [15] and shape/deformation synthesis approaches [13]. However, to the best of our knowledge, little work has been done on the evaluation and validation of such tools as related to clinical applications that rely on morphometric quantifications. Specifically, we believe that understanding the consequences of different SSM tools on the final analysis is critical for the careful choice of the tool to be deployed in real clinical scenarios. To address this lack of validation in a clinical scenario, we systematically assess the outcome of widely used off-the-shelf SSM tools, namely ShapeWorks [5], SPHARM-PDM [23], and Deformetrica [11], in the context of designing closure devices for left atrium appendage (LAA) in atrial fibrillation (AF) patients to prevent stroke.

Closure Device Design – A Potential Clinical Application: LAA closure is performed in AF patients to reduce the risk of stroke [24]. LAA morphology is complex and mainly divided into four types: cauliflower, chicken wing, wind sock, and cactus [24]. The geometric design and patient-specific selection of closure devices are typically performed by clinical experts with subjective decisions based on the morphology [24]. Nonetheless, obtaining these measurements manually for large cohorts of patients is a subjective, tedious, and error-prone process. SSM could thus provide an automated approach for developing less subjective categorizations of LAA morphology and measurements that can be used to make more objective clinical decisions regarding suitability for LAA closure. Hence, this study is motivated by the potential role of SSM in the geometric design of closure devices, which could be informed by population-level statistics, and patient-specific device selection, which is driven by anatomical measurements that could be automated by relating patient-level anatomy to population-level morphometrics. To validate different SSM tools, we present a semiautomated approach that makes use of shape models to estimate the LAA measurements to aid the patient-specific closure device selection process; a clinical application that needs consistent and accurate measurement estimation to avoid adverse outcomes that could result from incomplete appendage closure [20].

2   Methods

The crux of statistical shape modeling is defining a shape representation that allows performing shape statistics. To this end, *landmarks* are the most popular choice as a light-weight shape representation that is easy to understand and that promotes visual communication of the results [22,25]. To perform shape arithmetics (e.g., averaging), landmarks should be defined consistently within a given population to refer to the same anatomical position on every shape instance, a concept known as *correspondence*. Given an ensemble of shapes for a particular anatomy, these correspondences (or landmarks/points) are typically generated using some optimization process by defining an objective function to be minimized in a *pairwise* (w.r.t. a shape atlas/template or predefined surface parameterization, e.g., sphere) or *groupwise* (w.r.t. all shape samples where each shape provides new information about shape variability) manner. Different SSM tools implement different objective functions [15], raising the need to evaluate and validate their resulting shape models in clinical applications that rely on shape-based measurements. As such, we present a semiautomated approach to validate the results of widely used SSM tools in one such clinical application.

2.1 Statistical Shape Models

Statistical shape models consist of (1) a detailed 3D geometrical representation of the *average anatomy* of a given population and (2) a representation of the population-level *geometric variability* of such an anatomy, often in the form of a collection of principal modes of variation. Principal modes of variation define reduced degrees of freedom for representing a high-dimensional and thus complex variation in anatomical shapes. In particular, consider a cohort of shapes $\mathcal{S} = \{z_1, z_2, \ldots, z_N\}$ of N surfaces, each with its own set of M corresponding point $z_n = [z_n^1, z_n^2, \ldots, z_n^M] \in \mathbb{R}^{dM}$ where the ordering of each point $z_n^m \in \mathbb{R}^d$ implies a correspondence among shapes. For statistical modeling, shapes in $\mathcal{S}$ should share the same world coordinate system. Hence, a rigid transformation matrix T_n can be estimated to transform the points in the $n-$th shape local coordinate x_n^m to the world common coordinate z_n^m such that $z_n^m = T_n x_n^m$. Using principal component analysis (PCA), this high-dimensional point distribution model (PDM) can be reduced to a compact set of K modes of variations.

2.2 SSM Tools

Here is a brief summary of the SSM tools considered in this study.

ShapeWorks [5] is a groupwise correspondence approach that implements the particle-based modeling method (PBM) [6], which constructs compact statistical landmark-based models of shape ensembles that do not rely on any specific surface parameterization. It uses a set of interacting particle systems, one for each shape, using mutually repelling forces to optimally cover, and therefore describe, the surface geometry, thus avoiding many of the problems inherent in parametric representations, such as the limitation to specific topologies, processing steps necessary to construct parameterizations, and bias toward model initialization. PBM considers two types of random variables: a shape space variable $Z \in \mathbb{R}^{dM}$ and a particle position variable $X_n \in \mathbb{R}^d$ that encodes particles distribution on the $n-$th shape (configuration space). Correspondences are established by minimizing a combined shape correspondence and surface sampling cost function $Q = H(Z) - \sum_{n=1}^{N} H(X_n)$, where H is an entropy estimation assuming Gaussian shape distribution in the shape space and Euclidean particle-to-particle repulsion in the configuration space. This formulation favors a compact ensemble representation in shape space (first term) against a uniform distribution of particles on each surface for accurate shape representation (second term).

SPHARM-PDM [23] is a pairwise and parameterization-based correspondence method that maps each training sample to a unit sphere with an area preserving and distortion minimizing objective using spherical harmonics as basis functions. Hence, SPHARM is restricted to anatomies with spherical topology. Spherical parameterization is obtained by aligning the axes of first order ellipsoid fit of an input shape to the basis functions axes, The basis function of degree l and order m is given as, $Y_l^m(\theta\phi) = \sqrt{\frac{2l+1}{4\pi}\frac{(l-m)!}{(l+m)!}}P_l^m(\cos\theta)e^{im\phi}$, where $\theta \in [0; \pi]$ and $\phi \in [0; 2\pi]$. Every point on the surface is given by a parameter vector (θ_i, ϕ_i), which represents a location on the sphere. Each mesh's spherical parameterization is used in generation of the SPHARM description. Icosahedron subdivision of a sphere is performed to obtain homogeneous sampling of the parameter space and thereby obtain a point distribution model (PDM).

Deformetrica [11] is a deformation-based correspondence method that is based on the large deformation diffeomorphic metric mapping (LDDMM) framework. A deformation field $X(x)$ is generated using n control points $(q_i)_{i=1,2..,n}$ and momenta vectors $(\mu_i)_{i=1,2..,n}$, where $X(x) = \sum_{i=1}^p K(x, q_i)\mu_i$, x is the position at which the vector field is evaluated, and $K(x, y)$ is a Gaussian kernel with width σ. The deformation is obtained through the convolution between the control points and their momenta and the vertices of the input meshes. Varifold distance is used in estimating the distance between meshes. The transformation obtained by the deformation is denoted as $\phi_{q,\mu}$, where q and μ are the initial control points and momenta. The number of control points and the topology of the atlas are user-defined. The algorithm is initialized with the control points on the atlas and momenta vectors set to zero indicating no deformation. A path of deformations is estimated by mapping the atlas to the input shape. A final atlas is generated with the optimized control points and momenta vectors by considering the variability of all the input shapes. The deformations inform how different a shape is from the atlas and enable statistical shape analysis.

2.3   Evaluation Methodology

When the ground truth data of shape descriptors is not available, evaluation of shape models can be performed using *quantitative* metrics reported as a function of the number of principal modes of variation, namely [10]: (1) *compactness*, which encodes the percentage of variance captured by a specific number of modes (higher is better), and thus a compact shape model would express the shape variability with fewer parameters; (2) *generalization*, which assesses whether a learned model can represent unseen shape instances (using reconstruction error in a leave-one-out cross validation scheme) and quantifies the ability of the learned density function to spread out between and around the training shapes (lower is better); and (3) *specificity*, which reveals the ability of the model to generate plausible/realistic shapes, quantified as the Euclidean distance between a sampled shape and its closest training sample based on ℓ_2 norm (lower is better).

A *qualitative* analysis can be performed by analyzing the mean (average) anatomy and learned modes of variation. Furthermore, when the given population exhibits natural clustering (e.g., LAA), SSM tools can be evaluated by performing clustering analysis on the resulting correspondences to analyze which tool can help discover the intrinsic variability in the data.

2.4   Validation Methodology

Shape models for different SSM tools can be validated using manually defined landmarks. However, defining manual correspondences is time-consuming, especially when dealing with large cohorts, and requires significant human resources with sufficient domain-specific expertise. To address the issue of validation with the ground truth correspondences, we have designed a semiautomated approach to test the robustness of shape models in the context of the LAA closure process. Closure devices are available in different sizes and device design and selection is made by a clinician using manual analysis of a patient's LAA and the ostium (opening of LAA) [24]. The manual analysis can be automated by estimating the anatomical measurements of patient-specific LAA by relating it to the population-level statistics informed by shape models. The anatomical measurement estimation process is performed by (1) marking the correspondences of LAA ostium on the mean shape obtained from the shape model of an SSM tool, (2) warping the marked ostium to the individual samples (using mean-sample correspondences to construct a thin-plate spline (TPS) warp [3]) to obtain the geometry of a single sample LAA ostium, and (3) computing anatomical measurements using sample-specific ostium points. Measurements obtained by this SSM-based semiautomated process are then compared against ground truth measurements (defined by clinical experts) to estimate the accuracy of correspondences established by an SSM tool.

3   Results

3.1   Experimental Setup

SSM tools were evaluated and validated using a dataset of 130 LAA (isotropic resolution of 0.625 mm) that was obtained retrospectively from an AF patient image database at the University of Utah's Comprehensive Arrhythmia Research and Management (CARMA) Center. The MRI volumes were served with a single-handed segmentation by an expert. A preprocessing pipeline of rigid registration to a representative sample to factor out translational and rotational variations, cropping (using a largest bounding box of the dataset) to remove the unnecessary background that could slow down the processing, and topology-preserving smoothing were applied to the LAA shapes to generate signed distance transforms. The preprocessed shapes were then fed to ShapeWorks, SPHARM-PDM, Deformetrica with a mean LAA shape (distance tranform – μDT) as an atlas, and Deformetrica with a sphere shape as an atlas (similar to SPHARM-PDM). Resulting 3D point correspondences from different SSM tools were then used for evaluation and validation of the tools.

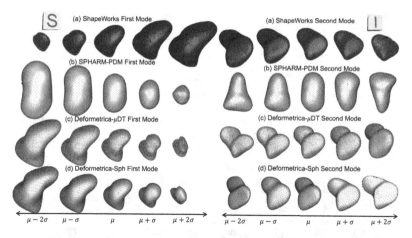

Fig. 2. The mean ±2 stds of the 1st and 2nd mode of LAA shape models (S: superior and I: inferior views) from (a) ShapeWorks [5], (b) SPHARM-PDM [23], (c) Deformetrica-μDT (mean LAA distance transform as the atlas) [11], and (d) Deformetrica-Sph (sphere shape as the atlas) [11].

3.2   Shape Models Evaluation

Modes of Variation: Figure 2 illustrates the first two dominant modes from different tools. In contrast to SPHARM-PDM, shape models from ShapeWorks and Deformetrica capture clinically relevant variations: the elongation of the appendage and the size of LAA ostia. Of particular interest, the second dominant mode of variation from SPHARM-PDM reflects the ambiguity in axes mapping of first order ellipsoid fit of the input shape to the axes in the parameter space.

Evaluation Metrics: Figure 3 shows the quantitative metrics from each SSM tool in comparison. ShapeWorks produces the most compact shape model whereas SPHARM-PDM yielded the least compact one. Neither Deformetrica nor SPHARM-PDM attempt to learn the underlying shape distribution, their generalization was inferior with few prinicipal modes as compared to Shape-Works, which reveals their tendency to overfit with sparse training samples in high-dimensional shape spaces. Furthermore, generated samples for ShapeWorks models preserved the shape characteristics of the given population, leading to a better specificity compared to shape models from the other tools. For Deformatrica models, the gap in the specificity performance indicated that selection of an atlas directly impacts the shape modeling process.

Clustering Analysis: LAA has natural clustering in which the shapes are mainly categorized into four types: cauliflower, chicken wing, wind sock, and cactus [24]. K-means clustering was performed on the correspondences from each SSM tool to generate four clusters. For comparison, k-means was also performed on the preprocessed distance transforms. The mean shapes of the four clusters from each tool were analyzed in comparison with the mean shapes of clustering

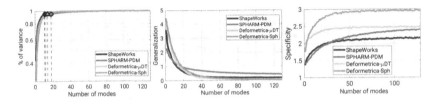

Fig. 3. Compactness (higher is better), generalization (lower is better), and specificity (lower is better) analysis of LAA shape models

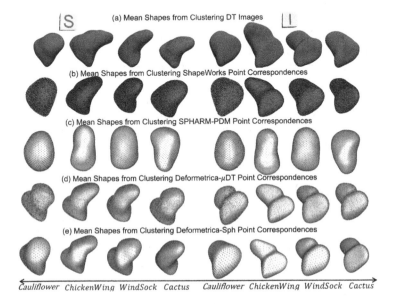

Fig. 4. The mean shapes from k-means clustering (S: superior and I: inferior views) from (a) Distance Transform (DT) images, (b) ShapeWorks, (c) SPHARM-PDM, (d) Deformetrica-μDT, and (e) Deformetrica-Sph. Cluster centers from ShapeWorks and Deformetrica models are closely aligned with the centers from distance transforms.

from the distance transform images to explore the capability of the SSM tool to capture the intrinsic variability and the underlying clustering in the given population. Figure 4 demonstrates that cluster centers from ShapeWorks and Deformetrica shape models better matched those from distance transforms.

3.3 Shape Models Validation

For the 130 LAA shapes, the anatomical landmarks on the LAA ostia were obtained manually (and validated by a clinical expert) using Corview (Marrek inc., Salt Lake City, UT) to serve as a ground truth. From the manual landmarks, the clinical measurements of LAA ostia such as minimum diameter, maximum diameter, area and circumference [24] were obtained by fitting an ellipse to the

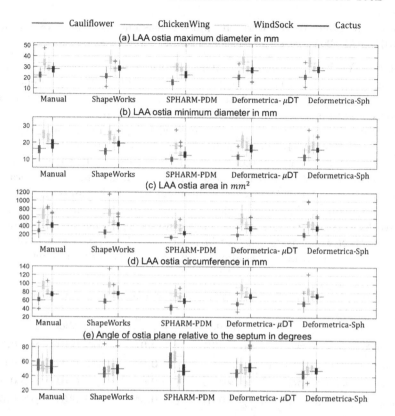

Fig. 5. Box plots of LAA ostia measurements (a) maximum diameter in mm, (b) minimum diameter in mm, (c) area in mm^2, (d) circumference in mm, and (e) angle of ostia plane relative to the septum in degrees.

manual landmarks. To account for different LAA clusters, validation was performed by comparing measurements estimated based on shape models from SSM tools with the measurements estimated from manual landmarks after clustering the preprocessed distance transforms into four clusters. The measurements from the SSM tools were calculated semiautomatically by clustering the point correspondences from each tool into four categories. The mean shape from every cluster of each tool was used to manually mark the shape of the LAA ostia contour using Paraview [2]. A clinical expert reviewed these contours. The point correspondences obtained on the ostium contour of the cluster mean shape were then warped back to the individual shape samples belonging to that cluster to generate the ostium contours of individual samples. An ellipse was fit on the points on the ostium contour of each shape, and the measurements were computed. The manual and semiautomated measurements from each SSM tool were then compared to quantify the accuracy of the learned shape models in estimating the anatomical measurements. Figure 5 illustrates that the measurements obtained from ShapeWorks were the most consistent whereas those obtained from SPHARM-PDM were the least consistent.

Statistical Testing: The manual and semiautomated measurements from each SSM tool were compared using a paired t-test to identify if the differences were statistically significant. A paired t-test takes in measurements obtained by manual and semiautomated means and assumes a null hypothesis that both the recordings come from normal distributions with equal means and equal but unknown variances. The result of the test is rejected when the p-value < 0.01 and is accepted when the p-value > 0.01. Hence, for p-values > 0.01, the measurement differences are not statistically significant. Tables 2, 3, 4, 5 and 6 enumerate the p-values of a paired t-test for each measurement obtained from each tool's cluster in comparison to the manual measurements. Measurements obtained from ShapeWorks were more consistent as the p-values were always greater than 0.01. SPHARM-PDM was least consistent in most cases. The performance of Deformetrica for both the atlases was almost same for all the measurements.

Table 2. p-values for LAA ostia maximum diameter measurement

Comparison	Cauliflower	ChickenWing	WindSock	Cactus
Manual vs ShapeWorks	**p > 0.01**	**p > 0.01**	**p > 0.01**	**p > 0.01**
Manual vs SPHARM-PDM	$p < 0.01$	**p > 0.01**	**p > 0.01**	$p < 0.01$
Manual vs Deformetrica-μDT	**p > 0.01**	**p > 0.01**	**p > 0.01**	**p > 0.01**
Manual vs Deformetrica-Sph	**p > 0.01**	**p > 0.01**	**p > 0.01**	**p > 0.01**

Table 3. p-values for LAA ostia minimum diameter measurement

Comparison	Cauliflower	ChickenWing	WindSock	Cactus
Manual vs ShapeWorks	**p > 0.01**	**p > 0.01**	**p > 0.01**	**p > 0.01**
Manual vs SPHARM-PDM	$p < 0.01$	**p > 0.01**	**p > 0.01**	$p < 0.01$
Manual vs Deformetrica-μDT	$p < 0.01$	$p < 0.01$	$p < 0.01$	$p < 0.01$
Manual vs Deformetrica-Sph	$p < 0.01$	$p < 0.01$	$p < 0.01$	$p < 0.01$

Table 4. p-values for LAA ostia area measurement

Comparison	Cauliflower	ChickenWing	WindSock	Cactus
Manual vs ShapeWorks	**p > 0.01**	**p > 0.01**	**p > 0.01**	**p > 0.01**
Manual vs SPHARM-PDM	$p < 0.01$	$p < 0.01$	$p < 0.01$	$p < 0.01$
Manual vs Deformetrica-μDT	$p < 0.01$	**p > 0.01**	**p > 0.01**	$p < 0.01$
Manual vs Deformetrica-Sph	$p < 0.01$	$p < 0.01$	**p > 0.01**	**p > 0.01**

Table 5. p-values for LAA ostia circumference measurement

Comparison	Cauliflower	ChickenWing	WindSock	Cactus
Manual vs ShapeWorks	**p > 0.01**	**p > 0.01**	**p > 0.01**	**p > 0.01**
Manual vs SPHARM-PDM	$p < 0.01$	$p < 0.01$	$p < 0.01$	$p < 0.01$
Manual vs Deformetrica-μDT	$p < 0.01$	**p > 0.01**	**p > 0.01**	$p < 0.01$
Manual vs Deformetrica-Sph	**p > 0.01**	**p > 0.01**	**p > 0.01**	**p > 0.01**

Table 6. p-values for angle of LAA ostia plane relative to septum measurement

Comparison	Cauliflower	ChickenWing	WindSock	Cactus
Manual vs ShapeWorks	**p > 0.01**	**p > 0.01**	**p > 0.01**	**p > 0.01**
Manual vs SPHARM-PDM	**p > 0.01**	$p < 0.01$	$p < 0.01$	**p > 0.01**
Manual vs Deformetrica-μDT	$p < 0.01$	**p > 0.01**	**p > 0.01**	**p > 0.01**
Manual vs Deformetrica-Sph	$p < 0.01$	**p > 0.01**	**p > 0.01**	**p > 0.01**

4   Conclusion

We presented an evaluation and a clinically driven validation framework for open-source statistical shape modeling (SSM) tools. SSM tools were evaluated quantitatively and qualitatively using measures such as compactness, generalization, specificity, modes of variation and intrinsic clustering discovery. ShapeWorks and Deformetrica shape models were shown to capture clinically relevant population-level variability compared to SPHARM-PDM models. With lack of ground truth shape descriptors/correspondences, validating resulting shape models from different SSM tools becomes a challenge. To address this challenge, we have designed a semiautomated approach that is driven by learned shape models in the context of a clinical application to estimate clinically relevant anatomical measurements. Results emphasized the different levels of consistencies exhibited by different SSM tools. Yet, ShapeWorks – by virtue of its optimized groupwise shape correspondences – yields the most consistent anatomical measurements. In the future, we will extend this study to other publicly available tools and clinical scenarios to benchmark SSM tools in different applications and to provide a blueprint for developing computational tools for shape models.

Acknowledgment. This work was supported by NIH [grant numbers R01-HL135568-01 and P41-GM103545-19] and Coherex Medical.

References

1. Ashburner, J.: SPM: a history. Neuroimage **62**(2), 791–800 (2012)
2. Ayachit, U.: The paraview guide: a parallel visualization application (2015)
3. Bookstein, F.L.: Principal warps: thin-plate splines and the decomposition of deformations. IEEE Trans. PAMI **11**(6), 567–585 (1989)

4. Carlier, A., Geris, L., Lammens, J., Van Oosterwyck, H.: Bringing computational models of bone regeneration to the clinic. Wiley Interdiscip. Rev.: Syst. Biol. Med. **7**(4), 183–194 (2015)
5. Cates, J., Elhabian, S., Whitaker, R.: ShapeWorks: particle-based shape correspondence and visualization software. In: Statistical Shape and Deformation Analysis, pp. 257–298. Elsevier (2017)
6. Cates, J., Fletcher, P.T., Styner, M., Shenton, M., Whitaker, R.: Shape modeling and analysis with entropy-based particle systems. In: Karssemeijer, N., Lelieveldt, B. (eds.) IPMI 2007. LNCS, vol. 4584, pp. 333–345. Springer, Heidelberg (2007). https://doi.org/10.1007/978-3-540-73273-0_28
7. Dalal, P., Shi, F., Shen, D., Wang, S.: Multiple cortical surface correspondence using pairwise shape similarity. In: Jiang, T., Navab, N., Pluim, J.P.W., Viergever, M.A. (eds.) MICCAI 2010. LNCS, vol. 6361, pp. 349–356. Springer, Heidelberg (2010). https://doi.org/10.1007/978-3-642-15705-9_43
8. Davies, R., Taylor, C., et al.: Statistical Models of Shape: Optimisation and Evaluation. Springer, London (2008). https://doi.org/10.1007/978-1-84800-138-1
9. Davies, R.H.: Learning shape: optimal models for analysing shape variability. Ph.D. thesis, University of Manchester (2002)
10. Davies, R.H., Twining, C.J., Cootes, T.F., Waterton, J.C., Taylor, C.J.: 3D statistical shape models using direct optimisation of description length. In: Heyden, A., Sparr, G., Nielsen, M., Johansen, P. (eds.) ECCV 2002. LNCS, vol. 2352, pp. 3–20. Springer, Heidelberg (2002). https://doi.org/10.1007/3-540-47977-5_1
11. Durrleman, S., et al.: Morphometry of anatomical shape complexes with dense deformations and sparse parameters. NeuroImage **101**, 35–49 (2014)
12. Fischl, B., Sereno, M.I., Tootell, R.B., Dale, A.M., et al.: High-resolution intersubject averaging and a coordinate system for the cortical surface. Hum. Brain Mapp. **8**(4), 272–284 (1999)
13. Gao, Y., Riklin-Raviv, T., Bouix, S.: Shape analysis, a field in need of careful validation. Hum. Brain Mapp. **35**(10), 4965–4978 (2014)
14. Goebel, R., Esposito, F., Formisano, E.: Analysis of functional image analysis contest (FIAC) data with brainvoyager QX: from single-subject to cortically aligned group general linear model analysis and self-organizing group independent component analysis. Hum. Brain Mapp. **27**(5), 392–401 (2006)
15. Gollmer, S.T., Kirschner, M., Buzug, T.M., Wesarg, S.: Using image segmentation for evaluating 3D statistical shape models built with groupwise correspondence optimization. Comput. Vis. Image Underst. **125**, 283–303 (2014)
16. Jenkinson, M., Beckmann, C.F., Behrens, T.E., Woolrich, M.W., Smith, S.M.: FSL. Neuroimage **62**(2), 782–790 (2012)
17. Kohara, S., Tateyama, T., Foruzen, A.H.: Preliminary study on statistical shape model applied to diagnosis of liver cirrhosis. IEEE (2011)
18. Markelj, P., Tomaževič, D., Likar, B., Pernuš, F.: A review of 3D/2D registration methods for image-guided interventions. Med. Image Anal. **16**(3), 642–661 (2012)
19. Oguz, I., et al.: Entropy-based particle correspondence for shape populations. Int. J. Comput. Assist. Radiol. Surg. **11**, 1–12 (2015)
20. Regazzoli, D., et al.: Left atrial appendage: physiology, pathology, and role as a therapeutic target. BioMed (2015)
21. Rodriguez-Florez, N., et al.: Statistical shape modelling to aid surgical planning: associations between surgical parameters and head shapes following spring-assisted cranioplasty. Int. J. Comput. Assist. Radiol. Surg. **12**(10), 1739–1749 (2017)
22. Sarkalkan, N., Weinans, H., Zadpoor, A.A.: Statistical shape and appearance models of bones. Bone **60**, 129–140 (2014)

23. Styner, M., et al.: Framework for the statistical shape analysis of brain structures using SPHARM-PDM. Insight J., 242 (2006)
24. Wang, Y., Di Biase, L., Horton, R.P., Nguyen, T., Morhanty, P., Natale, A.: Left atrial appendage studied by computed tomography to help planning for appendage closure device placement. J. Cardiovas, Electrophys **21**(9), 973–982 (2010)
25. Zachow, S.: Computational planning in facial surgery. Facial Plast. Surg. **31**(05), 446–462 (2015)
26. Zadpoor, A.A., Weinans, H.: Patient-specific bone modeling and analysis: the role of integration and automation in clinical adoption. J. Biomech. **48**(5), 750–760 (2015)

Characterizing Anatomical Variability and Alzheimer's Disease Related Cortical Thinning in the Medial Temporal Lobe Using Graph-Based Groupwise Registration and Point Set Geodesic Shooting

Long Xie[1]([✉]), Laura E. M. Wisse[1], Sandhitsu R. Das[1,3],
Ranjit Ittyerah[1], Jiancong Wang[1], David A. Wolk[2,3],
Paul A. Yushkevich[1], and for the Alzheimer's Disease
Neuroimaging Initiative

[1] Penn Image Computing and Science Laboratory (PICSL),
Department of Radiology, University of Pennsylvania, Philadelphia, USA
lxie@seas.upenn.edu
[2] Penn Memory Center, University of Pennsylvania, Philadelphia, USA
[3] Department of Neurology, University of Pennsylvania, Philadelphia, USA

Abstract. The perirhinal cortex (PRC) is a site of early neurofibrillary tangle (NFT) pathology in Alzheimer's disease (AD). Subtle morphological changes in the PRC have been reported in MRI studies of early AD, which has significance for clinical trials targeting preclinical AD. However, the PRC exhibits considerable anatomical variability with multiple *discrete variants* described in the neuroanatomy literature. We hypothesize that different anatomical variants are associated with different patterns of AD-related effects in the PRC. Single-template approaches conventionally used for automated image-based brain morphometry are ill-equipped to test this hypothesis. This study uses graph-based groupwise registration and diffeomorphic landmark matching with geodesic shooting to build statistical shape models of discrete PRC variants and examine variant-specific effects of AD on PRC shape and thickness. Experimental results demonstrate that the statistical models recover the folding patterns of the known PRC variants and capture the expected shape variability within the population. By applying the proposed pipeline to a large dataset with subjects from different stages in the AD spectrum, we find (1) a pattern of cortical thinning consistent with the NFT pathology progression, (2) different patterns of the initial spatial distribution of cortical thinning between anatomical variants, and (3) an effect of AD on medial temporal lobe shape. As such, the proposed pipeline could have important utility in the early detection and monitoring of AD.

Data used in preparation of this article were obtained from the Alzheimer's Disease Neuroimaging Initiative (ADNI) database (adni.loni.usc.edu). As such, the investigators within the ADNI contributed to the design and implementation of ADNI and/or provided data but did not participate in analysis or writing of this report. A complete listing of ADNI investigators can be found at: http://adni.loni.usc.edu/wp-content/uploads/how_to_apply/ADNI_Acknowledgement_List.pdf.

© Springer Nature Switzerland AG 2018
M. Reuter et al. (Eds.): ShapeMI 2018, LNCS 11167, pp. 28–37, 2018.
https://doi.org/10.1007/978-3-030-04747-4_3

1 Introduction

The human brain is highly variable in terms of its folding pattern and cytoarchitectural boundaries. Current leading paradigms in population studies using brain structural MRI are primarily based on normalization techniques that use a single template to capture variability between all subjects in a population, even when one to one correspondence between anatomies might not exist. Failing to account for the anatomical variability in the analysis degrades our ability to reliably localize and accurately quantify brain regions in individual subjects. Although characterizing anatomical variability of the brain "on a whole" is desirable, it might not be feasible given an almost infinite number of anatomical configurations. However, when focusing on specific local brain regions, regional anatomical variability can often be described by a few anatomical variants. A recent study by Ding and Van Hoesen [1] found that in the human perirhinal cortex (PRC), two major anatomical variants account for 97% of the cases. The PRC, consisting of Brodmann areas 35 and 36 (BA35/36), plays an important role in memory and is a site of early neurofibrillary tangle (NFT) pathology, which is linked to synaptic loss and cell death in Alzheimer's disease (AD). The two variants are characterized by the morphology of the collateral sulcus (CS) (continuous vs. discontinuous CS). Given the early involvement of the PRC in AD, there is considerable interest in using MRI-based measures of its atrophy as biomarkers, e.g., for tracking the effectiveness of future drugs targeting NFT pathology in preclinical AD stages. However, it is important to ensure that such biomarkers take into account the anatomical variability of the PRC, since the extents of AD-related pathology in the PRC are likely to differ between the different anatomical variants due to the sheet-like organization of the cerebral cortex. For example, for subjects with deeper CS, early NFT deposition may occur more medially than for subjects with a shallow CS.

In our prior work [2, 3], we showed that graph-based multi-template analysis better accounts for the existence of discrete PRC variants and improves the quality of template fitting and sensitivity to AD effects. The current paper goes further to show that, by coupling with geodesic shooting for diffeomorphic shape matching [4, 5], the graph-based multi-template analysis is able to characterize PRC anatomical variability that is more meaningful than a conventional single-template approach. Furthermore, our paper compares patterns of AD-related change between PRC anatomical variants. Disambiguating these patterns using multi-template analysis may lead to more sensitive MRI-based measurements of early AD-related changes in the PRC, which may in turn provide more effective biomarkers for monitoring change in preclinical AD research and clinical trials.

2 Materials and Method

2.1 Dataset

This paper uses two MRI datasets. A publicly available dataset described in [6] (referred to as **T1-atlas**) with manual segmentations of BA35, BA36, entorhinal cortex (ERC), CS and meninges is used for multi-atlas segmentation and to define shape models of anatomical variants of the PRC. It consists of 29 [14 mild cognitive impairment (MCI), 15 normal control (NC)] 1.0 mm^3 MPRAGE T1-weighted MRI scans (T1w) upsampled to 0.5 × 0.5 × 1 mm^3 using a super-resolution technique [7] (SR-T1w).

Shape models derived from the T1-atlas are used to analyze a large dataset of baseline T1w MRIs from the Alzheimer's Disease Neuroimaging Initiative (ADNI). ADNI subjects (n = 603, see Table 1) were grouped into five severity categories based on diagnosis, cognitive symptoms and PET evidence of amyloid pathology: amyloid negative controls (AN-CN, n = 180) and amyloid positive controls, (AP-NC, n = 94), early MCI (AP-EMCI, n = 130), late MCI (AP-LMCI, n = 109), and AD (AP-AD, n = 81). These categories reflect the continuum from cognitively normal to mild AD.

Table 1. Demographics of the ADNI dataset

	AN-CN	AP-CN	AP-EMCI	AP-LMCI	AP-AD
N	180	94	130	109	81
Age (yrs.)	72.0 (6.0)	74.5 (5.7)***	73.0 (6.9)	71.7 (6.8)	74.9 (7.8)***
Gender (M/F)	94/86	32/62**	80/59	57/52	47/34
Education (yrs.)	16.9 (2.4)	16.1 (2.7)*	15.7 (2.9)***	16.6 (2.6)	15.4 (2.6)**
MMSE	29.0 (1.3)	29.0 (1.1)	28.0 (1.7)***	27.2 (1.9)***	23.2 (2.1)***

Note: All statistics are in comparison to AN-CN. Two-sample t-test (age, education and MMSE) and χ^2 test (gender) are used. *$p < 0.05$; **$p < 0.01$; and ***$p < 0.001$. MMSE = mini-mental state examination.

2.2   Construction of Statistical Models of Anatomical Variants of the PRC

To boost the size of the T1-atlas, images were flipped across the midsagittal plane, yielding a total of 58 samples. Manual segmentations were assigned by visual inspection to one of two variants (1: continuous CS vs. 2: discontinuous CS, [1]). Then, a statistical model for each variant was constructed using the following steps.

2.2.1   Template Construction Using Graph-Based Groupwise Registration

A graph-based groupwise registration method similar to [8] is used to construct a population template of each anatomical variant (variant-template). First, we construct an undirected complete graph with the samples as vertices and edge weights indicative of dissimilarity between pairs of samples. To obtain the weights, affine and coarse-scale deformable diffeomorphic registration is performed between each pair of multi-label manual segmentations in the atlas. This uses a fast greedy diffeomorphic implementation adapted from [9, 10][1], with the sum of normalized cross correlation computed separately for each label as the image similarity metric. Importantly, a large spatial regularization term (the smoothing Gaussian kernel size is set to a 2.0 mm, which is a

---

[1] "Greedy" tool (https://github.com/pyushkevich/greedy).

large value considering the PRC is a small structure) is applied during diffeomorphic registration to limit the amount of deformation that is allowed. Then, the weight of each pair of segmentations is measured as the one minus the generalized Dice similarity coefficient (GDSC) [11] of labels BA35, BA36 and CS between the warped moving segmentation and the segmentation of the target sample. Due to strong regularization, deformable registration can only correct for coarse-scale differences in shape, which makes the residual disagreement measured by one minus GDSC indicative of anatomical dissimilarity. Once the graph is generated, we construct a minimum spanning tree that includes all the nodes in the graph [12] and mark as its "root" the sample that has the shortest path along the tree to all the nodes. The shortest path from each sample to the MST root corresponds to a sequence of affine and deformable registrations that involves the least amount of deformation at each step. A unique path from each sample to the root is then identified. For each sample, a second set of finer-scale deformable registrations (with the smoothing kernel size set to 0.8 mm) are performed between each pair of samples along the unique path. Then, we compose the sequence of affine transforms and finer-scale deformations (rather than the coarse deformations) along these unique paths and warp the segmentations of all the samples to the space of the root sample. In order to further align all the samples, at the end of this step, a population template is built from the warped multi-label segmentations in the space of the root sample using the same metric as in the pairwise coarse registration by applying the iterative unbiased template building algorithm [9].

2.2.2 Quantifying Shape Variability Using Pointset Geodesic Shooting

Subsequent shape analysis uses a large deformation diffeomorphic metric mapping (LDDMM) on point landmarks via geodesic shooting [4, 5, 13]. This provides several benefits: (1) diffeomorphic transformations of the template shape toward each of the subject shapes can be represented compactly using the initial momentum vector field; (2) linear statistics such as PCA can be applied to the initial momenta to characterize variability and to generate statistically plausible shapes; (3) landmark matching is simpler and more efficient than image-based geodesic shooting, and makes particular sense for matching multi-label images; (4) landmark correspondences can be easily interpolated to yield diffeomorphic transformations of the entire image domain. Using geodesic shooting in Sect. 2.2.1 will make the pipeline more consistent. However, performing N^2 registrations in the pairwise registration step using geodesic shooting is not efficient and impractical. Since we aim to develop an efficient pipeline for our application, we choose to use a fast implementation of the greedy registration approach instead.

For each variant-template, we first generate a dense surface mesh (M^T, 10^4 vertices) for the union of ERC, BA35 and BA36 labels, on which we uniformly sample a sparse set of L point landmarks $X^T = \{X_1^T, \ldots, X_L^T\}$ (about 2500 landmarks are sampled.) using Poisson Disk Sampling [14]. The landmarks are then warped to the space of each sample i of the N samples using the deformation field generated in Sect. 2.2.1, denoted as $X_i = \{X_{i,1}, \ldots, X_{i,L}\}$. The Procrustes algorithm [15] is applied to rigidly align X_i to X^T, denoted as $\hat{X}_i$. Then geodesic shooting is performed between $\hat{X}_i$ and X^T to generate the initial momenta of all the subjects. We follow the notation of the geodesic shooting method in [4]. Let α be a $L \times 3$ matrix of the landmarks' initial momenta. Let $q(t; \alpha) = \{q_1(t; \alpha), \ldots, q_L(t; \alpha)\}$ describe the evolution of landmark positions over time

$t \in [0,1]$ and let $p(t;\alpha) = \{p_1(t;\alpha),\ldots,p_L(t;\alpha)\}$ be the corresponding evolving momenta at time point t, with $q(0;\alpha) = X^T, p(0;\alpha) = \alpha$. The Hamiltonian $H(p,q) = \sum_j \sum_k e^{-|q_j-q_k|^2/2\sigma^2} p_j^T p_k$ describes the kinetic energy of the evolving landmark system and is constant over time; evolution is given by the system of equations $\{\frac{dq}{dt} = \frac{\partial H(q,p)}{\partial p}, \frac{dp}{dt} = -\frac{\partial H(q,p)}{\partial q}\}$ [16]. With this notation, the landmark-matching process can be formulated as an optimization problem for each sample i

$$\alpha_i^* = \arg\min_{\alpha \in \mathbb{R}^{3L}} H(X^T, \alpha) + \lambda \cdot ||q(1;\alpha) - \hat{X}_i|| \tag{1}$$

where λ is the weight of the fidelity term. The optimization problem is solved using a gradient-descent method as described in [4]. After optimization, a smooth time-varying velocity field over the entire spatial domain can be obtained from the optimal landmark trajectories $q(t;\alpha_i^*)$ and the corresponding momenta $p(t;\alpha_i^*)$ using Eq. 2 and the diffeomorphic transformation over the image domain $\phi_i(x,t)$ can be derived by integrating the corresponding time points of the velocity field.

$$\frac{d\phi_i(x,t)}{dt} = v_i(x,t) = \sum_{l=1}^{L} G_\sigma(||q_l(t;\alpha_i^*) - x||) \cdot p_l(t;\alpha_i^*), x \in \mathbb{R}^3 \tag{2}$$

A drawback of the graph-based groupwise registration approach (Sect. 2.2.1) is that the template is very similar in shape to the root sample and may not be a good representation of the groupwise mean. We use an iterative approach to perform shape correction. Let $X^{T,0}$ be the landmark locations in the root template. At iteration k, we perform the following steps: (1) for each sample i, we rigidly align X_i to $X^{T,k}$ to generate $\hat{X}_i^k$, and α_i^k is obtained by geodesic shooting from $X^{T,k}$ to $\hat{X}_i^k$ (Eq. 1), (2) we compute the average initial momentum $\bar{\alpha}^k = \frac{1}{N}\sum_{i=1}^{N} \alpha_i^k$, (3) the template landmarks $X^{T,k}$ are deformed by geodesic shooting in the direction of $\bar{\alpha}^k$ to generate $\hat{X}^{T,k+1}$, (4) to avoid expansion or shrinkage of the landmark configurations due to global scaling, $X^{T,k}$ are rigidly aligned to $\hat{X}^{T,k+1}$ to generate the updated template landmarks positions $X^{T,k+1}$ and the template surface mesh $M^{T,k}$ is updated to $M^{T,k+1}$ using the same rigid transformation. This process is repeated until the template becomes stable yielding the final template landmarks $X^{T,K}$ and the final template surface mesh $M^{T,K}$.

PCA is applied to the initial velocity fields, computed from the corresponding initial momenta generated in the last iteration, to quantify anatomical variability. Principal modes are visualized by applying geodesic shooting to $M^{T,K}$ along the principal eigenvectors in both the positive and negative directions.

2.3   Fitting the Templates to a New Target Image

(1) Automatic Segmentation and Template Assignment. A multi-atlas segmentation method [17] is used to generate automatic segmentations of bilateral MTL

substructures in ADNI T1w MRI scans, using the T1-atlas as the atlas set. For a given target T1w MRI scan, let S_{tg} denote its segmentation. To automatically determine the anatomical variant of S_{tg}, similar to the pairwise registration step in Sect. 2.2.1, S_{tg} is coarsely registered to all the 58 samples in the T1-atlas and the GDSCs of labels BA35, BA36 and CS are computed. The six samples with the highest GDSCs are used to perform weighted (by GDSC) voting and the variant that gets the highest vote is assigned to the target sample.

(2) Template Fitting. The sample in the atlas set that belongs to the same anatomical variant with S_{tg} and yields the highest GDSC is identified, referred to as S_{bdg}. Then, the landmarks in the corresponding variant-template space, i.e. $X^{T,K}$, are warped to the space of the target sample, referred to as X_{tg}, using the deformation field generated by composing the deformations from the variant-template to S_{bdg} (obtained in Sect. 2.2.1) and from S_{bdg} to S_{tg} [generated in step (1) above]. Similar to that in Sect. 2.2.2, we (1) rigidly align X_{tg} to $X^{T,K}$ using Procrustes algorithm [15] to generate $\hat{X}_{tg}$, (2) compute the optimal α_{tg} by matching $X^{T,K}$ to $\hat{X}_{tg}$ and (3) deform $M^{T,K}$ to the space of each subject by applying the velocity field derived from α_{tg} using Eq. 2.

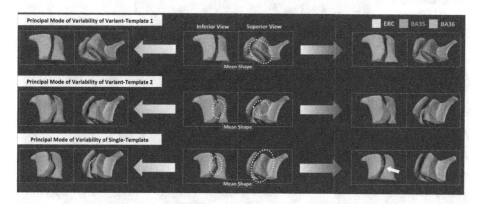

Fig. 1. The variant-templates (the first and second rows) and single-template (the third row), and their corresponding principal modes of variability. Yellow dashed circles highlight the regions with the most variability. White arrow indicates the anatomically implausible structure in the single-template. Videos are available in Supplementary Videos S1 (variant templates 1 and 2) and S2 (single template).

3   Experiments and Results

3.1   Statistical Shape Models

In the T1-atlas, 24 cases were assigned to variant 1 and 34 samples to variant 2. Figure 1 shows the smooth variant-template meshes (first two rows, middle column) and the principal mode of variations of the two statistical models (Supplementary Videos S1). As expected, the two variant-templates resemble anatomical variants with continuous and discontinuous CS, respectively, and appear to be consistent with the anatomical subtypes described in [1]. The first PCA mode of variant 2 captures variation in the relative length of anterior and posterior CS. This variability makes anatomical sense, as variant 2 has been further dichotomized in anatomy literature into two subtypes based on the relative length of anterior and posterior CS [1]. This shows that the graph-based template-building approach is able to align subjects with discontinuous CS. The first PCA mode of variant 1 captures variation in the depth of the CS, which is also a recognized source of variability in this region [1].

To compare our multi-template pipeline with the conventional approach, we also build a statistical shape model for all the samples without grouping by anatomical variants (the third row in Fig. 1, Supplementary Video S2). This single-template approach has two major limitations: (1) An anatomically implausible shape is observed in the middle of the CS (white arrow in Fig. 1); (2) The first PCA mode appears to be less meaningful anatomically, capturing a combination of variability in depth of the CS and the relative length of anterior and posterior CS.

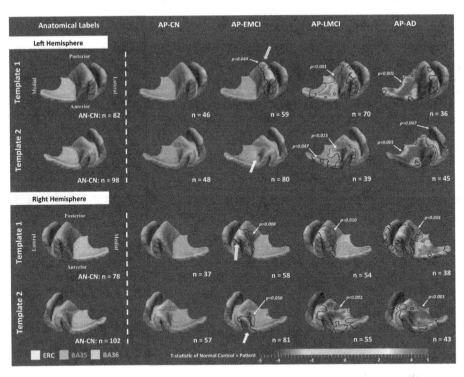

Fig. 2. t-statistical maps of the contrast between AN-CN and four disease groups. Black contours outline significant clusters and the corrected p-values are indicated by the white arrow and text. The corresponding anatomical labels are shown in the first column.

3.2   AD-Related Cortical Thinning

In the ADNI dataset, the number of subjects assigned to different anatomical variants by group is shown in Fig. 2. Across all groups and both hemispheres, 558 (46%) samples were classified into variant 1 and 648 (54%) into variant 2. The proportion of variants between left and right is not significantly different ($\chi^2 = 2.6, p > 0.1$).

To evaluate the patterns of cortical thinning, regional thickness analyses were performed between the control group (AN-CN) and the 4 patient groups separately. Regional thickness is measured by first extracting the pruned Voronoi skeleton [18] of the fitted template mesh and computing the distance between each vertex and the closest point on the skeleton. A general linear model is fit at each vertex with thickness as the dependent variable, group membership as the factor of interest, and age, education as covariates. To account for multiple statistical comparisons, cluster-level familywise error rate correction is used [19] (empirical threshold: uncorrected $p = 0.05$). Permutation testing with 1000 iterations is used to assign a corrected p-value to each cluster. Analysis is performed separately for each variant of each hemisphere.

As shown in Fig. 2, we observed a consistent pattern of disease progression across variant-templates of both hemispheres: initiating largely in BA35 as early as in the AP-EMCI stage and progressing to ERC and BA36 in later stages. This is consistent with neuropathological staging of NFT progression [20]. Cluster size, spatial distribution, and magnitude of significance increase along with disease severity. Also, significant clusters at later stages almost always cover the ones in the corresponding previous stages. No significant effects are observed in AP-CN. Being able to replicate the patterns of disease progression in the MTL observed in *ex vivo* pathology studies using *in vivo* MRI (Fig. 2) has great potential significance for tracking the early neurodegenerative stages of disease critical for measurement of intervention effects in clinical trials.

A novel aspect in this study is that we examine the relationship between the spread of AD-related atrophy and PRC variants. The first site of cortical thinning in variant 1 appears to be located at the fundus of the CS (gray arrows in Fig. 2), whereas in variant 2, it is located more medially, at the boundary of ERC and BA35 (yellow arrows in Fig. 2). There is not much difference between anatomical variants in later stages, probably because the majority of the MTL cortex is affected by the disease.

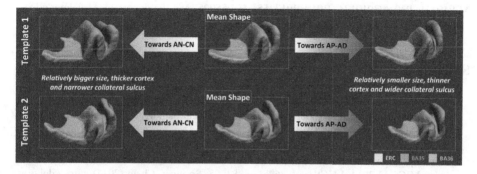

Fig. 3. The effect of AD on medial temporal lobe cortex shape of the anatomical variants. Videos are available in Supplementary Videos S3.

3.3   Effect of AD on MTL Shape

To investigate the effect of AD on MTL shape, for each variant, the initial momenta of subjects from the opposite ends of the AD spectrum, i.e. AN-CN and AP-AD (excluded cases from the other groups), are converted to initial velocity fields and projected to the first m PCA modes that account for 95% of the total variance of the corresponding statistical model ($m = 19/26$ for variant 1/2 respectively) and a support vector machine (SVM) with a linear kernel [21] is trained on the PCA loadings to discriminate the two groups. The vector orthogonal to the SVM hyperplane, which is assumed to be the direction that best discriminates the two groups, is shown in Fig. 3 (Supplementary Videos S3). The result shows that AD is associated with decrease in overall size of the MTL, cortical thinning and widening of the CS. It will be interesting to investigate in future studies whether these shape features provide complementary information in identifying disease groups.

4   Conclusion

In this study, we propose a novel analysis pipeline to quantify shape variability of anatomical variants of the PRC. Experimental results demonstrate that the statistical models recover the folding patterns of the known anatomical variants of the PRC defined in the neuroanatomy literature and capture the expected shape variability within the population. In addition, when applied to a large dataset with subjects from different stages in the AD spectrum, the novel shape analysis reveals a progression of cortical thinning and shape that is consistent with known progression of NFT pathology within the MTL cortex related to AD. Also, different patterns of the spatial distribution of cortical thinning are observed between anatomical variants. Summary thickness measurements extracted from the significant clusters (Fig. 2) and the features associated with shape changes may be useful markers for early detection and tracking disease progression. As such, we believe the proposed method may have important utility in the early detection and monitoring of AD and the findings in this study may help us better understand the effect of AD on the shape of MTL substructures.

Acknowledgements. This work was supported by NIH (grant numbers R01-AG056014, R01-AG040271, P30-AG010124, R01-EB017255, AG055005) and the donors of Alzheimer's Disease Research, a program of the BrightFocus Foundation (L.E.M.W.).

References

1. Ding, S.-L., Van Hoesen, G.W.: Borders, extent, and topography of human perirhinal cortex as revealed using multiple modern neuroanatomical and pathological markers. Hum. Brain Mapp. **31**(9), 1359–1379 (2010)
2. Xie, L., et al.: Automatic clustering and thickness measurement of anatomical variants of the human perirhinal cortex. In: Golland, P., Hata, N., Barillot, C., Hornegger, J., Howe, R. (eds.) MICCAI 2014. LNCS, vol. 8675, pp. 81–88. Springer, Cham (2014). https://doi.org/10.1007/978-3-319-10443-0_11

3. Xie, L., et al.: Multi-template analysis of human perirhinal cortex in brain MRI: explicitly accounting for anatomical variability. Neuroimage **144**, 183–202 (2017)
4. Allassonnière, S., Trouvé, A., Younes, L.: Geodesic shooting and diffeomorphic matching via textured meshes. In: Rangarajan, A., Vemuri, B., Yuille, A.L. (eds.) EMMCVPR 2005. LNCS, vol. 3757, pp. 365–381. Springer, Heidelberg (2005). https://doi.org/10.1007/11585978_24
5. Vaillant, M., Miller, M.I., Younes, L., Trouvé, A.: Statistics on diffeomorphisms via tangent space representations. Neuroimage **23**(Suppl 1), S161–S169 (2004)
6. Xie, L., et al.: Accounting for the confound of meninges in segmenting entorhinal and perirhinal cortices in T1-weighted MRI. In: Ourselin, S., Joskowicz, L., Sabuncu, M.R., Unal, G., Wells, W. (eds.) MICCAI 2016. LNCS, vol. 9901, pp. 564–571. Springer, Cham (2016). https://doi.org/10.1007/978-3-319-46723-8_65
7. Manjón, J.V., Coupé, P., Buades, A., Fonov, V., Collins, L.D., Robles, M.: Non-local MRI upsampling. Med. Image Anal. **14**(6), 784–792 (2010)
8. Wu, G., Jia, H., Wang, Q., Shen, D.: SharpMean: groupwise registration guided by sharp mean image and tree-based registration. Neuroimage **56**(4), 1968–1981 (2011)
9. Joshi, S., Davis, B., Jomier, M., Gerig, G.: Unbiased diffeomorphic atlas construction for computational anatomy. Neuroimage **23**(Suppl 1), S151–S160 (2004)
10. Avants, B.B., Epstein, C.L., Grossman, M., Gee, J.C.: Symmetric diffeomorphic image registration with cross-correlation: evaluating automated labeling of elderly and neurodegenerative brain. Med. Image Anal. **12**(1), 26–41 (2008)
11. Crum, W.R., Camara, O., Hill, D.L.G.: Generalized overlap measures for evaluation and validation in medical image analysis. IEEE Trans. Med. Imaging **25**(11), 1451–1461 (2006)
12. Prim, R.C.: Shortest connection networks and some generalizations. Bell Syst. Tech. J. **36**(6), 1389–1401 (1957)
13. Miller, M.I., Trouvé, A., Younes, L.: Geodesic shooting for computational anatomy. J. Math. Imaging Vis. **24**(2), 209–228 (2006)
14. Corsini, M., Cignoni, P., Scopigno, R.: Efficient and flexible sampling with blue noise properties of triangular meshes. IEEE Trans. Vis. Comput. Graph. **18**(6), 914–924 (2012)
15. Dryden, I.L., Mardia, K.V.: Statistical Shape Analysis, with Applications in {R}, 2nd edn. Wiley, Chichester (2016)
16. Ott, E.: Chaos in dynamical systems. Cambridge University Press, Cambridge (2002)
17. Yushkevich, P.A., et al.: Automated volumetry and regional thickness analysis of hippocampal subfields and medial temporal cortical structures in mild cognitive impairment. Hum. Brain Mapp. **36**(1), 258–287 (2015)
18. Ogniewicz, R.L., Kübler, O.: Hierarchic Voronoi skeletons. Pattern Recognit. **28**(3), 343–359 (1995)
19. Nichols, T., Hayasaka, S.: Controlling the familywise error rate in functional neuroimaging: a comparative review. Stat. Methods Med. Res. **12**(5), 419–446 (2003)
20. Braak, H., Braak, E.: Staging of Alzheimer's disease-related neurofibrillary changes. Neurobiol. Aging **16**(3), 271–278 (1995)
21. Vapnik, V.N.: Statistical Learning Theory. Wiley, Hoboken (1998)

Interpretable Spiculation Quantification for Lung Cancer Screening

Wookjin Choi[1], Saad Nadeem[1], Sadegh Riyahi[1], Joseph O. Deasy[1], Allen Tannenbaum[2], and Wei Lu[1(✉)]

[1] Department of Medical Physics, Memorial Sloan Kettering Cancer Center, New York, USA
luw@mskcc.org
[2] Departments of Computer Science and Applied Mathematics, Stony Brook University, Stony Brook, USA

Abstract. Spiculations are spikes on the surface of pulmonary nodule and are important predictors of malignancy in lung cancer. In this work, we introduced an interpretable, parameter-free technique for quantifying this critical feature using the area distortion metric from the spherical conformal (angle-preserving) parameterization. The conformal factor in the spherical mapping formulation provides a direct measure of spiculation which can be used to detect spikes and compute spike heights for geometrically-complex spiculations. The use of the area distortion metric from conformal mapping has never been exploited before in this context. Based on the area distortion metric and the spiculation height, we introduced a novel spiculation score. A combination of our spiculation measures was found to be highly correlated (Spearman's rank correlation coefficient $\rho = 0.48$) with the radiologist's spiculation score. These measures were also used in the radiomics framework to achieve state-of-the-art malignancy prediction accuracy of 88.9% on a publicly available dataset.

1 Introduction

Lung cancer is the leading cause of cancer death in the United States [12]. The National Lung Cancer Screening Trial showed a clear survival benefit for screening with a low-dose computed tomography (CT) in current and former smokers. Recently radiomics studies [1,2,4], which extract a large number of quantitative features from medical images and subsequently perform data mining, have been proposed for various clinical applications. For instance, radiomics has been studied for the prediction of tumor responses and patient outcomes, resulting in more accurate prediction of local control and overall survival.

Lung cancer screening using radiomics has also been studied. Hawkins *et al.* [4] proposed a random forest classifier using 23 stable radiomic features.

W. Choi and S. Nadeem—The first two authors contributed equally to this work.

© Springer Nature Switzerland AG 2018
M. Reuter et al. (Eds.): ShapeMI 2018, LNCS 11167, pp. 38–48, 2018.
https://doi.org/10.1007/978-3-030-04747-4_4

Buty *et al.* [1] developed a random forest classifier using 4096 appearance features extracted with a pre-trained deep neural network and 400 shape features extracted with spherical harmonics; spherical harmonics are a decomposition of frequency-space basis for representing functions defined over the sphere. The decomposition is applicable to describe overall shape of the object, but it cannot provide local features for a given region on a shape (e.g. spiculation). However, the area distortion metric from the spherical conformal (angle-preserving) parameterization can accurately provide local spiculation features. Kumar et al. [5] developed a deep neural network model using 5000 features. Liu et al. [6] proposed a linear classifier based on 24 image traits visually scored by physicians. Choi *et al.* [2] developed a model using support vector machine and least absolute shrinkage and selection operator (SVM-LASSO) to predict malignancy of pulmonary nodules (PNs) with only two CT radiomic features (shape and texture). Although these radiomics studies have improved prediction accuracy, there still remains a limitation with respect to the lack of clinical/biological interpretation of the features.

Radiographic edge characteristics of a PN, especially spiculation, influence the probability of malignancy [13]. Typically, benign nodules have well-defined and smooth boundaries while malignant nodules have blurred and irregular boundaries. The Lung Imaging Reporting and Data System (Lung-RADS) was developed by the American College of Radiology (ACR) to standardize the screening of lung cancer on CT images using size, appearance type and calcification [7]. For more accurate prediction, spiculation was suggested as an additional image finding that increases the suspicion of malignancy. The McWilliams model [9] was introduced to compute the probability of lung cancer. This model uses nine variables, such as age, sex, family history of lung cancer, emphysema, size, type, location, count, and spiculation. PN size and spiculation were the major malignancy predictors in both models.

Spiculation quantification has been previously studied in a number of papers, but not in the context of malignancy prediction. Niehaus *et al.* [11] developed a computer-aided diagnosis (CAD) system and investigated the size dependence of shape features for quantifying spiculation. Dhara *et al.* [3] reported a differential geometry-based technique for quantifying spiculation using the binary mask of the segmented nodule.

In this work, we presented a comprehensive method to quantify spiculation using spherical parameterization and evaluate its importance in malignancy prediction. The contributions are as follows:

1. A novel interpretable spiculation feature is introduced, computed using the area distortion metric from spherical conformal parameterization;
2. Improved malignancy prediction using radiomics (shape and texture) + proposed spiculation quantification with accuracy 88.9%;
3. Achieved higher Spearman's correlation, $\rho = 0.48$ between our spiculation measures and radiologist's spiculation score than previous methods.

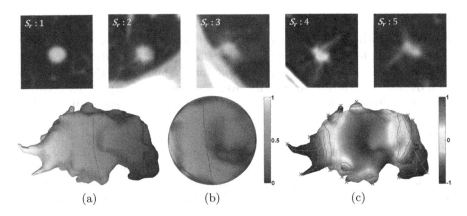

Fig. 1. Radiologist's spiculation score, s_r, for different PNs (top row) and our spiculation quantification pipeline (bottom row). (a) First non-trivial eigenfunction of the Laplace-Beltrami operator is computed for a given mesh. The zeroth-level set (red curve) of this eigenfunction is used to divide the mesh into two topological disks, which are conformally welded and stereographically projected to a sphere (b), which in angle-preserving spherical parameterization [10]. (c) The area distortion metric of the spherically parameterized surface is used to detect apex (red x's), and compute heights (yellow curves) for each spike/spiculation. (Color figure online)

2   Method

In this section, we introduce some background for using area distortion metric and spherical conformal parameterization in spiculation quantification, followed by a novel spiculation score based on the quantified measures. Finally, we talk about spiculation classification and malignancy prediction in the radiomics analysis subsection.

2.1   Conformal Mappings and Area Distortion

We first give a theoretical overview of the distortion of area in conformally mapping a genus zero Riemannian surface S to the unit sphere $\mathcal{S}^2$ to motivate the pipeline in spiculation; see [10] for the relevant mathematical references. By the *Theorema Egregium* of Gauss, one cannot find a diffeomorphism from S with non-constant Gaussian curvature to $\mathcal{S}^2$ which preserves both angles and area. Further, by a general result in complex analysis (uniformization), S and $\mathcal{S}^2$ are conformally equivalent, that is, there exists a diffeomorphism $\phi : S \to \mathcal{S}^2$ that preserves angles. ϕ is unique up to Möbius transformation on $\mathcal{S}^2$. By rescaling, we may assume that the surface area of S is 4π. This is the **spherical parameterization** of a compact genus 0 surface for which we want to measure area distortion.

The first approach does not use the explicit mapping ϕ. Namely, let g_0 be the Riemannian metric on S with corresponding Gaussian curvature K_0. Let K_u be the curvature on the conformally equivalent surface with metric $g_u = e^{2u} g_0$. Then it is well-known that $\Delta u + K_u e^{2u} = K_0$. This equation gives a specific measure of the distortion in area in any spherical parameterization procedure. Indeed, for the unit sphere $K_u = 1$, and thus u satisfies the Poisson equation $\Delta u = K_0 - e^{2u}$. u is called the *conformal distortion factor*, and e^{2u} measures the distortion in area in going from the surface S to the sphere S^2. If one examines the latter Poisson equation, one qualitatively sees that the more $K_0(x)$ varies, the greater the variation in u, and from the maximum principle, ***spikes/spiculations may be identified by the greatest negative variation in area distortion.***

The second approach explicitly employs the conformal mapping $\phi : S \to S^2$, to give a measure of area distortion. (Via Gauss-Bonnet it is equivalent to the first approach.) We can quantify the change of area as a density function μ at each point of the sphere S^2, so that the integral on the unit sphere will give us the area measure of the original surface: $\int_{\phi^{-1}(U)} dy = \int_U \mu(x) \, dx$, $\forall U \subset S^2$ measurable. By change of variables, it is easy to see that this density function is the determinant of the Jacobian of ϕ^{-1}, i.e., $\mu = \det(\nabla \phi^{-1})$.

2.2   Spiculation Quantification Pipeline

In the paper [10], the above program is carried out in a discrete setting with respect to a triangulated surface $S = (V, E, F)$, where V denotes the vertices, E the edges, and F the faces. Here, one may measure the area distortion on each triangle. Using this discrete version of spherical parameterization, the pipeline of spiculation detection (with height and width detection; see Fig. 1), is as follows:

1. Compute conformal (angle-preserving) spherical parameterization [10]: First non-trivial eigenfunction of the Laplace-Beltrami operator is computed for a given mesh (Fig. 1a). The zeroth-level set (red curve in Fig. 1a) of this eigenfunction is used to divide the mesh into two topological disks, which are conformally welded and stereographically projected to a sphere (Fig. 1b).
2. Compute the normalized area distortion. For each vertex v_i, the *area distortion* is defined as

$$\epsilon_i := \log \frac{\sum_{j,k} A([\phi(v_i), \phi(v_j), \phi(v_k)])}{\sum_{j,k} A([v_i, v_j, v_k])}$$

   where $A(.)$ represents the area of a triangle, and $[v_i, v_j, v_k]$ is the triangle formed by v_i, v_j, v_k.
3. Find all the baselines where normalized area distortion is zero.
4. Recursively traverse closed curves toward the negative distortion values until an apex with the most negative area distortion vertex is reached. During the recursion, the closed curves can break into multiple closed curves and move towards different spikes. The spikes and the corresponding closed curves are assigned unique IDs to track their progression and for height computation in the next step.
5. The sum of the distances between the successive centroids of the traversed closed curves give the height of the spike from the baseline. The spike width is the largest distance between the baseline vertices.

NOTE: Comparisons with other state-of-the-art spherical mapping algorithms are provided in [10]. The lowest angle distortion achieved in [10] provides a unique opportunity to exploit the corresponding area distortion metric effectively in our context.

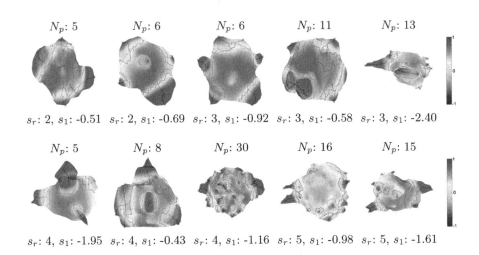

Fig. 2. Spiculation spikes and heights computed via area distortion metric. s_r: radiologist's spiculation score, s_1: proposed spiculation score and N_p: no. of spikes.

2.3   Spiculation Score

Here, we described a novel spiculation score normalized by height, s_1, which summarizes sharpness and height of spikes for each PN,

$$s_1 = \frac{\sum_i \mathrm{mean}(\epsilon_{\mathrm{p}(i)}) * h_{\mathrm{p}(i)}}{\sum_i h_{p(i)}},$$

where $p(i)$ is spike i, $h_{p(i)}$ is height of spike $p(i)$, and $\mathrm{mean}(\epsilon_{p(i)})$ is the mean of the area distortion of all the vertices (sharpness) in $p(i)$. Figure 2 show the results of our spiculation quantification, its measures (no. of spikes N_p and spiculation score s_1) and radiologist's score (s_r). We compared our spiculation score with Dhara's spiculation scores s_a and s_b in [3],

$$s_a = \sum_i e^{-\omega_{p(i)}} h_{p(i)}, s_b = \frac{\sum_i h_{p(i)} \cos \omega_{p(i)}}{\sum_i h_{p(i)}}$$

where $\omega_{p(i)}$ is the solid angle subtended at apex of spike $p(i)$.

2.4   Spiculation Classification and Malignancy Prediction

We evaluated our spiculation measures (N_p and s_1) and radiomic features for classifying spiculation because the current clinical standard (Lung-RADS and McWilliams model) uses binary classification of spiculation. Dhara's spiculation scores (s_a and s_b) were also evaluated. We extracted 103 radiomic features from each PN to quantify its intensity, shape, and texture [2]. Moreover, we extracted features from the mesh model, such as shape features (size - average of longest and its perpendicular diameters, volume, equivalent volume sphere's diameter, and roundness) and statistical features of the area distortion metric ϵ. We performed a univariate analysis using Wilcoxon rank-sum test, the area under the receiver operating characteristic curve (AUC), and Spearman's correlation coefficient ρ to evaluate the significance of each feature to classify spiculation. p-values were adjusted by Bonferroni correction, because we tested multiple features for a single outcome.

For multivariate analysis, we developed a binary classification model using a radial basis kernel SVM ($\gamma = 0.001$ and cost $= 64$). We divided our data into three groups (training 60%, validation 20%, and test 20%), and the details of model construction are as follows:

1. Training set: distinctive features were identified based on hierarchical clustering [2], and then fed to the SVM classifier training.
2. Validation set: The best feature set was selected by a backward selection (recursive feature elimination) to optimize the SVM classification which was trained using the training set.
3. Test set: The performance of the optimized binary classification model was evaluated.

To predict malignancy of PNs, we applied the SVM-LASSO model [2] which uses two CT radiomic features: Bounding Box Dimension of Anterior Posterior axis (BB_AP), and Standard Deviation of Inverse Difference Moment (SD_IDM). We evaluated the original SVM-LASSO model and combinations of the model and spiculation classifications using our spiculation measures and radiologist's spiculation score (s_r), respectively.

3   Results

The Lung Image Database Consortium image collection (LIDC-IDRI) contains 1018 cases with low-dose screening thoracic CT scans and marked-up annotated lesions [8]. Four experienced thoracic radiologists performed contouring and image annotation including spiculation, lobulation, texture, margin and malignancy. Spiculation scoring ranged between 1 (non-spiculated) and 5 (highly spiculated). *We binarized the score (1 as 0, non-spiculated and 2 to 5 as 1, spiculated) because the current clinical standard uses binary classification.* 883 cases (585 non-spiculated vs. 298 spiculated) in the dataset have PNs with contours.

We divided the dataset into two subsets depending on whether diagnostic data (pathological malignancy) was available (72 cases) or not (811 cases). The

811 cases (266 spiculated) were used for training of the spiculation classification, and the 72 cases (32 spiculated) were used for validation of the classification. On the other hand, the 72 cases were used for training of the malignancy prediction, and the 811 cases were used for validation of the prediction. For the validation, we used malignancy score (1 highly unlikely, 2 moderately unlikely, 3 indeterminate likelihood, 4 moderately suspicious, and 5 highly suspicious for cancer) determined radiologically since pathological malignancy is not available.

3.1 Spiculation Classification

We generated synthetic PNs with spiculations (2 mm and 5 mm height) to validate spiculation quantification as shown in Fig. 3. Three of four isolated 2 mm and all four 5 mm synthetic spiculations were detected. The measured average heights were 3.8 and 6.5 mm respectively.

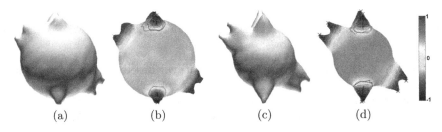

(a)   (b)   (c)   (d)

Fig. 3. Spiculation quantification validation using synthetic pulmonary nodules. (a, b) 2 mm height spiculation, (c, d) 5 mm height spiculation.

In univariate analysis, 23 features were identified as significant features (adjusted p-value < 0.05) to classify spiculation. Two roundness features from mesh model and voxel-based mask image respectively were the best features. All statistical features of ϵ (minimum, variance, maximum, mean, skewness, kurtosis, and median) and most spiculation scores (s_1 and s_b) were significant. In addition, five shape features and seven texture features were significant. Table 1 shows the univariate analysis results of the ten most significant features. Our spiculation score (s_1: 0.67 AUC, P $= 4.29$E-08, $\rho = -0.33$) outperformed Dhara's (s_a: 0.59 AUC, P $= 0.068$, $\rho = 0.22$ and s_b: 0.66 AUC, P $= 1.47$E-07, $\rho = 0.29$). Figure 4 compares our method and Dhara's mean curvature based method. Mean curvature based method detects all critical points on the surface first and then find the baseline of each critical point to detect spikes. So it generated too many spike candidates at a single spike and baseline detection was not accurate. On the other hand, the proposed method can directly detect spikes as a whole.

Table 1. Ten most significant features in univariate analysis for Spiculation classification.

Rank	Feature name	AUC	Corr	P
1	Roundness (Mesh)	0.72	-0.42	$1.82\mathrm{E}{-14}$
2	Roundness (Voxel)	0.70	-0.40	$2.64\mathrm{E}{-11}$
3	Minimum ϵ	0.69	-0.37	$2.93\mathrm{E}{-10}$
4	Long Run Emphasis	0.67	-0.28	$9.40\mathrm{E}{-09}$
5	Variance ϵ	0.67	0.33	$1.48\mathrm{E}{-08}$
6	Maximum ϵ	0.67	0.32	$2.22\mathrm{E}{-08}$
7	s_1	0.67	-0.33	$4.29\mathrm{E}{-08}$
8	s_b	0.66	0.29	$1.47\mathrm{E}{-07}$
9	Mean ϵ	0.66	-0.33	$1.64\mathrm{E}{-07}$
10	2D Roundness	0.65	-0.33	$1.33\mathrm{E}{-06}$

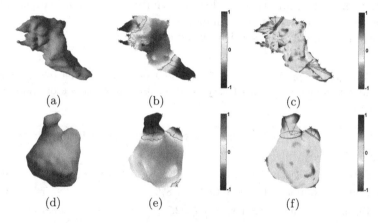

(a)   (b)   (c)

(d)   (e)   (f)

Fig. 4. Comparison with mean curvature method. (a, d) original model, (b, e) spiculation apex and height results computed via area distortion metric, and (c, f) spiculation apex and height results computed via mean curvature method [3].

The number of spikes N_p and spiculation score s_1 were selected to classify PNs into spiculated or non-spiculated in multivariate analysis, and the classification performance is shown in Table 2. The spiculation classification achieved an accuracy of 76.70%, and the validation on the 72 cases showed comparable results (73.61% accuracy). Texture and intensity features were not good predictors. Statistical features of area distortion metric showed similar performance to our spiculation measures.

Table 2. Spiculation classification results

	Sensitivity	Specificity	Accuracy	AUC
Training on 811 cases	73.3%	77.9%	76.7%	0.80
Validation on 72 cases	75.0%	72.5%	73.6%	0.82

3.2 Malignancy Prediction

As shown in Table 3, our spiculation measures (in addition to shape and texture features [2]) improved the malignancy prediction. The prediction accuracy was comparable to using radiologist's spiculation score (Spearman's $\rho = 0.48$) not only on the 72 cases (10 × 10 fold cross-validation) but also on the 811 cases (independent validation of the model trained by the 72 cases). Malignancy was defined as moderately suspicious to highly suspicious (malignancy score > 3) on radiologic readings. Many moderately suspicious PNs were mis-classified as benign (false negative) and thus the low sensitivity 47%. When malignancy was defined as highly suspicious (malignancy score > 4), which was closer to true pathological malignancy, the sensitivity increased to 73.7%.

Table 3. Malignancy prediction by SVM-LASSO radiomics model (shape and texture) [2] and combining with predicted spiculations by radiologist's score (s_r) and our measures ($N_p + s_1$)

	Sensitivity	Specificity	Accuracy	AUC
Training on 72 cases				
Shape+Texture	87.2%	81.2%	84.6%	0.89
Shape+Texture+Radiologist's score (s_r)	87.8%	87.1%	87.5%	0.91
Shape+Texture+Our measures ($N_p + s_1$)	92.7%	83.9%	88.9%	0.92
Validation on 811 cases (malignancy score > 3)				
Shape+Texture	34.6%	93.3%	74.2%	0.81
Shape+Texture+Radiologist's score (s_r)	40.3%	93.8%	76.5%	0.81
Shape+Texture+Our measures ($N_p + s_1$)	47.5%	89.8%	76.1%	0.81
Validation on 811 cases (malignancy score > 4)				
Shape+Texture	63.2%	82.1%	79.4%	0.79
Shape+Texture+Radiologist's score (s_r)	73.7%	64.1%	65.5%	0.77
Shape+Texture+Our measures ($N_p + s_1$)	73.7%	80.9%	79.9%	0.82

Table 4 shows the comparisons with recently reported lung cancer screening radiomic studies. Our method showed better or comparable performance, and its sensitivity, specificity, accuracy, and AUC were well balanced. The malignancy prediction performance was improved when combining spiculation quantification into the radiomics model (shape and texture)[2].

Table 4. Comparison with lung cancer screening radiomic studies

	Dataset	Sensitivity	Specificity	Accuracy	AUC
Hawkins *et al.* (2016) [4]	Baseline CT scans of 261 patients in NLST	51.7%	92.9%	80.0%	0.83
Buty *et al.* (2016) [1]	LIDC 2054 PNs Ground-truth by radiologists assessment			82.4%	
Kumar *et al.* (2015)[5]	LIDC 97 patients Including metastatic tumors	79.1%	76.1%	77.5%	
Liu *et al.* (2016)[6]	172 patients Two independent cohorts 102 and 70 patients	71.4%	83.7%	80.0%	0.81
Choi *et al.* (2018) [2]	LIDC 72 patients	87.2%	81.2%	84.6%	0.89
Proposed Method	LIDC 72 patients	**86.6%**	**84.5%**	**88.9%**	**0.92**

4 Conclusion and Future Work

We presented a novel method for quantification of pulmonary nodule spiculation in lung cancer using the spherical conformal parameterization. The quantitative spiculation measures were found to be highly correlated with the radiologist's spiculation score and lead to state-of-the-art malignancy prediction results with accuracy of 88.9%. A current limitation of our work is the use of manual segmentations from the LIDC datasets, which do not precisely delineate the spiculations. We plan to use semi-automatic segmentation to extract more accurate and reliable mesh models for spiculation quantification. Moreover, we will test this new measure in breast cancer datasets where spiculation again is a good malignancy predictor.

References

1. Buty, M., Xu, Z., Gao, M., Bagci, U., Wu, A., Mollura, D.J.: Characterization of lung nodule malignancy using hybrid shape and appearance features. In: Ourselin, S., Joskowicz, L., Sabuncu, M.R., Unal, G., Wells, W. (eds.) MICCAI 2016. LNCS, vol. 9900, pp. 662–670. Springer, Cham (2016). https://doi.org/10.1007/978-3-319-46720-7_77
2. Choi, W., et al.: Radiomics analysis of pulmonary nodules in low-dose CT for early detection of lung cancer. Med. Phys. **45**, 1537–1549 (2018)
3. Dhara, A.K., Mukhopadhyay, S., Saha, P., Garg, M., Khandelwal, N.: Differential geometry-based techniques for characterization of boundary roughness of pulmonary nodules in CT images. Int. J. Comput. Assist. Radiol. Surg. **11**(3), 337–349 (2016)
4. Hawkins, S., et al.: Predicting malignant nodules from screening CT scans. J. Thorac. Oncol. **11**(12), 2120–2128 (2016)
5. Kumar, D., Shafiee, M.J., Chung, A.G., Khalvati, F., Haider, M.A., Wong, A.: Discovery radiomics for computed tomography cancer detection. arXiv preprint arXiv:1509.00117 (2015)
6. Liu, Y., et al.: Radiological image traits predictive of cancer status in pulmonary nodules. Clin. Cancer Res. **23**, 1442–1449 (2016). clincanres-3102

7. McKee, B.J., Regis, S.M., McKee, A.B., Flacke, S., Wald, C.: Performance of ACR Lung-RADS in a clinical CT lung screening program. J. Am. Coll. Radiol. **12**(3), 273–276 (2015)
8. McNitt-Gray, M.F., Armato, S.G., Meyer, C.R., Reeves, A.P., et al.: The lung image database consortium (LIDC) data collection process for nodule detection and annotation. Acad. Radiol. **14**(12), 1464–1474 (2007)
9. McWilliams, A., Tammemagi, M.C., Mayo, J.R., Roberts, H., et al.: Probability of cancer in pulmonary nodules detected on first screening CT. New Engl. J. Med. **369**(10), 910–919 (2013)
10. Nadeem, S., Su, Z., Zeng, W., Kaufman, A., Gu, X.: Spherical parameterization balancing angle and area distortions. IEEE Trans. Vis. Comput. Graph. **23**(6), 1663–1676 (2017)
11. Niehaus, R., Raicu, D.S., Furst, J., Armato, S.: Toward understanding the size dependence of shape features for predicting spiculation in lung nodules for computer-aided diagnosis. J. Dig. Imaging **28**(6), 704–717 (2015)
12. Siegel, R.L., Miller, K.D., Jemal, A.: Cancer statistics, 2016. CA: Cancer J. Clin. **66**(1), 7–30 (2016)
13. Swensen, S.J., Silverstein, M.D., Ilstrup, D.M., Schleck, C.D., Edell, E.S.: The probability of malignancy in solitary pulmonary nodules: application to small radiologically indeterminate nodules. Arch. Intern. Med. **157**(8), 849–855 (1997)

Shape and Facet Analyses of Alveolar Airspaces of the Lung

Roman Grothausmann[1,2,3(✉)], Christian Mühlfeld[1,2,3], Matthias Ochs[1,2,3], and Lars Knudsen[1,2,3]

[1] Institute of Functional and Applied Anatomy, Hannover Medical School, Hannover, Germany
grothausmann.roman@mh-hannover.de
[2] REBIRTH Cluster of Excellence, Hannover, Germany
[3] Biomedical Research in Endstage and Obstructive Lung Disease Hannover (BREATH), Hannover, Germany

Abstract. Changes in lung volume during the breathing cycle and also lung diseases are likely to deform even the smallest airspace units, the alveoli. This study reports general ideas to investigate such changes with 3D digital image processing. It comprises morphological characterizations like volume and surface, an evaluation of the angle distribution between facets formed by the septal walls, the number of neighboring alveoli and a shape analysis of the alveolar airspace. The software used is open-source and custom programs are available at:
http://github.com/romangrothausmann/.

1 Introduction

The mammalian lung supplies a huge surface area within a limited space, the thoracic cage, to accommodate its central function which is the up-take of oxygen into the blood and at the same time the elimination of carbonic acid gas. [43] In order to meet the requirements for gas exchange, lung parenchyma is composed of so-called acini [12,41] which can be described as alveolated airways, encompassing the alveolar ducts (acinar airway) and the alveoli. The alveolar ducts are surrounded by alveolar entrances by which the ductal airspaces communicate directly with the alveolar airspaces. The alveoli can therefore be described as air-filled bulges of the alveolar duct. Alveoli are separated from each other by thin interalveolar septa which contain a very dense capillary network. [9,30] The interalveolar septa protrude into the alveolar duct and form at their edges the alveolar entrance rings separating the ductal airspace from the alveolar airspace. [29] These entrance rings form a network and thereby a "fisherman's net"-like boundary of the alveolar duct. Alveoli are arranged in series side-by-side along the axis of the alveolar duct but they are also arranged

Electronic supplementary material The online version of this chapter (https://doi.org/10.1007/978-3-030-04747-4_5) contains supplementary material, which is available to authorized users.

© Springer Nature Switzerland AG 2018
M. Reuter et al. (Eds.): ShapeMI 2018, LNCS 11167, pp. 49–64, 2018.
https://doi.org/10.1007/978-3-030-04747-4_5

back-to-back, e.g. if they belong to different acinar airways. One interalveolar septum is shared by the adjoining alveoli and one alveolus has several neighboring alveoli so that its boundary is usually formed by a diversity of interalveolar septa. Therefore, the alveolar parenchyma forms a 3D network consisting of quasi-planar interalveolar septa. [3] A healthy lung is ventilated homogeneously and the stresses acting on the interalveolar septa are balanced. Heterogeneous ventilation occurs in lung diseases when alveoli become unstable and collapse to form so-called microatelectases. Microatelectases exert tethering forces on interalveolar septa of neighboring alveoli so that stresses and strains are no longer balanced. These forces are likely to deform the local microarchitecture resulting in changes in alveolar sizes and shapes as well as the distribution of angles between neighboring quasi-planar septa. [24, 28] These model-based predictions might play a role for disease progression and are therefore of high clinical relevance but have never been validated empirically using 3D analyses. This was most likely due to a lack of appropriate imaging techniques and analytical methods. Therefore, the present study was designed to close this methodological gap by advancing image data processing tools applied to 3D datasets of lung tissue with the following specific aims:

1. morphometric data of individual alveoli such as size, diameter and surface area using automated image analyses, Sect. 3.1
2. angle distribution between adjoining quasi-planar interalveolar septa, characterized as individual facets forming the interface between alveolar airspace and the confining interalveolar septa, Sect. 3.2
3. distribution of the number of neighboring alveoli per alveolus in comparison to the number of facets, Sect. 3.3
4. shape of individual alveolar airspaces based on their 3D representation Sect. 3.4.

2   Methods

2.1   Sample Preparation, Data Acquisition and Reconstruction

The analyses are based on a 3D dataset that was obtained by serial histological sectioning of lung tissue, subsequent scanning and alignment of the resulting image stack to reconstruct the lost spatial correspondence, for details see [9], the raw data is available at http://osf.io/hy6r9/. The sample was taken from the control group of the study published by [23]. Air-filled rat lungs were fixed in-situ by vascular perfusion at a defined airway opening pressure of 13 cmH_2O with the goal to be as close as possible to the in-vivo situation. The alignment was done with Fiji's "Register Virtual Stack" [4], a script to employ Elastix [17, 25] with optional manual intervention for such a task is available at http://github.com/romangrothausmann/elastix_scripts/.

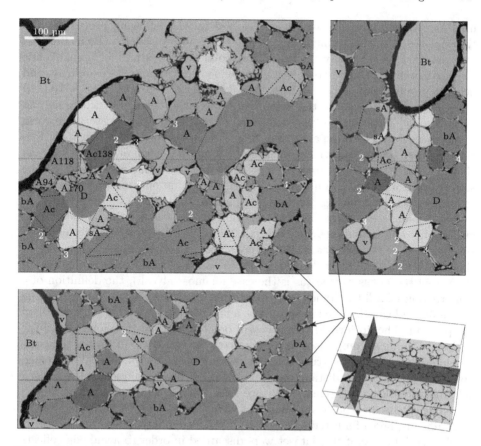

Fig. 1. Slices of the dataset overlaid with label image

The labels are colored arbitrarily and are partially transparent, except label 0 is fully transparent and label 1 is red and used for the airspace to be excluded, consisting of the ductal airspace (D) and labels that touch the borders (bA). Some (but not all) structures are annotated:

A: single alveolus (surface extents correspond to stereological decision, slightly dashed lines indicate stereological "lid" line, further explained in Sect. 2), Ac: alveolar cluster (with stereological subdividing lines), sA: sub-alveolus (with stereological lid line), bA: border alveoli, D: ducts, Bt: terminal bronchiolus, v: vessels (artery, arterioles, venules, veins), s: septa (consisting of blood capillaries enclosed by tissue), A94, A118, Ac138, A170 are referenced in Fig. 2, some 2D junctions of septa are marked in white with their degree (2, 3, 4).

The 3D view shows the arrangement of the slices (blue cross-hair in the slice images). (Color figure online)

2.2   Segmentation, Partition Creation and Processing

The full segmentation of the dataset, i.e. air, blood and tissue, as obtained for Ref. [9] with conventional, morphological methods such as opening/closing, distance maps and watershed transforms combining 2D and 3D processing, was used as a base. Only the air segment is used for the following processing and the analyses. The sub-segmentation of the terminal bronchiolus (Bt in Ref. [9]) was removed so that only ductal and alveolar airspaces are regarded. While the distinction of these two is not well defined and represents a difficult and delicate problem [18], a mere morphological closing with a 3D ball ($\varnothing = 70$ µm) was chosen here to enable the demonstration of the developed programs and their results. This can be regarded as a general means to create some form of subspace (alveolar airspace) that is not separated by tissue (in regard to the ductal airspace) and which consists of sub-units (alveoli or alveolar cluster) that are mostly separated from each other by tissue. In this way alveoli can be seen as for example a "foam cell" or "cavities" with an opening to a connecting tree-like space (conducting airways) comparable to a "sponge". In contrast to a closed "foam cell", these openings of the sub-units make this a challenging evaluation. The boundaries that are missing in order to form a fully enclosed sub-unit can be regarded as a lid to a pot. They are constrained (by the rim of the pot) but not uniquely defined, e.g. a lid can be convex, concave or flat. If the rim of the pot is ragged (as is the case for most alveoli), the definition of a construction of a lid becomes even more difficult. Using morphological closing with a 3D ball can then be interpreted as a lid creation by placing a large ball on the pot rim. The lid formed this way will be concave, and therefore reduce the enclosed volume in comparison to a flat or convex lid. In case of ragged rims, the still missing parts are constructed from the borders of a morphological watershed applied to an Euclidean distance map, which also brings a unique labeling of each sub-unit (alveolus or alv. cluster) [2], see Figs. 1 and 2. This approach alone was not sufficient because most alveoli do not have a constriction, i.e. they cover less than a hemisphere of a fitted sphere. Sub-units (commonly referred to as labels) touching the border of the dataset were discarded in order to avoid edge effects such as cropped shapes and extra lid parts. However, this simple method can lead to a bias, which is further discussed in Sect. 4. The processing was limited to a sub-region (because the border in the original dataset is defined by a mask) with a voxel size of 1 µm. This yielded 152 labeled alveoli/cluster.

2.3   Quantities per Alveoli and Histograms

Each labeled alveoli/cluster was characterized with the following determined quantities (see Fig. 3), which were then accumulated to plot histograms to visualize their distributions in Sect. 3.

Volume V, diameter of a sphere with equal volume (d_v), the closed surface S_c, the sphericity Ψ, the ellipsoidity η and the number of adjacent labels Ξ can be gathered from the voxel representation. [21,22] The number of adjacent labels was determined with MatImage [19] and does not distinguish between neighboring alveoli of the same duct and those of another duct or even acinus.

The surface of the tissue surrounding alveoli (S_o), i.e. that of a label without the surface of the closing lid (S_l) and the ratio of S_l/S_o were deduced from a mesh representation. The mesh i.e. surface representation was generated by the discrete marching cubes filter from VTK. An extension to the filter [6] was created in order to open the mesh of each label where it is not touching tissue (Figs. 2 and 11).

The sphericity ($\Psi = S_s/S_c = \sqrt[3]{36\pi V^2/S_c^3}$) relates the surface of a sphere of equal volume (S_s) to the surface of the object (S_p) and is a measure that is equal to 1 for a sphere and lower the more the object deviates from a sphere. The ellipsoidity ($\eta = S_e/S_c$) is defined in a similar way, i.e. in regard to the surface of a fitted ellipsoid of equal volume (S_e). For example, an object in the shape of a very prolate or oblate ellipsoid would have a low sphericity but the ellipsoidity would be 1.

2.4   Facet Analysis of Alveoli

The facet analysis (FA) determines planar partitions of the surface mesh of each label and is insensitive to some degree of roughness (i.e. noise). A direction vector for each planar region (facet) is computed which can be regarded as the normal of a fitting plane. An interplanar angle θ_e is the angle between the normals of two adjacent facets (for details see Ref. [7,8]). In general, each label has multiple facets (colored arbitrarily, Figs. 3 and 11) and multiple interplanar angles which can be characterized by a histogram or the median (Fig. 3). The mesh does not have to be closed and it is possible to allow non-faceted regions (colored gray) or not. The number of facets of a label Υ is not necessarily equal to the number of adjacent labels Ξ.

2.5   Shape Analysis of Alveoli

The shape type analysis (STA, Fig. 9) uses the principal axes of each label to fit an ellipsoid of equal volume (Figs. 3 and 11). The three principal axes lengths are sorted ($a < b < c$), interpreted as point coordinates and projected onto the unit sphere (to make the analysis independent of the size). The sorting makes the naming distinct and restricted the points to a spherical triangle of $1/8 \times 1/6$ of the unit sphere (Fig. 9). A separation line is defined by $a/b = b/c$ and allows the distinction of prolate (red) and oblate (green) ellipsoids. Points, whose error box (uncertainty of the axes lengths) intersects with the separation line, indicate a shape that is uncertain (yellow) within the error limits. If however the error box includes the sphere point ($a = b = c$) the corresponding alveolus is regarded as spherical (blue) within the error limits (for further details see Ref. [10]).

2.6   Processing Dependencies, Source Code and Reproduction

The digital processing used in this paper is defined and documented in source-code, scripts and Makefiles, their dependencies are governed by `git`. The general shape and facet analyses applied to lung tissue and alveolar clusters are in a git repository http://gitlab.com/romangrothausmann/SA-alv.git. It combines the general shape analysis [10] with the facet analysis [7,8] (http://github.com/romangrothausmann/ell_eval.git and http://github.com/romangrothausmann/

FacetAnalyser.git, both also applicable to other data e.g. from material sciences). Its specific application to the dataset from Ref. [9] and the results (referred to in this article) are stored in http://gitlab.com/romangrothausmann/SA_h3d_res.git. The Makefiles in this repository reproduce data, images and analyses reported in this article. GNU/Linux (Debian 9) was used as operating system, making use of various open-source tools, e.g. ITK, VTK, ParaView, octave, gnuplot, GNU parallel and many others. [5, 14, 33, 39, 42, 44]

3 Results

Figure 2 selectively highlights some of the results like the generated lid, neighborhood, facet detection and fit ellipsoid with its categorization. These are explained further in the following section.

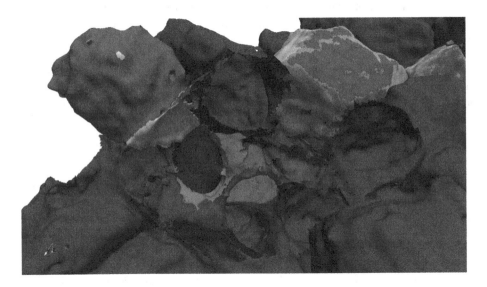

Fig. 2. Alveoli along a duct
3D render viewed along a duct at the border of the dataset to reduce occlusion. The dark magenta colored alveolus is A118 in Fig. 1, where the cross-hair is positioned. Its 5 neighboring labels are colored, all others are gray. The detected facets are colored arbitrarily for the alveolar cluster Ac138 that is dark blue in Fig. 1. The fit ellipsoid (transparent blue) is rendered for A170. The lid of A94 is shown in white. (Color figure online)

The various distributions of possible measurements were plotted as a histogram with absolute (bars filled blue) and relative frequency (dotted frame, scaled to be identical with blue bars), which allows the histogram to be correlated with a kernel-density plot (accumulation of Gaussian distribution, $\sigma = $ bin, relative frequency) allowing consideration of uncertainties in the measurements.

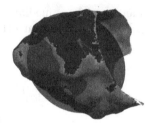
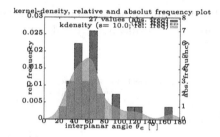

Fig. 3. Exemplary individual results of a typical alveolus

The results of the analyses for each individual label consist of integral measures (table on the left), a 3D render of the opened surface (S_o, facets colored arbitrarily as in Fig. 2) with the fit ellipsoid (here transparent blue, i.e. sphere type, see Fig. 9) and the closed surface (S_c, transparent gray, hardly visible here), and a plot of the distribution of the interplanar angles (θ_e, see Fig. 7). The quantities and the analyses are further described in the text. (Color figure online)

Figure 3 shows one of the results generated for each individual label. The complete catalog for the 152 labels can be found in the supplemental data (Fig. 10). The catalog data were used for the following figures, which can be regarded as overall evaluations.

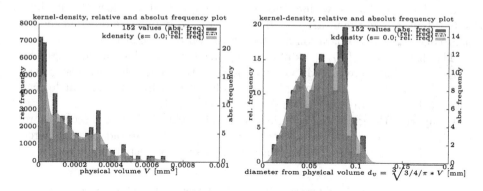

Fig. 4. Volume (closed) and diameter of sphere with equal volume

3.1 Morphometric Data of Individual Alveoli

The distribution of volume (V) and diameter of a volume equivalent sphere (d_v) were plotted in Fig. 4. The asymmetric volume distribution exhibits some slight peaks, which should not be interpreted as long as the uncertainty in the way of separating and closing alveoli in 3D is not well defined. The value of the comparable measurement $\bar{v}_a(alv)$ of 308×10^3 $\mu m^3 \approx 0.0003$ mm^3 from Table 2 of [23] is within the distribution but below the median (≈ 0.00013 mm^3) and the mean (≈ 0.00017 mm^3), which can be expected due to the concave lids used here in contrast to 2D linear line lids used during the stereological evaluation.

The distribution of d_v tends to be more symmetric with a median ($\approx$ 0.062 mm) and a mean ($\approx$ 0.061 mm) close to but below values from other studies.

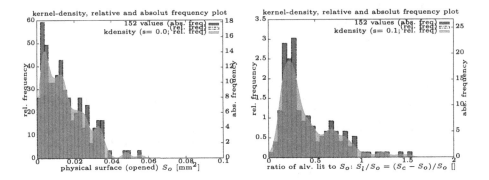

Fig. 5. Surface (opened, lid/opened)

The surface of the tissue surrounding alveoli (S_o) together with the ratio of S_l/S_o were plotted in Fig. 5. The value of the comparable measurement $S(alvepi, ventilpar)/N(alv, lung) = 1.46 \times 10^3/7.32 \times 10^6$ [cm^2] ≈ 0.02 [mm^2] from Table 2 of [23] is within the distribution but also below the median (≈ 0.013 mm^2) and the mean (≈ 0.015 mm^2), probably due to a different judgement concerning the separation of adjacent alveoli or alveolar cluster.

The distribution of S_l/S_o exhibits two peaks below 1, which might originate from alveoli that were already nearly closed by the morphological closing, i.e. with a ball, and alveoli whose lid had a significant part from the morphological watershed, which can lead to values above 1, see Fig. 1.

Comparing the graphs of sphericity and ellipsoidity in Fig. 6, it seems more alveoli or alveolar clusters are better approximated by ellipsoids than spheres (see also Fig. 10), which motivates the shape analysis of Sect. 3.4.

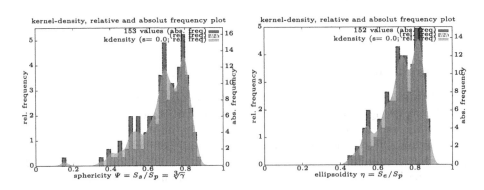

Fig. 6. Sphericity, Ellipsoidity

3.2 Angle Distribution Between Interalveolar Septa

The distribution of interplanar angles of adjacent facets (θ_e, angle between face normals) found by the facet analysis (FA) was plotted in Fig. 7. It has a well defined peak at about 60° (which corresponds to 120° between septa) and tends towards the shape of a log-normal distribution. The angular uncertainty was estimated to be around 10° which is also used as σ for the kernel density plot. Since each alveolus has 5 to 15 facets (see Υ in Fig. 8) there are far more adjacent facet pairs (> 3000) than labels (152).

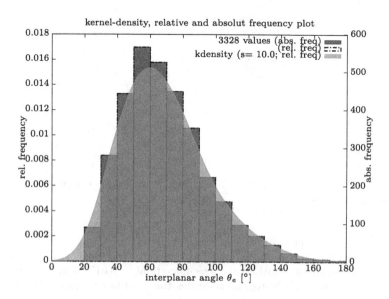

Fig. 7. Accumulated interplanar angle distribution

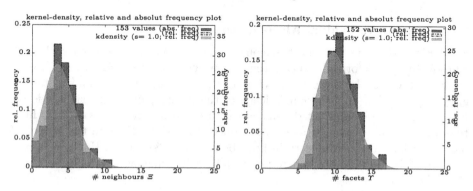

Fig. 8. # neighbors, # facets (per alveolus, excluding ducts)

3.3   Distribution of the Number of Neighboring Alveoli

The number of adjacent labels Ξ (i.e. neighboring alveoli) seems to be about half the number of facets of a label Υ, as can be seen in Fig. 8. This could mean that the septal wall towards a neighboring alveolus has a crease or fold and that on average this part of the septal wall has 2 facets, which is further discussed in Sect. 4 and is annotated with a white 2 in Fig. 1.

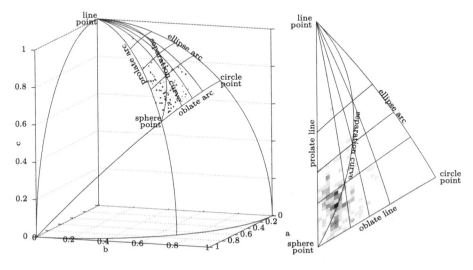

Fig. 9. Shape Type Analysis (STA)
sphere-type (blue): 52; oblate-type (green): 13; prolate-type (red): 12; uncertain-type (yellow): 76; oblate/prolate ratio: 1.08; axes-uncertainty : 0.015 mm. The gray value of the overlaid sheared 2D histogram indicates the local point density. (Color figure online)

3.4   Shape of Individual Alveolar Airspaces

Since Fig. 6 suggests that most alveoli/cluster are better approximated by an ellipsoid, i.e. a deformed sphere, the shape type analysis (STA, Fig. 9) was applied. It yields the 3D plot of a, b, c on the left side of Fig. 9 and a stereographic projection of this triangle leads to the planar plot on the right side of Fig. 9, where the local point density is indicated by sheared fields of a 2D histogram. With an estimated axes uncertainty of about 0.015 mm, the shape of most alveolar clusters is uncertain but about 1/3 are spherical. However, most axes ratios lie between the sphere point and the 2/3 line, as visible in Fig. 9 on the right.

4   Discussion

The present study was designed to advance image data processing tools with the potential to characterize the 3D alveolar microarchitecture with regard to alveolar morphometric data, shape and the distribution of angles between neighboring quasi-planar septa. The latter form a pre-stressed network within the lung, providing stability and thereby laying the foundation for relatively homogeneous ventilation essential for effective gas exchange. [36] Model predictions suggest that in the case of homogeneous ventilation stresses acting on interalveolar septa are balanced and evenly distributed within lung parenchyma and would then primarily depend on the elastic recoil pressure which is the gradient between pleural pressure and alveolar pressure. [28] Oldmixon and co-workers identified junctions of 3 quasi-planar interalveolar septa on 2D histological sections of healthy lungs and found a mean angle between neighboring quasi-planar septa of 120°, which was in line with the model predictions of balanced and evenly distributed stresses within the lung mentioned above. [32] According to model predictions, non-homogeneity in ventilation e.g. due to microatelectases would lead to a considerable local increase of stresses which might result in undue deformation and local volume increase of adjacent alveoli. [45] These increased stresses and strains resulting from interdependence of the network of interalveolar septa have long been discussed as playing important roles in pathogenesis e.g. in the context of ventilation induced lung injury. However, empirical validations of these model predictions in lung parenchyma in 3D are very limited in part due to a lack of appropriate image data analyzing tools.

We used a 3D data set of a healthy, air-filled rat lung, fixed in-situ by vascular perfusion at a defined airway opening pressure of 13 cmH$_2$O in order to close this methodological gap. In a first step distributions of individual morphometric data of those alveoli which were identified by the automatic image processing were generated (Figs. 4 and 5). Both the mean alveolar volume and surface area per alveolus were lower compared to previously published stereological data. Design-based stereology is the current gold standard for quantitative assessment of lung structure and, based on a consent statement, recommended by the American Thoracic Society and European Respiratory Society in this context. [13] Design-based stereological methods provide unbiased and representative data of individual lungs, meaning that the sampling of tissue is also very critical and follows standardized, unbiased procedures to make sure that every part in the lung has the same chance of being included in the analyses. In the present study only one tissue block within one lung was analyzed and this piece of lung parenchyma might not be representative of the group of healthy rat lungs. This aspect might at least in part explain the difference between stereological data and those generated in the current study. In human lungs it has been described that the microarchitecture including, for example the alveolar size is significantly dependent on the region where samples are taken [27] and this might also be the case in rat lung. However, the strength of the approach applied in the current study is that local distributions of alveolar sizes can be generated which might be of relevance if investigators are interested in questions of interdependences, e.g. the effects of microatelectases on the surrounding alveolar microarchitecture. Another source of bias derives from the approach we chose to identify the alveoli included in this study. A sphere of a certain diameter was used to define ductal airspaces and identify individual alveoli. The alveoli which were touching the edges of the dataset in a way that their boundaries were missing were excluded from analyses. Larger alveoli have a higher probability to touch and even go beyond the edges of the dataset, which results in a bias called the edge effect. [11] So larger alveoli have a higher probability of being excluded, so that the analyses in their current form under-represent alveoli with larger volumes. This issue is likely to play a major role regarding the differences between stereological data presented in Ref. [23] and those illustrated in the current study. This source of bias, however, can in principle be controlled by the implementation of a 3D guard area (based on the diameter of the largest alveolus) and an unbiased counting frame. [31,38]. The strength of the present analytical method is the fact that distributions of alveolar sizes can be generated, which goes beyond currently available analytical techniques in this context including design-based stereological methods.

Oldmixon and co-workers identified a mean angle between neighboring septa of 120° for junctions of 3 quasi-planar interalveolar septa and concluded even distributions of stresses acting on these adjoining septa. The investigators used histological sections for their analyses and ignored junctions of less or more than 3 quasi-planar interalveolar septa (annotated with a white 3 in Fig. 1) as well as the presence of a larger vessel in the corresponding junction. In the present study, a 3D approach was used to identify quasi-planar surfaces of interalveolar septa which we defined as facets and which were generating the direct boundary of the corresponding alveolar airspace. In a mathematical sense, a plane was fitted to each facet, whose orientation is defined by a perpendicular vector (pointing outwards from the label). The angle between these adjacent facet normals was determined independently of the number of adjoining facets of neighboring alveoli. Figure 7 illustrates the corresponding angle distribution which shows a peak at 60° in line with previous observations published in Ref. [32]. However, while Oldmixon and co-workers described very low standard deviations of 2° to 7° the distribution in the current study was much more skewed with interplanar angles ranging between 20° and 160°. These differences can, aside from differences in the analytical approach (e.g. using unique facet-defining vectors in 3D), best be explained that all junctions between facets were considered independent of the number of facets which come together at a junction. In this context Butler and co-workers analyzed a type of junction in which only 2 quasi-planar septa (annotated with a white 2 in Fig. 1) were involved and observed in these cases values clearly above 120°. [3] Such junctions were included in the present study and likely contribute to the much more skewed distribution of angles presented in Fig. 7, and also cause a higher number of facets for an alveolus than the number of its neighbors. The angles of such folds in the septa are most likely to change during inflation/deflation during the breathing cycle when the volume of the lung constantly changes. Also junctions with a higher degree than 3 can be found in Fig. 1. By fitting ellipsoids to alveolar airspaces we also analyzed individual alveolar shapes. These shapes were categorized as spheres-type, oblate-type and prolate-type. To the best of the authors' knowledge this is the first study using this kind of shape analysis of alveolar airspaces based on 3D data sets. Alveoli of uncertain shape between oblate and prolate-type dominated the distribution. Among those alveolar airspaces which could be categorized, the sphere-type was the most frequent form. Changes in alveolar shape have been discussed as representing a very important mechanism by which alveolar airspace can increase their volume without undue and potential harmful stretching of the interalveolar septa during inspiration although studies addressing this important question in lung physiology are very limited. [34] Therefore, the effects of lung volume changes on the distribution of these types of alveolar shape might add important new insight for our understanding of the dynamical changes of alveoli during a respiratory cycle.

5 Conclusion

In the present study an image-analyses approach of a 3D dataset was used to characterize the acinar microarchitecture. The strength of this tool was the generation of a distribution of the angles between neighboring interalveolar septa, a feature which might be dependent on stress and strain distribution within the lung and therefore affected by the occurrence of so-called stress concentrators such as microatelectases. Hence, the methods presented are promising for studies aiming at evaluating alveolar interdependence and stress-strain distributions.

Acknowledgement. Many thanks go to David Legland for his `MatImage` [19] support and for helping to use it also within `octave` [5] and to Sheila Fryk for polishing the English language as native speaker.

A Catalogue

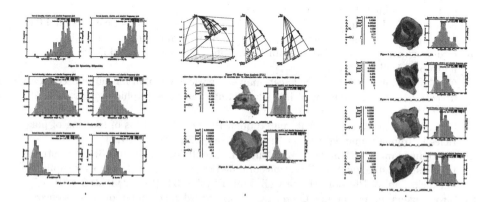

Fig. 10. Catalog of all analyzed alveoli/cluster

Excerpt from the catalog comprising integral measures (such as in Fig. 4) and all individually analyzed alveoli/cluster (such as in Fig. 3). The full catalog can be found as a separate PDF in the supplementary data.

B   Video

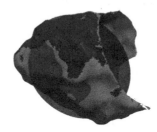

Fig. 11. Rotating view of alveolus

Video of the rotating alveolus shown in Fig. 3, visualizing the shape, the fitted ellipsoid (blue), the detected facets, the opening and its lid (transparent gray).

References

1. Ayachit, U.: The ParaView Guide. Kitware Inc., Clifton Park (2016)
2. Beare, R., Lehmann, G.: The watershed transform in ITK - discussion and new developments. Insight J. (2006)
3. Butler, J.P., Oldmixon, E.H., Hoppin, F.G.: Dihedral angles of septal "bend" structures in lung parenchyma. J. Appl. Physiol. **81**(4), 1800–1806 (1996)
4. Cardona, A., Arganda-Carreras, I., Saalfeld, S.: Register Virtual Stack Slices (Fiji). http://imagej.net/Register_Virtual_Stack_Slices
5. Eaton, J.W., Bateman, D., Hauberg, S., Wehbring, R.: GNU Octave version 4.0.0 manual: a high-level interactive language for numerical computations (2015)
6. Grothausmann, R.: Providing values of adjacent voxel with vtkDiscreteMarchingCubes. VTK J. (2016)
7. Grothausmann, R., Beare, R.: Facet analyser: paraview plugin for automated facet detection and measurement of interplanar angles of tomographic objects. MIDAS J. (2015)
8. Grothausmann, R., et al.: Automated quantitative 3D analysis of faceting of particles in tomographic datasets. Ultramicroscopy **122**, 65–75 (2012)
9. Grothausmann, R., Knudsen, L., Ochs, M., Mühlfeld, C.: Digital 3D reconstructions using histological serial sections of lung tissue including the alveolar capillary network. Am. J. Physiol. - Lung Cell. Mol. Physiol. **312**(2), L243–L257 (2017)
10. Grothausmann, R., et al.: Quantitative structural assessment of heterogeneous catalysts by electron tomography. J. Am. Chem. Soc. **133**(45), 18161–18171 (2011)
11. Gundersen, H.: Estimators of the number of objects per area unbiased by edge effects. Microscopica Acta **81**(2), 107–117 (1978)

12. Haefeli-Bleuer, B., Weibel, E.R.: Morphometry of the human pulmonary acinus. Anat. Rec. **220**(4), 401–414 (1988)
13. Hsia, C.C.W., Hyde, D.M., Ochs, M., Weibel, E.R.: An official research policy statement of the American Thoracic Society/European Respiratory Society: standards for quantitative assessment of lung structure. Am. J. Respir. Criti. Care Med. **181**(4), 394–418 (2010)
14. ITK development team: ITK, see [15, 46]. Kitware Inc. http://www.itk.org
15. Johnson, H.J., McCormick, M.M., Ibáñez, L., the Insight Software Consortium: The ITK Software Guide. Kitware Inc. (2018)
16. Klein, S., Staring, M., Murphy, K., Viergever, M.A., Pluim, J.P.: elastix: a toolbox for intensity-based medical image registration. IEEE Trans. Med. Imaging **29**(1), 196–205 (2010)
17. Klein, S., Staring, M.: elastix, see [16, 37]. Image Sciences Institute, University Medical Center Utrecht. http://elastix.isi.uu.nl/
18. Knudsen, L., Ochs, M.: A critical comment on a recent publication using parenchymal airspace profiling. Am. J. Respir. Cell Mol. Biol. **57**(1), 132–132 (2017)
19. Legland, D.: MatImage, see [20]. https://github.com/mattools/matImage
20. Legland, D., Kiêu, K., Devaux, M.-F.: Computation of minkowski measures on 2D and 3D binary images. Image Anal. Ster. **26**(2), 83–92 (2007)
21. Lehmann, G.: Label object representation and manipulation with ITK. Insight J. (2008)
22. Lehmann, G., Legland, D.: Efficient n-dimensional surface estimation using crofton formula and run-length encoding. Insight J. (2012)
23. Lutz, D., et al.: Alveolar derecruitment and collapse induration as crucial mechanisms in lung injury and fibrosis. Am. J. Respir. Cell Mol. Biol. **52**(2), 232–243 (2015)
24. Makiyama, A., Gibson, L., Harris, R., Venegas, J.: Stress concentration around an atelectatic region: a finite element model. Respir. Physiol. Neurobiol. **201**, 101–110 (2014)
25. Marstal, K.: SimpleElastix, see [26]. Image Sciences Institute, University Medical Center Utrecht. http://simpleelastix.github.io/
26. Marstal, K., Berendsen, F., Staring, M., Klein, S.: SimpleElastix: a userfriendly, multi-lingual library for medical image registration. In: Schnabel, J., Mori, K. (eds.) International Workshop on Biomedical Image Registration (WBIR). IEEE Conference on Computer Vision and Pattern Recognition Workshops, Las Vegas, Nevada, USA, pp. 574–582 (2016)
27. McDonough, J.E., Knudsen, L., Wright, A.C., Elliott, W.M., Ochs, M., Hogg, J.C.: Regional differences in alveolar density in the human lung are related to lung height. J. Appl. Physiol. **118**(11), 1429–1434 (2015)
28. Mead, J., Takishima, T., Leith, D.: Stress distribution in lungs: a model of pulmonary elasticity. J. Appl. Physiol. **28**(5), 596–608 (1970)
29. Mercer, R.R., Laco, J.M., Crapo, J.D.: Three-dimensional reconstruction of alveoli in the rat lung for pressure-volume relationships. J. Appl. Physiol. **62**(4), 1480–1487 (1987)
30. Mühlfeld, C., Wrede, C., Knudsen, L., Buchacker, T., Ochs, M., Grothausmann, R.: Recent developments in 3D reconstruction and stereology to study the pulmonary vasculature. Am. J. Physiol. - Lung Cell. Mol. Physiol. (2018)
31. Ochs, M., et al.: The number of alveoli in the human lung. Am. J. Respi. Crit. Care Med. **169**(1), 120–124 (2004)
32. Oldmixon, E.H., Butler, J.P., Hoppin, F.G.: Dihedral angles between alveolar septa. J. Appl. Physiol. **64**(1), 299–307 (1988)

33. ParaView development team: ParaView, see [1]. Kitware Inc. http://www.paraview.org

34. Roan, E., Waters, C.M.: What do we know about mechanical strain in lung alveoli? Am. J. Physiol.-Lung Cell. Mol. Physiol. **301**(5), L625–L635 (2011)

35. Schroeder, W., Martin, K., Lorensen, B.: The Visualization Toolkit: An Object-Oriented Approach to 3D Graphics. Kitware Inc., Clifton Park (2006)

36. Schürch, S., Bachofen, H., Possmayer, F.: Surface activity in situ, in vivo, and in the captive bubble surfactometer. Comp. Biochem. Physiol. Part A: Mol. Integr. Physiol. **129**(1), 195–207 (2001)

37. Shamonin, D., Bron, E., Lelieveldt, B., Smits, M., Klein, S., Staring, M.: Fast parallel image registration on CPU and GPU for diagnostic classification of alzheimer's disease. Front. Neuroinformatics **7**, 50 (2014)

38. Sterio, D.C.: The unbiased estimation of number and sizes of arbitrary particles using the disector. J. Microsc. **134**(2), 127–136 (1984)

39. Tange, O.: GNU Parallel - The Command-Line Power Tool, see [40]. http://www.gnu.org/s/parallel

40. Tange, O.: GNU parallel - the command-line power tool. USENIX Mag. **36**(1), 42–47 (2011)

41. Vasilescu, D.M., et al.: Assessment of morphometry of pulmonary acini in mouse lungs by nondestructive imaging using multiscale microcomputed tomography. Proc. Natl. Acad. Sci. **109**(42), 17105–17110 (2012)

42. VTK development team: VTK, see [35]. Kitware Inc. http://www.vtk.org

43. Weibel, E.R.: What makes a good lung? Swiss Med. Wkly. **27**(139), 375–386 (2009)

44. Williams, T., Kelley, C.: gnuplot. http://gnuplot.sourceforge.net/docs_4.4/gnuplot.pdf

45. Wu, Y., Kharge, A.B., Perlman, C.E.: Lung ventilation injures areas with discrete alveolar flooding, in a surface tension-dependent fashion. J. Appl. Physiol. **117**(7), 788–796 (2014)

46. Yoo, T., et al.: Insight into Images: Principles and Practice for Segmentation, Registration, and Image Analysis. A K Peters Ltd., Natick (2004)

SlicerSALT: Shape AnaLysis Toolbox

Jared Vicory[1]([✉]), Laura Pascal[1], Pablo Hernandez[1], James Fishbaugh[3],
Juan Prieto[2], Mahmoud Mostapha[2], Chao Huang[2], Hina Shah[1], Junpyo Hong[2],
Zhiyuan Liu[2], Loic Michoud[4], Jean-Christophe Fillion-Robin[1], Guido Gerig[3],
Hongtu Zhu[2], Stephen M. Pizer[2], Martin Styner[2], and Beatriz Paniagua[1]

[1] Kitware, Inc., Clifton Park, USA
jared.vicory@kitware.com
[2] University of North Carolina at Chapel Hill, Chapel Hill, USA
[3] New York University, New York City, USA
[4] Univeristy of Michigan, Ann Arbor, USA

Abstract. SlicerSALT is an open-source platform for disseminating
state-of-the-art methods for performing statistical shape analysis. These
methods are developed as 3D Slicer extensions to take advantage of its
powerful underlying libraries. SlicerSALT itself is a heavily customized
3D Slicer package that is designed to be easy to use for shape analysis
researchers. The packaged methods include powerful techniques for creating and visualizing shape representations as well as performing various
types of analysis.

Keywords: Shape analysis · Statistics · Software

1 Introduction

Statistical shape analysis is an active area of research in the medical imaging
community with many groups working on novel methods of representing and
analyzing the shape of anatomical structures. Unfortunately, due to the sheer
number of data formats and software packages created in a variety of program-
ming languages, it can be difficult to pull together pipelines making use of methods created by different groups. In addition, much of the available software is
written only to be used by other computer scientists, making it difficult for the
wider medical community to make use of these powerful analysis techniques.

SlicerSALT [3] is an open-source platform for the dissemination of state-of-
the-art methods for performing statistical shape analysis. The goal of SlicerSALT
is to provide an easy to use end-to-end solution for performing statistical shape
analysis of anatomical objects. As shown in Fig. 1, SlicerSALT provides methods
for importing segmentation data in several formats, performing a variety of pre-
processing and quality control tasks, deriving shape representations with good
correspondences from these segmentations, and performing statistical analysis

---

SlicerSALT development is funded by NIH R01EB021391.

© Springer Nature Switzerland AG 2018
M. Reuter et al. (Eds.): ShapeMI 2018, LNCS 11167, pp. 65–72, 2018.
https://doi.org/10.1007/978-3-030-04747-4_6

using a variety of powerful techniques. SlicerSALT is a heavily customized version of 3D Slicer [1,5] that is designed to streamline the importing and running of the included methods to make it easy for even non-experts to perform powerful shape analysis studies as well as remove the non-relevant modules of 3D Slicer to avoid confusion.

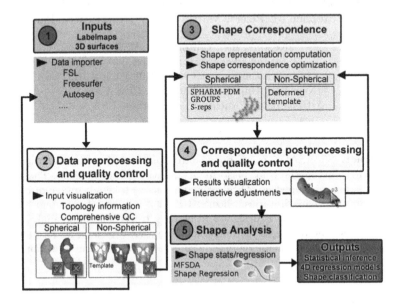

Fig. 1. The SlicerSALT workflow

SlicerSALT is built as a series of extensions to 3D Slicer. This enables Slicer-SALT to leverage the power of Slicer's underlying toolkits as well as its large and active developer community. It also makes contributing to SlicerSALT easy, as additional functions can be created as indepednent Slicer extensions and incorporated into SlicerSALT's build system. This is combined with a strong software infrastructure including automatic building, unit testing, and dashboards. The end result is a robust software package that is easy to both extend and maintain as new methodology continues to be developed.

2 Available Extensions

This section describes the extensions developed as part of SlicerSALT. These are available as part of the SlicerSALT distribution as well as individually in 3D Slicer via the Slicer Extension Manager. Because the methods are packaged as 3D Slicer modules, non-expert users are able to run them through the SlicerSALT UI while advanced users could also run them from the command line.

2.1   Home

SlicerSALT starts by default on the home module shown in Fig. 2. This module describes a basic workflow from data loading through the creation and analysis of the target shapes. It also features links to jump directly to each module. This module is designed to guide new and inexperienced users through a typical workflow.

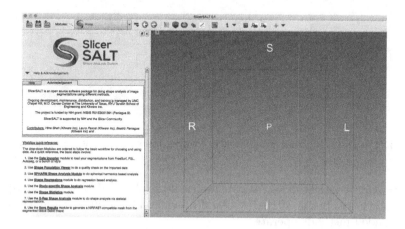

Fig. 2. The SlicerSALT home module with direct links to the available extensions.

2.2   Data Importer

This extension is designed to make it easy for the user to import data in multiple different formats and perform quick visualizations and quality control prior to analysis. Data can be imported as either binary label maps or surfaces. The Data Importer also has special logic to deal with importing data output from popular segmentation applications such as Autoseg [14], FSL [9], and FreeSurfer [6]. Figure 3 shows the Data Importer interface with an example dataset.

2.3   SPHARM-PDM

SPHARM-PDM [13] is a tool that uses spherical harmonics to compute point distribution models (PDMs) using a parametric boundary description for use in shape analysis. The SPHARM-PDM extension takes one or more binary images as input. The binary images are first processed to ensure spherical topology, then converted to surface meshes using marching cubes. The spherical parameterization was computed from the surface meshes using area-preserving, distortion-minimizing spherical mapping. The SPHARM description was then computed from the mesh and its spherical parameterization. Using icosahedron subdivison on the spharm description, a set number of points is sampled to create correspondent PDMs. These resulting PDMs have been shown to provide a strong

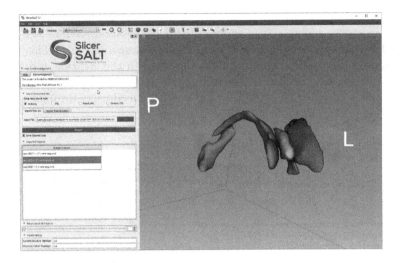

Fig. 3. The Data Importer module after loading lateral ventricle segmentations.

foundation for a variety of statistical studies of the shape of anatomical objects, particularly in the brain. SPHARM-PDM provides a basis on which many of the other included methods operate.

Also included is ShapePopulationViewer [2], shown in Fig. 4, for visualizing the resulting PDMs and their parameterizations to ensure good correspondence.

2.4   Group-Wise Registration for Shape Correspondence (GROUPS)

GROUPS [11] is a method for improving correspondence of a population of PDMs, such as those resulting from SPHARM-PDM, using a group-wise registration and optimization strategy. This optimization works by minimizing the entropy of the distribution of curvedness of the surface at corresponding point locations, ensuring that corresponding points are in positions with similar geometric features across the population. This method is particularly helpful in improving correspondences on objects with complicated geometry where the standard SPHARM-PDM correspondences may prove inadequate.

2.5   Multivariate Functional Shape Data Analysis (MFSDA)

MFSDA [10] packages a powerful set of advanced statistical tools that can efficiently correlate shape data with clinical and demographic variables such as age, gender, and genetic markers. Users can load in sets of additional data corresponding to each input shape and determine whether there is a statistically significant morphological difference caused by some combination of the covariates.

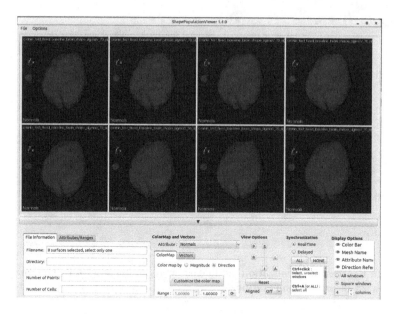

Fig. 4. ShapePopulationViewer visualizing a set of brain segmentations

2.6 Shape Regression

This extension allows for modeling the continuous evolution of anatomical objects via geodesic regression and creates a 4D shape model [7]. There are two separate modules as part of this extension: RegressionComputation for computing the regression and RegressionVisualization for visualizing the resulting shape model. A visualization of a regression on a set of brain data is shown in Fig. 5.

2.7 Shape Evaluator

The Shape Evaluator module is designed to take in a set of corresponding PDMs such as those generated by SPHARM-PDM or GROUPS and use principal component analysis (PCA) to compute a mean shape and its major modes of variation. The user can then visualize the mean shape as well as how moving along each principal component changes the shape of the object. This module allows for a quantitative comparison of the generated shape space to those created by other methods by examining the percent of variation explained by the modes of variation as well as computing generalization, specificity, and compactness measures on the distribution.

2.8 Skeletal Representations (S-reps)

This module packages methods for creating and visualizing skeletal representations, known as s-reps, of anatomical objects. S-reps are powerful shape representations that have been shown to have beneficial properties compared to pure boundary models [12] in applications such as classification and segmentation.

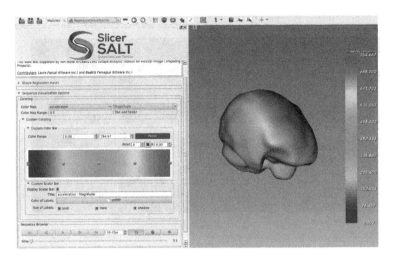

Fig. 5. The RegressionVisualization module showing the result of a regression computation on a set of brain segmentations.

Currently only s-rep visualization is included, but there will soon be support
for fitting s-reps to objects and eventually for estimating probability distributions and performing classification. These statistical methods are designed to
work on s-reps as data from a non-Eucliean manifold and will be applicable to
other representations such as PDMs as well. An example of an s-rep loaded into
SlicerSALT is shown in Fig. 6.

3   Software Infrastructure

SlicerSALT is set up with a modern open-source software infrastructure. In addition to information about the individual methods available in the package, the
SlicerSALT website [3] has a variety of information on using and contributing to
SlicerSALT. The code for SlicerSALT itself is hosted on GitHub [4] and includes
information on how to build the software locally as well as guidelines for contributing to SlicerSALT.

The main SlicerSALT repository has code for pulling in and building a
lightweight version of 3D Slicer and its dependencies as well as links to the
external repositories where the code for the various included methods is stored.
During the building of SlicerSALT, the code for each method is checked out from
its own Git repository and built as a 3D Slicer extension. During packaging these
extensions are then pulled in along with the customized version of 3D Slicer to
create the final SlicerSALT package.

SlicerSALT is built nightly and the results of these builds are uploaded to
a dashboard to track and diagnose problems with building Slicer or any of the
individual extensions. Additionally each extension has its own set of tests to
ensure they are functioning correctly as well as documentation and tutorials.

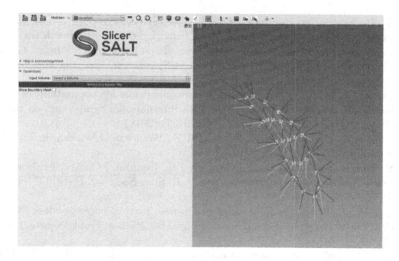

Fig. 6. An example skeletal model (s-rep) loaded into SlicerSALT.

4   Discussion

The first release of SlicerSALT packages a number of powerful tools for performing statistical shape analysis with an easy-to-use interface. It is designed as a platform for disseminating these methods to the broader medical community.

SlicerSALT development is ongoing. Several of the methods described here are still under active development and we will continue to improve the existing modules as well as introduce new methods for representing and analyzing shape.

In particular, there is ongoing work [8] to establish correspondence between shapes with complex geometry, including those with non-spherical topology, that cause traditional methods such as SPHARM-PDM to fail. This work establishes correspondences by using a diffeomorphic registration technique to deform a template shape representation into each member of a population.

SlicerSALT is open to contributions of other shape representation and analysis methods. New methods can be contributed by packaging them as 3D Slicer extensions. Detailed contribution guidelines can be found in the SlicerSALT GitHub repository.

Future work will also include user evaluations and usability testing of the software to ensure that it is easily usable by both expert and non-expert users.

References

1. 3D Slicer. http://www.slicer.org
2. Shape population viewer. https://www.nitrc.org/projects/shapepopviewer/
3. SlicerSALT. http://salt.slicer.org
4. SlicerSALT GitHub. https://github.com/Kitware/SlicerSALT
5. Fedorov, A., et al.: 3D slicer as an image computing platform for the quantitative imaging network. Magn. Reson. Imaging **30**(9), 1323–1341 (2012)

6. Fischl, B.: FreeSurfer. Neuroimage **62**(2), 774–781 (2012)
7. Fishbaugh, J., Durrleman, S., Gerig, G.: Estimation of smooth growth trajectories with controlled acceleration from time series shape data. In: Fichtinger, G., Martel, A., Peters, T. (eds.) MICCAI 2011. LNCS, vol. 6892, pp. 401–408. Springer, Heidelberg (2011). https://doi.org/10.1007/978-3-642-23629-7_49
8. Fishbaugh, J., et al.: Estimating shape correspondence for populations of objects with complex topology. In: 2018 IEEE 15th International Symposium on Biomedical Imaging (ISBI 2018), pp. 1010–1013. IEEE (2018)
9. Jenkinson, M., Beckmann, C.F., Behrens, T.E., Woolrich, M.W., Smith, S.M.: FSL. Neuroimage **62**(2), 782–790 (2012)
10. Li, Y., Zhu, H., Shen, D., Lin, W., Gilmore, J.H., Ibrahim, J.G.: Multiscale adaptive regression models for neuroimaging data. J. R. Stat. Soc.: Ser. B (Stat. Methodol.) **73**(4), 559–578 (2011)
11. Lyu, I., et al.: Robust estimation of group-wise cortical correspondence with an application to macaque and human neuroimaging studies. Front. Neurosci. **9**, 210 (2015)
12. Pizer, S.M., et al.: Nested sphere statistics of skeletal models. In: Breuß, M., Bruckstein, A., Maragos, P. (eds.) Innovations for Shape Analysis. MATHVISUAL, pp. 93–115. Springer, Berlin (2013)
13. Styner, M., et al.: Framework for the statistical shape analysis of brain structures using SPHARM-PDM. Insight J. (1071), 242 (2006)
14. Wang, J., et al.: Multi-atlas segmentation of subcortical brain structures via the AutoSeg software pipeline. Front. Neuroinf. **8**, 7 (2014)

3D Shape Analysis for Coarctation of the Aorta

Lina Gundelwein[1]([⊠]), Heiko Ramm[1], Leonid Goubergrits[2], Marcus Kelm[3], and Hans Lamecker[1]

[1] 1000shapes GmbH, Berlin, Germany
info@articardio.de
[2] Biofluid Mechanics Laboratory, Charité-Universitätsmedizin Berlin, Berlin, Germany
[3] Department of Congenital Heart Disease, German Heart Centre Berlin, Berlin, Germany

Abstract. A population of 54 cases diagnosed with coarctation of the aorta (CoA) was investigated for correlations between complex 3D shape and clinical parameters. Based on a statistical shape model (SSM) of the aortic arch (AA) including supra-aortic branches, clustering was performed. The result confirmed the current clinical classification scheme (normal/crenel or gothic). Furthermore, another 3D shape class related to age of the patient was identified.

Keywords: Statistical shape model · Aortic arch
Cardiovascular disease · Coarctation of the aorta · Shape clustering

1 Background

Classification using complex morphometric data can complement current clinical diagnostics and possibly identify new relationships between the manifestations of a disease and the morphology of the affected organ. Such knowledge can also be beneficial for designing and optimizing individual treatment planning.

Previous works based on SSM methodology have already revealed several insights into aortic morphology related to normal and abnormal cases: (a) vessel size, arch unfolding and symmetry are principal modes of variation in normal thoracic aorta morphology [5], (b) valve regurgitation in transcatheter aortic valve replacement patients can be linked to aortic shape [1], and (c) cavopulmonary connection outcome is correlated with the AA shape [4].

For post-op CoA cases it has been shown that the clinical assessment of abnormality can be associated with AA shape variations [2]. Furthermore, post-op CoA cases can be discriminated via the AA shape from other groups (normal or arterial switch operation cases) [3], and sub-groups seem to exist. Hence, in this work, we analyze such subgroups of - in our case - pre-op CoA cases with respect to AA shape/size and clinical characterization. Furthermore, a clinical

© Springer Nature Switzerland AG 2018
M. Reuter et al. (Eds.): ShapeMI 2018, LNCS 11167, pp. 73–77, 2018.
https://doi.org/10.1007/978-3-030-04747-4_7

study [6] has shown that the artery branches play an important role in this respect, so in contrast to earlier works we include them into our analysis.

2 Methods

Thoracic magnetic resonance imaging (MRI) of 54 CoA patient (age 21.5 ± 12.6, 36 male, 18 female) as well as measurement of AA width, height and height/width (H/W) ratio were provided by Charité Berlin.

All AAs were manually segmented from MRI including ascendens, three supra-aortic branches and descendens cut at the height of the apex of the heart. Centerlines were computed with the local radius mapped onto the lines to reflect the vessel thickness, see Fig. 1.

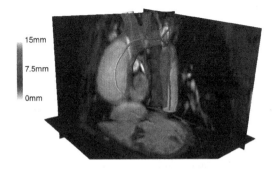

Fig. 1. The surface of a thoracic aorta, reconstructed from the centerline and inscribed radii. Local vessel radii are color coded on the centerline. (Color figure online)

The models were rigidly registered using the centerlines of the AA with a uniform scale adjustment to reduce the influence of large size variations in the training population related to age differences. Radii were scaled accordingly to preserve relative difference in thickness. 3D point correspondence was established by equidistantly resampling each AA region (ascendens, branch region and descendens) and the branches.

Principal component analysis was performed on the centerline geometry of the aligned aorta models. The radii were interpolated using the found principal modes as a new basis.

Agglomerative hierarchical clustering using correlation distance metric and a weighted linkeage method was performed on the shape vectors of the training data consisting of the weights for each PCA mode.

3 Results

Three clusters of similar cluster size (20, 17 and 17) and inner cluster distance were found (see Fig. 2a). A scatter plot of the weights associated with the first two PCA shape modes shows that the first two modes suffice already to discriminate between the three clusters (see Fig. 2b). The first two modes describe arch unfolding and symmetry, confirming the results from [5].

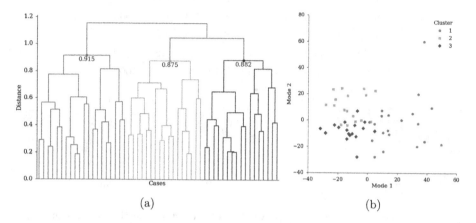

(a)   (b)

Fig. 2. (a) Dendogram showing shape clustering on weights of the PCA modes with annotated distances for the three shape clusters. (b) Scatter plot of 3D shape space described by subject-specific PCA shape vector entries. (Color figure online)

The statistically significant differences between the clusters with respect to age, width and H/W ratio were assessed using Kruskal-Wallis H-test and are reported in Table 1.

Qualitative differences in the shape of each cluster are shown in Fig. 3. Cluster I includes aortas with a strong curve in the descendens. The mean age and AA width are significantly higher ($p < 0.01$) than in the other two clusters and the H/W ratio lower. The highest inner cluster variance is introduced by the valve orientation and in the upper part of the descendens, where several cases show a kinking, resulting in an S-curve in severe cases. Cluster II consists of gothic aortas and therewith a significantly higher H/W ratio ($p < 0.05$) than the two other clusters. The strongest shape variation in this cluster encodes the different lengths of the ascendens. Cluster III covers a similar age group and AA width as cluster II, but comprises mostly normal and crenel AA shapes, i.e. aortas with lower H/W ratio than in cluster II.

4   Discussion

Clustering on the PCA modes of a CoA SSM was able to discriminate gothic arch (high H/W ratio) from normal and crenel cases (low H/W ratio). Confirming the finding of [6], we could not find a statistically significant relationship between age and current clinical arch type classification. However, an additional third group of aortas with a curved descendens and tendency to kinking was found, with

Table 1. Comparison of patient age, AA width, height and H/W ratio and differences between the three clusters. Statistical significance is marked with a star.

Cluster	Mean			SD			P-Value
	I	II	III	I	II	III	
Age	29.5	15.8	17.9	14.2	5.39	10.9	0.003*
Width	56.3	53.1	54.2	8.35	5.53	8.25	0.015*
Height	36.0	39.0	34.7	6.55	5.86	5.24	0.160
H/W ratio	0.60	0.73	0.65	0.14	0.08	0.14	0.006*

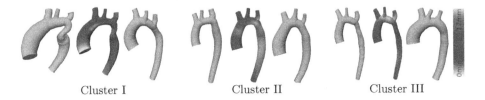

Cluster I   Cluster II   Cluster III

Fig. 3. First principal modes of shape variation for clusters I to III each. Mean shape with color coded local variation and min. and max. shape variation (left and right). (Color figure online)

a statistically significant higher age. The analysis of shape features in relation to other clinical parameters such as hemodynamic measurements are topic of future work, as well as investigating whether the subgroups found in post-op CoA cases [3] match our clusters. Furthermore, we want to study the sensitivity of our results with respect to different shape modeling techniques (e.g. the LDDMM framework) and analyze the shape variance in the supra-aortic branches.

Acknowledgements. This work is sponsored by the German Federal Ministry of Education and Research program "Medizintechnische Lösungen für die digitale Gesundheitsversorgung" under the contract number 13GW0208C, see www.articardio.de.

References

1. Bosmans, B., et al.: Statistical shape modeling and population analysis of the aortic root of TAVI patients. J. Med. Dev. **7**(4), 040925–2 (2013)
2. Bruse, J.L., et al.: A non-parametric statistical shape model for assessment of the surgically repaired aortic arch in coarctation of the aorta: how normal is abnormal? In: Camara, O., Mansi, T., Pop, M., Rhode, K., Sermesant, M., Young, A. (eds.) STACOM 2015. LNCS, vol. 9534, pp. 21–29. Springer, Cham (2016). https://doi.org/10.1007/978-3-319-28712-6_3
3. Bruse, J.L., et al.: Detecting clinically meaningful shape clusters in medical image data: metrics analysis for hierarchical clustering applied to healthy and pathological aortic arches. IEEE Trans. Biomed. Eng. **64**(10), 2373–2383 (2017)

4. Bruse, J.L., et al.: Looks do matter! Aortic arch shape after hypoplastic left heart syndrome palliation correlates with cavopulmonary outcomes. Ann. Thorac. Surg. **103**(2), 645–654 (2017)
5. Casciaro, M.E., et al.: Identifying the principal modes of variation in human thoracic aorta morphology. J. Thorac. Imag. **29**(4), 224–232 (2014)
6. Demertzis, S., et al.: Aortic arch morphometry in living humans. J. Anatomy **217**(5), 588–596 (2010)

Morphometric Sex Estimation from the Hip Bone by Means of the HIP 1.1 Software

Miroslav Králík[1]([envelope]) [iD], Ondřej Klíma[2] [iD], Petra Urbanová[1] [iD],
Lenka Polcerová[1] [iD], and Martin Čuta[1] [iD]

[1] Laboratory of Morphology and Forensic Anthropology, Department of
Anthropology, Masaryk University, Kotlářská 2, 611 37 Brno, Czech Republic
{kralik,urbanova,cuta}@sci.muni.cz, 394630@mail.muni.cz
[2] IT4Innovations Centre of Excellence, Brno University of Technology,
Božetěchova 1/2, 612 66 Brno, Czech Republic
iklima@fit.vutbr.cz

Abstract. Estimation of biological sex from an unknown human skeleton is an important step in analyses of forensic and archaeological skeletal cases. Traditionally, the hip bone (pelvic or innominate bone) is preferentially used for this purpose due to its universal sexual dimorphism in shape resulting from its important reproductive functions of the bone in females. Despite much advancement in the field of sex estimation by means of modern morphometric approaches, no practical software had been available for sex estimation utilizing the shape analysis of the hip bone. We developed HIP 1.1 software (High-sensitive Innominate Processing) which is the second functional version of the software designed for morphometric estimation of sex of an unknown skeletal find based on the pelvic bone. The program works with standardized 2D images of bones from a desktop scanner and produces an assignment of sex to each case/skeletal remains using methods of traditional and geometric morphometry. One-dimensional and multi-dimensional statistics computing procedures and graphical procedures are based on the R software, distributed under the GNU (GPL) license, and its extending libraries from various authors.

Keywords: Sexual dimorphism · Hip bone
Linear discriminant analysis · Procrustes superimposition
Geometric morphometrics

1 Introduction

1.1 Sex Differences in the Human Pelvic Bone

An estimation and assignment of biological sex to an unknown human skeleton is among the first important steps within each osteological analysis in archeological and forensic cases. Sex can be assessed, and traditionally is, from the skeleton

© Springer Nature Switzerland AG 2018
M. Reuter et al. (Eds.): ShapeMI 2018, LNCS 11167, pp. 78–89, 2018.
https://doi.org/10.1007/978-3-030-04747-4_8

itself. One option is to base the estimation on typical size differences between sexes [13]. However, in most of the skeletal elements, males and females overlap substantially in size (a proportion of males are of smaller bodies than an average female and *vice versa*) and, additionally, differences between human populations might be higher than the typical sex difference within a population. This taken together makes sex estimation of an unknown skeleton according to the size of bones very unreliable.

On the contrary, sex differences in the bony pelvis reflect fundamental differences in function of the pelvic girdle in reproduction. In both sexes the pelvic girdle serves as a biomechanical transmitter of forces (weight) from the trunk to the lower appendages in bipedal up-right locomotion. In females, however, it is also a bony support structure for the growing fetus in pregnancy and a birth channel in labor. Therefore, the male pelvis is adapted solely by biomechanical forces of locomotion, whereas female pelvis is an expression of a compromise (trade-off) between the needs of bipedal locomotion and the needs of reproduction. Therefore, a male pelvic bone is more robust in widths (caused by higher weight of the upper body, more robust skeleton and musculature) and larger in the vertical direction, while the female pelvic bone is more gracile, smaller in vertical direction but it possesses larger dimensions in the parts important for supporting the fetus in pregnancy and passing the fetus during parturition [8,18,21]. These proportional (or shape) differences are universally present in all human populations (Fig. 1) and it is also the reason why the pelvic bone (other names: hip bone, innominate bone) is preferentially used for sex estimation in human osteology.

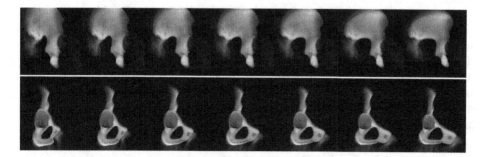

Fig. 1. Seven positions in the male (left) to female (right) range of variations of reconstructed models of the hip bone shape from the iliac (upper row) and pubic (lower row) view. The middle position represents an average shape, the immediate neighbors are average male and female shapes. The second and sixth positions represent extremely masculine and feminine shapes within the natural range of variations and the ends are exaggerated (artificial) shapes beyond the limits of natural variation. The models were created by means of regression analysis in the software tpsRegr [23] and morphing in the software tpsSuper [23].

1.2   Previously Developed Software for Estimating Sex by Skeleton

Despite a long history of human osteology, sex estimation according to the human bones mostly relies on visual assessment and/or manual measurements of distances directly on bones. Software applications enhancing these methods by e.g. automatic computations of discriminant analyses are relatively rare. As an example we can mention FORDISC® 1.0 [15], now available in version 3.1.312, allowing the estimation of sex of the individual based on cranial measurements. As far as the pelvic bone is concerned, the only available software known to us is the DSP software: *Diagnose Sexuelle Probabiliste* [20] (and its preliminary unpublished versions). Murail *et al.* [20] based their program on a worldwide hip bone metrical database that involved 2040 adult specimens of known sex (from 12 different reference populations) and it was recently updated from MS Excel Macro to a stand-alone computer program [6]. All these programs work just with linear measurements (distances, traditional osteometric measures) but do not analyse bone shape. Regarding the skull, shape analysis for routine sex assessment has been introduced in the COLIPR [25] and 3D-ID [24] computer programs using landmark-based approach together with discriminant and canonical variates analysis. For the hip bone, no similar shape-oriented software was available although some articles showed great potential of shape analysis of the hip bone for sex estimation [2, 3, 7, 14, 26]. It was the reason we started to develop HIP (abbreviation of *High-sensitive Innominate Processing*) software in 2012 and today proceeded to the version HIP 1.1 [17].

2   HIP Software

The software allows sex estimation according to the standardized images of the hip bone by means of both traditional and geometric morphometrics. The main advantages of the software are two. (1) On the contrary to the other software, HIP does not operate with predefined range of discriminant functions but constructs – each time – a new discriminant function *ad hoc* according to the size and shape variables available in the analysed case. (2) The second advantage is represented by the possibility of shape sex estimation by means of geometric morphometrics.

2.1   Included Reference Bone Collections

Sex estimation of an unknown case is based on a comparison with documented reference bone collections, that is, the bones of people whose sex was documented during their lives and is known for certain. The recent version of the program contains data from three documented collections of pelvic bones:

- **Athens**: pelvic bones of 102 males and 84 females from the modern Greek population from the collection of The University of Athens Human Skeletal Reference Collection, National and Kapodistrian University of Athens, Greece. The bones were obtained by exhuming the tombs from several cemeteries in the area of Athens [11].

- **Brno**: pelvic bones of 23 males and 6 females from the autopsy collection from the Department of Anatomy, Faculty of Medicine, Masaryk University, Brno, Czech Republic. The bone collection originated from the autopsies of the bodies of the deceased which are used in the education of medical students.
- **Prague**: pelvic bones of 54 males and 46 females from Czech premodern population [16] deposited at the Institute of Anatomy, First Faculty of Medicine, Charles University, Prague, Czech Republic. The skeletal remains are autopsy material. The majority of individuals (90 individuals) are part of the so-called Pachner Collection - skeletons macerated at the Czech anatomical institute during the 1930s.

In total, there are 611 pelvic bones from 315 human individuals (179 males, 136 females) included in the reference data of the software.

2.2 Image Recording and Landmark Definitions

Since a wide applicability using a simple device was one of the requirements and the bone is relatively flat in some views, the bones were scanned by a flat desktop scanner (CanoScan 4400) which provides 2D images of properties suitable for 2D shape analysis. The orientation of the bones on the scanner board/glass was standardized and the bones were scanned in 2 different views:

- (A) Pubic view – scanning of the outer surface of the *os pubis*.
- (B) Iliac view – scanning of the outer surface of the iliac wing.

The bones were recorded into full-color TIF files, 100% in size, resolution 150 dpi in both directions. The program also loads JPG and PNG files. On the standardized images, measuring points were defined for the subsequent morphometric application based on the landmark methods. On the pubic and iliac view we defined 24 and 21 points, respectively (Fig. 2). Some of the points represent true landmarks (respecting borders between anatomical structures) but most of them are extremal or geometrically defined points.

2.3 Programming, Technical Issues and Availability

The program was written in C++ and R, and created in QtToolkit framework, version 4.8.2, the user interface was created in QtDesigner. It uses R environment, version 2.15.1. Rtools were used to compile Qt libraries and the entire application, Rtpp, Rinside, and examples from QtDensity (under the GPL licence) were used for compiling Qt and R. Qt itself is licensed under LGPL. During the creation of the program, the computational and graphic functions of the following packages of the program R [22] and packages working in this environment (cited below) were used. HIP 1.1 is designed for Windows operating system, versions Vista and higher. The program was not tested on lower versions of the Windows operating system (Windows XP, NT, 98, 95) and probably will not work properly. The HIP 1.1 can be downloaded at the web site: https://sourceforge.net/projects/hip-project/. The software is freely available and is distributed under the GPLv3 license. The official license text is available at http://gnu.org/licenses/gpl.html.

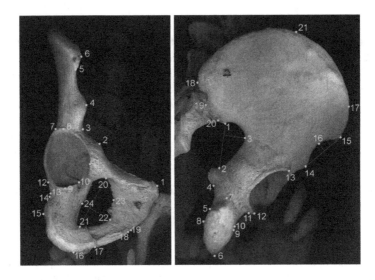

Fig. 2. Landmarks defined on the images of the pelvic bone in the pubic view (left) and the iliac view (right).

3   Using the HIP 1.1 Software

3.1   Digitizing Landmarks and Selecting the Data

After loading an image of a bone in the standardized position, the user must manually specify/measure the defined measuring points. HIP provides some automatic tools for delimiting positions of points in a deepest position, points positioned on a line lying in an upright direction to another line and points positioned in the farthest distance from another point. Precise definitions of osteometric points are stated in the manual of the HIP software and each user should familiarize with them before measurements. During the measurement, the program offers both text definitions of the points and visual examples (images) of digitized points on various cases of the hip bone. If some parts of the bone are destroyed or abraded the user can omit the point and proceed to the following one. However, the more points available the more detailed descriptions of its shape and the better data for the analysis. The program automatically checks the available points for subsequent analyses. If the position of a point is not certain, the option is to deactivate the point and compare the results of the analyses with and without the point. Recorded Cartesian coordinates *(x, y)* of the measured points represent raw data for subsequent computations and can be saved into a file of TPS format [23] with 3D array data structure. HIP can save and also open the file again and work with the data included. An important option (in the right menu) is a reference sample selection for the analysis (Fig. 3). The user can compare his/her analyzed bone with all three samples at once or select only one or two of them. At the same time, body side can be chosen automatically (right bones compared with right bones of the reference samples) or manually.

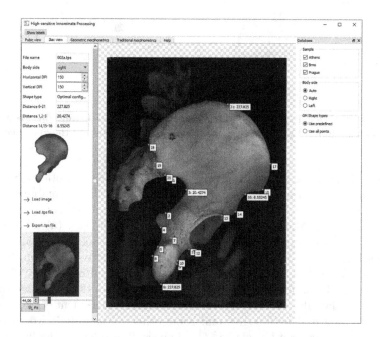

Fig. 3. Screenshot of the digitizing window of the HIP software (iliac view).

3.2 Traditional Morphometrics

The program allows automatic scale calibration according to metadata in the loaded image (visible in the left menu). After calibration the user can easily compute and visualize selected measurement (distance within a pair of selected points) and compare the computed value of the analyzed bone with male and female variation (histogram and boxplot) of the same measurement in a selected reference sample (Fig. 4). A simple visualizing of individual distances might be useful for selecting variables for traditional Linear Discriminant Analysis (LDA).

Sex estimation by means of traditional morphometrics represents LDA [12] computed on a set of traditional measurements (here distances between points). The method searches in a multidimensional space for a combination of variables that maximizes the differences between groups (in our case between the sexes). The LDA program calculates the *lda* function of the *MASS* package [27], the prediction of the unknown case sex is performed using the *predict* function from the *MASS* [27]. In this traditional sex discrimination, the program allows two options: (A) LDA on arbitrarily selected fixed set of distances or (B) stepwise LDA with automatic selection of distances by means of a permutation procedure.

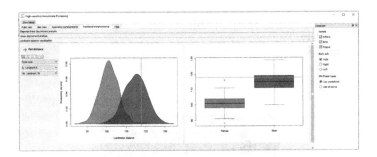

Fig. 4. Screenshot of a visualization of an example of a selected distance between points 8 and 16 in the pubic view. The green line points to the position of the analyzed case.

If the user chooses the arbitrary selection he/she has several options. Separate pubic or iliac view variables can be used or both views can be combined. Seminally, one body side or both body sides of the reference samples can be chosen for the comparison. Moreover, the program can compute with (a) all distances available on the analyzed bone, or (b) exclude some of all the distances (i.e., negative selection), or select only some distances (i.e. positive selection) from all the distances available. In the option (b) the program automatically disallows the calculation of discriminant analysis from the distances that were determined to be inappropriate due to small absolute size, high measurement error, frequent presence of connected pathologies and some other reasons. It is worth noting that, hence, the data can be selected for analysis at two levels, the first level is the activation and deactivation of the points in the measurement window, the second level is the blocking or the selection of the variables (distance between points) before the LDA. After calculating the LDA, the program returns a table including *prior probability* (i.e. the original probability of the case classification by sex even without an analysis that is set to the proportion of the given sex in the reference sample), *posterior probability* (indicating the likelihood of correct case classification and sex estimation), and a classification table with total number of males and females in the references sample and the number and percentages of misclassified cases. The second output table includes selected results of discriminant analysis and classification, e.g. the value of a discriminant score for the unknown case, the cut-off point, and the total number of cases and variables in the analysis. Other outputs contain the coefficients of the discriminant function for each dimension, the mean of each of the included distances for males and females, and the respective value of the unknown case variable (Fig. 5). The discriminant score value is also visualized in a probability density plot and the box and whisker plot of the reference cases (analogically to the plots of single distances in the Fig. 4).

The option (B) in the traditional morphometrics is the Stepwise LDA. Since LDA is very sensitive to the ratio between the sample size (number of cases) and number of variables, it is generally recommended that the ratio (case/variables) be at least 5:1 (5 cases per variable) or higher [19]. It is therefore appropriate to

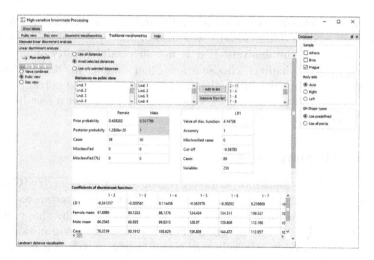

Fig. 5. Screenshot of a result from the LDA with arbitrarily selected variables. The analyzed case was compared with Prague reference sample of bones of the same body side, the distances computed on the pubic view only were used and avoiding predefined inappropriate distances was selected. The results of the estimation indicate clearly the male sex.

include only a few of the most effective variables (in traditional morphometrics: interlandmark distances) in the model. This is the purpose of Stepwise Linear Discriminant Analysis (Stepwise LDA). The program uses functions from the *MASS* [27] and *klaR* [28] packages, in particular the *stepclass* and *lda* functions. The prediction is again performed by the function *predict* from the *MASS* package [26]. The user can choose the distances from which the analysis is to be calculated and the stepwise procedure is then realized by a default setting of the function *stepclass* using the function *ucpm* from the *klaR* package [28] to calculate the criteria for assigning a variable to the resulting model. The calculation includes a leave-one-out randomization method, i.e. n-fold cross-validation, where n is the number of cases of the reference sample. The number of cases (and thus the number of cross-validated samples) will vary according to the selection of bone views and, above all, the selection of reference samples. One case is randomly selected from the reference sample and a discriminant function is computed on the rest of the sample (with $n-1$ number of cases). The pre-selected case is then used as validation (test) and the discriminant function is used on it. The whole process is repeated n-times. Details of the preconfigured stepwise procedure are described in the manual of the *klaR* package [28]. Due to the stepwise procedure and verifying, the calculation is time consuming and may take from a few tens of seconds to several tens of minutes depending on the number of cases (reference samples) and variables (preselected distances/measurements) included. The program lists results in the same structure as the classic LDA described above. In order to reach a compromise between the calculation speed and the estimation reliability, the preferred way of working with the program might be to use a classical LDA on a small number of selected variables, let's say deliberately chosen 3 individually well-discriminating distances in each view and use these six for the analysis. If it is not successful (posterior probability does not reach 0.95 or higher), choose a few other dimensions and perform the discriminant analysis again. Given the growth patterns of the pelvic bone, it is the preferred choice (if you have both views available) to select a few dimensions from each of the two views [21].

3.3   Geometric Morphometrics

An alternative to traditional morphometry is geometric morphometry (GM). GM procedures are most often based on data in the form of Cartesian coordinates of landmarks and have the advantage that we can address the shape and size of objects separately [1]. The program offers the same selection options of the reference sample and body side as in traditional morphometrics. In addition, the user can choose between calculations with all points or appropriate (predefined) configurations of points which adequately represent the shape being evaluated and at the same time do not contain redundant points. Selected point configurations are superimposed by Generalized Procrustes Analysis (GPA) [5,10] with size standardization on unit centroid size (CS). For the GPA calculation, the program uses the *procOPA* function from the *shapes* package [9]. Procrustes shape coordinates as shape variables and centroid size (CS) as a size variable are then used as input variables for LDA. It is possible to choose whether the user wants to discriminate based on the shape purely, which is the default setting, or to combine the shape variables with the centroid size. The results of sex discrimination have a similar structure to that of traditional morphometry, including graphs, as described above. In addition, this analysis shows graphically the shape of the unknown case in a superposition with the average shape (consensus) for males and females. The tps grid of this plot (Fig. 6) is calculated using the *tps.grid* function from the *Momocs* package [4].

3.4   Saving and Export of Results

All results are automatically saved in the program directory in the *outs* folder in separate subfolders, named by time (year-month-day hour-minute-second) when the analysis took place (e.g. 2017-11-02 22-23-41). The results are saved in the HTML format which can be viewed in any internet browser; data can be simply selected and copied for further use. Images are also stored separately in the PNG format.

4   Limitations and Future Development

One limitation of the software is the necessity of a relatively well preserved (non-destroyed) bone for scanning which favors application of these procedures in forensic cases rather than in archaeologically excavated skeletons. The next

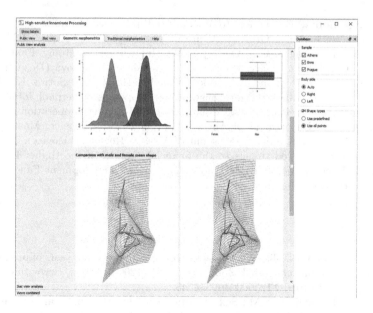

Fig. 6. Screenshot of a result from the GM analysis. The analyzed case is represented by a green line. In the tps grids, mean female shape is in red and mean male in blue. The largest shape differences are shown by thickening (darkening) or by diluting (lightening) of the grid.

limitation relates to the recording technique. The 2D desktop scanner was chosen because it is affordable for almost everyone and allows very fast estimations (in several minutes, which is not possible to reach while generating full 3D models) with high accuracy. Measurement preciseness, repeatability and estimation accuracy reached high values (comparable to or better than other software available today, especially thanks to the involvement of shape analysis) and will be part of a full-length paper on the software. However, different desktop scanners provide almost identical images of the configuration on the scanner plane, but the three-dimensional formations over the plate (above its plane) they convert into 2D image slightly differently. Therefore, as with any other recording device, it is always necessary to calibrate the images. Due to this, we have recorded all existing cases with the Canon CanoScan 4400 F scanner. For other scanners, the data need to be adjusted but an automatic calibration of the scanner is not yet part of this software. Therefore, it is strictly recommended to use HIP 1.1 only on images from this particular scanner (Canon CanoScan 4400F). We are working on creating a calibration feature for other scanners and cameras, and we expect it to be included in the program in one of the later versions. In the next version, we'd like to extend the program also by descriptive statistics of input variables (coordinates, dimensions), other indicators of prediction and reliability of discrimination, inclusion of other classification procedures (e.g. logistic regression), new reference samples and new plots and visualizations.

Acknowledgements. For access to documented reference samples and versatile help let us thank to Miloš Grim (Institute of Anatomy, First Faculty of Medicine, Charles University, Prague, CZ), Ondřej Naňka (Institute of Anatomy, First Faculty of Medicine, Charles University, Prague, CZ), Ladislava Horáčková (Department of Anatomy, Faculty of Medicine, Masaryk University, Brno, CZ), Sotiris K. Manolis (University of Athens, Greece), and Constantinos Eliopoulos (Liverpool John Moores University, GB). For assistance with organization and further cooperation we thank Tomáš Mořkovský (Department of Anthropology, Faculty of Science, Masaryk University) and Michaela Králíková (Museum of Vyškov Region, Bučovice). The computer program was created thanks to the financial support of the Higher Education Development Fund (project FRVS/2034/2012) and MU Development Fund (project UNI/FR/0284/2014).

References

1. Adams, D., Rohlf, F., Slice, D.: Geometric morphometrics: ten years of progress following the 'revolution'. Ital. J. Zool. **71**(1), 5–16 (2004). https://www.tandfonline.com/doi/abs/10.1080/11250000409356545
2. Ali, R.S., Maclaughlin, S.M.: Sex identification from the auricular surface of the adult human ilium. Int. J. Osteoarchaeol. **1**(1), 57–61 (1991). https://doi.org/10.1002/oa.1390010108
3. Anastasiou, E., Chamberlain, A.T.: The sexual dimorphism of the sacro-iliac joint: an investigation using geometric morphometric techniques. J. Forensic Sci. **58**(s1), S126–S134 (2012). https://doi.org/10.1111/j.1556-4029.2012.02282.x
4. Bonhomme, V., Picq, S., Gaucherel, C., Claude, J.: Momocs: outline analysis using R. J. Stat. Softw. **56**(13), 1–24 (2014). http://www.jstatsoft.org/v56/i13/
5. Bookstein, F.L.: Morphometric Tools for Landmark Data: Geometry and Biology (1991)
6. Brůžek, J., Santos, F., Dutailly, B., Murail, P., Cunha, E.: Validation and reliability of the sex estimation of the human os coxae using freely available DSP2 software for bioarchaeology and forensic anthropology. Am. J. Phys. Anthropol. **164**(2), 440–449 (2017)
7. Bytheway, J.A.: Ross: a geometric morphometric approach to sex determination of the human adult os coxa. J. Forensic Sci. **55**(4), 859–864 (2010). https://doi.org/10.1111/j.1556-4029.2010.01374.x
8. Correia, H., Balseiro, S., De Areia, M.: Sexual dimorphism in the human pelvis: testing a new hypothesis. HOMO - J. Compar. Hum. Biol. **56**(2), 153–160 (2005). http://www.sciencedirect.com/science/article/B7GW4-4GG8W5B-1/2/1f7349a5d67a076e7b026b68bdd8c4a4
9. Dryden, I.L.: Shapes: Statistical Shape Analysis. R package version 1.2.0. (2017). https://CRAN.R-project.org/package=shapes
10. Dryden, I., Mardia, K.: Statistical shape analysis. Wiley, Chisester (1998)
11. Eliopoulos, C., Lagia, A., Manolis, S.: A modern documented human skeletal collection from Greece. HOMO **58**(3), 221–228 (2007)
12. Fisher, R.A.: The use of multiple measurements in taxonomic problems. Ann. Eugenics **7**(2), 179–188 (1936)

13. Frayer, D.W., Wolpoff, M.H.: Sexual dimorphism. Ann. Rev. Anthropol. **14**(1), 429–473 (1985). http://www.annualreviews.org/doi/abs/10.1146/annurev. an.14.100185.002241

14. Gonzalez, P.N., Bernal, V., Perez, S.I.: Geometric morphometric approach to sex estimation of human pelvis. Forensic Sci. Int. **189**(1–3), 68–74 (2009). http://www.sciencedirect.com/science/article/B6T6W-4W8KHN0-1/2/8709c8c3c 338b93e8658f093e7cc0076

15. Jantz, R.L., Ousley, S.D.: FORDISC 3.1.312: Computerized Forensic Discriminant Functions (2005). http://math.mercyhurst.edu/~sousley/Fordisc/

16. Jurda, M., Urbanová, P., Králík, M.: The post-mortem pressure distortion of human crania uncovered in an early medieval Pohansko (Czech Republic) graveyard. Int. J. Osteoarchaeol. **25**(4), 539–549 (2013). https://doi.org/10.1002/oa. 2321

17. Králík, M., Urbanová, P., Klíma, O., Mikešová, T., Wagenknechtová, M., Jungerová, J.: HIP 1.1 - High-Sensitive Innominate Processing (2017). https:// sourceforge.net/projects/hip-project/

18. Leong, A.: Sexual dimorphism of the pelvic architecture: a struggling response to destructive and parsimonious forces by natural and mate selection. McGill J. Med.: MJM **9**(1), 61–66 (2006). http://www.ncbi.nlm.nih.gov/pmc/articles/ PMC2687900/

19. Meloun, M., Militký, J.: Kompendium statistického zpracování dat. Metody řešené úlohy včetně CD. Academia, Praha (2002)

20. Murail, P., Bruzek, J., Houët, F., Cunha, E.: DSP: a tool for probabilistic sex diagnosis using worldwide variability in hip-bone measurements. Bulletins et mémoires de la Société d'Anthropologie de Paris **17**(3–4), 167–176 (2005)

21. Novotný, V.: Sex determination of the pelvic bone: a systems approach. Anthropologie **24**, 197–206 (1986)

22. R Core Team: R: A Language and Environment for Statistical Computing. R Foundation for Statistical Computing, Vienna, Austria (2012). http://www.R-project. org/. ISBN 3-900051-07-0

23. Rohlf, F.: The TPS series of software. Hystrix. It. J. Mamm. **26**, 1–4 (2015). http://www.italian-journal-of-mammalogy.it/Issue-1-2015,2849

24. Slice, D.E., Ross, A.H.: 3D-ID: Geometric Morphometric Classification of Crania for Forensic Scientists (2009). http://www.3d-id.org/

25. Urbanová, P., Králík, M.: COLIPR 1.5.2 (2008). http://www.sci.muni.cz/lamorfa/ veda-a-vyzkum#projekty

26. Vacca, E., Novotný, V., Vančata, V., Delfino, V.: Shape analysis of incisura ischiadica major in sexing the human pelvis. Anthropologie **35**, 291–301 (1997)

27. Venables, W.N., Ripley, B.D.: Modern Applied Statistics with S, 4th edn. Springer, New York (2017). https://cran.r-project.org/doc/manuals/r-release/R-intro.pdf

28. Weihs, C., Ligges, U., Luebke, K., Raabe, N.: klaR Analyzing German Business Cycles. In: Baier, D., Decker, R., Schmidt-Thieme, L. (eds.) Data Analysis and Decision Support, pp. 335–343. Springer, Berlin (2005). https://doi.org/10.1007/ 3-540-28397-8_36

Shape Methods

Deformable Cubic Hermite Mesh Templates for Statistical Liver Shape Analysis

Hao Bo Yu[1], Yui Nakagawa[2], Harvey Ho[1(✉)], Atsushi Saito[2],
and Akinobu Shimizu[2]

[1] Auckland Bioengineering Institute, University of Auckland,
Auckland, New Zealand
`harvey.ho@auckland.ac.nz`
[2] Tokyo University of Agriculture and Technology, Koganei, Tokyo, Japan

Abstract. In this paper we present a novel statistical shape model for the liver based on a cubic Hermite mesh. With a small number of nodes (4, 12 or 20 for 1, 2 and 4 parametric cubic Hermite elements respectively) the complex liver shape can be captured with details. Such a model evolves from a generic ellipsoid-shaped template to fit to the data clouds of liver surfaces segmented from CT images. No landmarks on the data cloud are required to instruct the deformation of the parametric mesh. Through a Principle Component Analysis (PCA) for the nodal distribution on liver surfaces, a statistical shape model for the liver is generated. We found that 6 modes of the statistical model could interpret 96% of liver shape variations in 15 subject-specific livers. To evaluate the quality of node correspondence we devised a curvature criterion so that mis-alignments of nodes could be detected. In summary, a novel cubic Hermite mesh based statistical shape model is proposed. The mesh has a small set of nodes for PCA analysis, and the nodal correspondence across the shape database can be evaluated from a curvature criterion.

Keywords: Liver · Cubic Hermite mesh · Statistical shape analysis

1 Introduction

The liver is an organ with large inter-subject variations. A statistical shape model that bears some common features of the liver has many practical applications such as model-based image segmentation, liver shape analysis for a population, etc. [1]. The state-of-the-art statistical liver models include that proposed in [1] and [2]. Specifically, the statistical liver model in [1] follows the idea of Active Shape Models (ASM) proposed in [3], whereby a principal component analysis (PCA) is performed for the point (landmark) distribution on a deformable mesh. However, this approach requires a large number of landmarks (in the order of thousands) to represent the liver shape, and it is cumbersome to determine

© Springer Nature Switzerland AG 2018
M. Reuter et al. (Eds.): ShapeMI 2018, LNCS 11167, pp. 93–101, 2018.
https://doi.org/10.1007/978-3-030-04747-4_9

the landmark correspondence. In [4] a parametric surface is used to represent a deformable kidney model. The advantage of this approach is that a much smaller number of landmarks are required. However this method has not been applied to the statistical representation of the liver, which has a more complex shape. For example, the posterior aspect of the liver has imprints from the compression of other organs, which are difficult to model with a parametric mesh.

Moreover, the parameter mesh approach usually requires landmarks or labelled points on the mesh to guide the morphing. This process itself can be problematic, as the landmarkers need to be selected from the data cloud, e.g., the extremities of the shape, either manually or via complex algorithms.

In this paper we introduce a novel approach, in which a 3D deformable cubic Hermite mesh is fitted to the data clouds of liver surfaces, and the node correspondence is implicitly solved. The mesh, consisting of only a few elements, can capture salient features of the liver geometry since each node on the mesh contains a good set of geometric information. We apply the technology to the derivation of a statistical liver template trained from a set of 15 livers. We then devise a curvature based criterion to assess the quality of node correspondence. Next we will briefly introduce the workflow of this method, and present some initial results.

2   Methods

2.1   Semi-automatic Image Segmentation

The segmentation method for CT images (SIEMENS, Somatom Definition Flash) of resolution $0.67 \times 0.67 \times 3 \, \mathrm{mm}^3$ is based on the statistical shape model introduced in [5]. This requires two types of manual inputs of landmarks. The first type is on the surface of the liver including the endpoints of each plane (axial, coronal, and sagittal), and the second type is for specifying the center and radius of a sphere containing the liver.

Based on the manual inputs, four fully-automatic steps are executed. Firstly, the CT images are standardized using a bounding box specified by the endpoints. Then, a patient-specific probabilistic atlas is generated from the statistical shape model under the constraints applied by manual input of landmarks. Next, the parameters of Gaussian mixture models of the CT images are estimated by the expectation maximization algorithm [5] using the probabilistic atlas, followed by the Maximum a posteriori (MAP) based rough segmentation. Finally, graph cuts are applied for the final segmentation. Overall, the segmentation took 10–15 min to complete for each subject.

2.2   Individual Shape Representations

The use of Cubic-Hermite mesh to represent the human body and organs has been reported e.g. in [6], therefore its mathematical background is not stated here. The advantage of using a cubic Hermite mesh is that a small number of

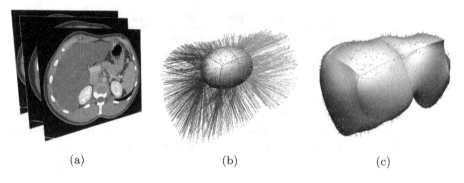

(a)   (b)   (c)

Fig. 1. Illustration of the work flow: (a) semi-automatic segmentation of the liver to generate a data cloud; (b) the initial ellipsoid-shaped cubic Hermite mesh and the projection vectors from the data cloud to the mesh surface; and (c) the mesh is fitted to the liver of a patient.

elements can capture complex geometric details of an organ, as we will demonstrate in this paper. Moreover, the indexes of the nodes on the mesh are identical across the liver dataset and thus the node correspondence is implicitly addressed. The problem to be solved is the quality of liver representation. To that end we adopt a mesh optimisation algorithm formulated in [6], whereby a generic cubic Hermite mesh is fitted to the data clouds of liver surfaces. This is performed by iteratively minimising the sum of the projection vectors, and updating consecutively the nodal positions on the mesh. The workflow is shown in Fig. 1(b) and (c). Here the mesh has two tri-cubic Hermite elements with total 12 nodes.

In the implementation, the optimisation algorithm consists of two functions with respect to mesh parameters, u. The first function is the squared sum $D(u)$ of all the projection vectors from the data cloud to the mesh (Fig. 1b), while the second function is a Sobelov smoothing function $G(u, \alpha, \beta)$ introduced to prevent the surface mesh from overfitting to the data cloud [6]. Hence, the optimisation problem is formed by summing up the projection error and the smoothing function terms:

$$\min_{u} \quad D(u) + G(u, \alpha, \beta) \tag{1}$$

Note, that the parameters α and β in the second term are tunable, with α controls the smoothness constraints, and β tunes convergence. The optimisation routine is implemented using the Least Squared Quasi Newton (LSQN) method in the OPT++ optimisation library. A typical fitting process takes 140 iterations, around 10 min to complete on a desktop computer (CPU@2.80 GHz).

2.3   Statistical Shape Model for the Liver

We applied the Principle Component Analysis (PCA) to the shape analysis similar to [1] and [3]. For node q on the mesh, the nodal information is stored in a vector:

$$I_q = \left[x_q, \frac{\partial x_q}{\partial s_1}, \frac{\partial x_q}{\partial s_2}, \frac{\partial x_q}{\partial s_3}, \frac{\partial x_q^2}{\partial s_1 \partial s_2}, \frac{\partial x_q^2}{\partial s_1 \partial s_3}, \frac{\partial x_q^2}{\partial s_2 \partial s_3} \right] \in \mathbb{R}^{21} \qquad (2)$$

where the vector x_i is a concatenation of the nodal positions (in physical space), and the physical derivatives with respect to the arc-length.

For a liver model with k nodes, the shape vector can be written as $X = [I_1, \ldots, I_k]$. For N shapes in the training set, the mean shape $\bar{I}$ is given by $\bar{I} = \frac{1}{N} \sum_{i=1}^{N} I_i$. For each shape in the training set, i, we find its deviation from the mean, $dI_i = I_i - \bar{I}$, then the covariance matrix S is given by:

$$S = \frac{1}{N} \sum_{i=1}^{N} dI_i dI_i^{\top} \qquad (3)$$

The principal axes, or the modes of variation, are described by the eigenvectors of S. A shape in the training set can be approximated using the mean shape and the product of the eigenvectors and weights:

$$I = \bar{I} + Pb \qquad (4)$$

where $P = (p_1, p_2, \ldots, p_k)$ is a matrix of the k eigenvectors that can explain most of the variations in the liver shape.

2.4   Assessing Nodal Correspondence Quality

As mentioned before, the nodal correspondence is implicitly addressed in the parametric mesh. However, the quality of such correspondence requires further investigation because the nodes are not bound to any feature points on the liver surface. We propose a curvature based criterion for the sake of its quantitative description of the smoothness/curvedness of liver shape. Such a criterion highlights the edges, sharp corners and imprints on a liver surface (Fig. 2).

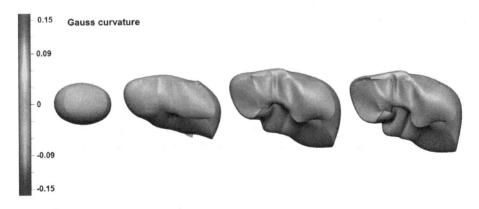

Fig. 2. Evolution of the Gauss curvature on the cubic Hermite mesh, starting from the initial ellipsoid to the final fitted liver. Note the imprints caused by the inferior vena cava and other organs are captured by the 2-element mesh.

The vector given in Eq. (2) contains the Cartesian coordinates, the first and second derivatives of each node. However these do not explicitly provide the curvature information. Hence, we evaluate the mean (κ_{mean}) and Gaussian ($\kappa_{Gaussian}$) curvatures for each node using the algorithm introduced in [7]. Further, we devise a *curvature space* composed of the κ_{mean} (y-axis) and $\kappa_{Gaussian}$ (x-axis). The nodal curvatures of the same node I from N liver surfaces can then be cast into this space to assess the quality of correspondence.

3   Results

3.1   Geometric Description of Liver Shapes

Applying the semi-automatic segmentation algorithm to the 15 livers resulted in 15 data clouds for the segmented liver surfaces. Each data cloud consists of approximately 2,000 points.

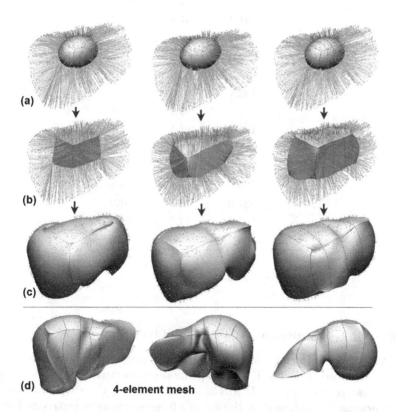

Fig. 3. Fitting procedure for 1, 2 and 4 elements shown in its respective columns. (a) Initial ellipsoid shaped elements; (b) intermediate step after 40 iterations; and (c) final fitted geometry after 140 iterations. (d) Fitting result using 4-element mesh with anterior, posterior and inferior views.

Figure 3 illustrates the scenario where the initial ellipsoid-shaped cubic Hermite mesh consisting of one, two and four elements were used to fit the data cloud of a liver surface. As can be seen, the 1-element mesh of eight nodes can already approximate the liver shape, and the 2- and 4-element mesh yield more details. In Fig. 3(d), the fitted 4-element mesh is viewed from different perspectives (anterior, posterior and inferior) where details of the liver such as the imprints from the inferior vena cava (IVC) are clearly visible. The summed fitting error for each of the 15 subjects by using the 1, 2, and 4 elements are shown in Table 1. Interestingly, the 2-element mesh had the least overall fitting error, and so it is used for the statistical shape analysis as described below.

Table 1. The sum of projection errors (mm) of 2,000 data points for 1, 2, 4 element mesh when applied to 15 subjects

Subject ID	1-element	2-element	4-element
1	95.8	61.8	65.7
2	121.2	87.6	94.4
3	87.4	59.2	70.5
4	92.5	62.4	68.5
5	98.4	80.6	76.5
6	132.1	105.2	114.6
7	117.6	89.4	122.6
8	102.8	68.1	87.7
9	111.7	70.9	75.6
10	103.8	62.4	105.4
11	124.7	88.8	91.8
12	237.0	93.0	91.9
13	102.3	77.2	86.8
14	134.3	80.0	98.9
15	98.6	79.5	67.4
Mean error	120.2	77.4	90.3

3.2   Principle Component Analysis for Liver Shapes

The 2-element cubic Hermite mesh was used to represent the fifteen livers using the method defined in Sect. 2.3. The shape modes were derived by evaluating the covariant matrix S in Eq. (3). It was found that 96% of the shape variations of the 15 livers can be explained by the leading 6 eigenvectors of matrix S. Figure 4 illustrates the transformation of the statistical liver by varying the leading two modes λ_1 and λ_2 by a factor of $\pm 2\sqrt{\lambda}$.

We cast the curvature of the nodes (total 12 in the liver mesh) of the fifteen livers into the curvature space separately, so that each plot contains 15 data

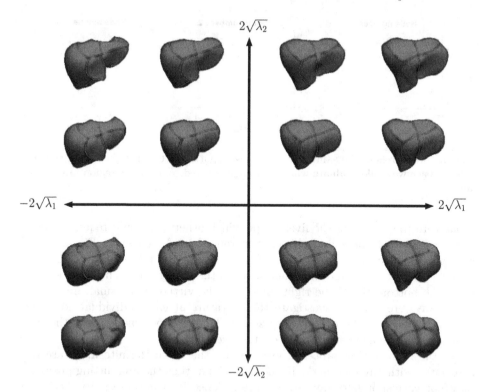

Fig. 4. Liver shapes generated by varying the two most significant eigenvectors. Horizontal and vertical variations, illustrates the first and second eigenvectors, respectively. The range is chosen such that $-2\sqrt{\lambda_i} \leq b_i \leq 2\sqrt{\lambda_i}$.

points from the nodes with the same index. Three such plots showing curvature distributions are listed in Fig. 5. Here node number 1 has a broader distribution implying a wider variance of surface appearance. This implies the location at node number 1 has a wide range of curvatures across the fifteen livers. In contrast, node number 6 has a consistent curvature distribution except in one liver. This means the mesh location at this node has a consistent shape. The liver with the unfitting node number 6 requires a closer investigation to check whether a manual fitting for that node is required.

4   Discussion

A novel statistical shape model for the liver is introduced in this paper. The model is based on the cubic Hermite mesh that evolves from an initial ellipsoid to a subject-specific liver. The drastic difference between our approach and the parametric mesh introduced before, e.g., in [8] is that the fitting template (i.e. the ellipsoid) does not assume any specific shape (in this case the liver), thus render the method versatile. The evolving high order cubic Hermite mesh is used

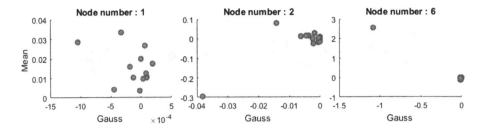

Fig. 5. Curvatures of the same nodes. By investigation of the distribution in the curvature space we could evaluate whether a node is fitted to a similar region in the liver surface.

to capture the details of the liver shape which otherwise would require a much larger number of nodes and elements to represent. As shown in Fig. 4, the 2-element cubic Hermite mesh of 12 nodes yield bountiful information of the liver shape, such as the left and right lobe septum, the corners at the liver extremities (e.g., the bottom tip of the right lobe). By the virtue of the small number of nodes, we were able to investigate the curvature at each individual node and their influences on the overall liver shape. To our knowledge, this is the first time a curvature analysis is made for the liver surface.

In the mesh fitting process the nodes on the cubic Hermite mesh are not associated with any landmarks in the data cloud, thus the final fitting positions may not correspond to any key features. Hence it is important to check the quality of node correspondence. To assist this task we designed a measure of curvature space, which is the combination of mean and Gaussian curvatures, and is another novelty of this work. For the future work we will investigate the use of this method in image segmentation, and compare it with other registration methods, e.g. [9].

The statistical liver carries the features common to the 15 livers and also can be used to approximate individual livers by varying the leading modes per Eq. (4), as shown in Fig. 4. It should be pointed out that the number of livers (15) used for the analysis is small. A larger number of livers would certainly require more principle modes to represent the statistic liver shape. In addition, both normal and abnormal livers need to be included in an augmented database, so that the method would be able to represent abnormal or post-mortem liver shapes [2].

5   Conclusion

A novel cubic Hermite mesh based method is introduced in this paper for statistical shape analysis of the liver. With only a few elements the mesh can capture the liver shape details and also facilitate curvature analysis.

Acknowledgments. We acknowledge the support of a Catalyst seed grant (Project number 3711560) from the Royal Society of New Zealand.

References

1. Heimann, T., Wolf, I., Meinzer, H.-P.: Active shape models for a fully automated 3D segmentation of the liver – an evaluation on clinical data. In: Larsen, R., Nielsen, M., Sporring, J. (eds.) MICCAI 2006. LNCS, vol. 4191, pp. 41–48. Springer, Heidelberg (2006). https://doi.org/10.1007/11866763_6
2. Saito, A., Yamamoto, S., Nawano, S., Shimizu, A.: Automated liver segmentation from a postmortem CT scan based on a statistical shape model. Int. J. Comput. Assist. Radiol. Surg. 12(2), 205–221 (2017)
3. Cootes, T.F., Taylor, C.J., Cooper, D.H., Graham, J.: Active shape models-their training and application. Comput. Vis. Image Underst. 61(1), 38–59 (1995)
4. Tsagaan, B., Shimizu, A., Kobatake, H., Miyakawa, K.: An automated segmentation method of kidney using statistical information. In: Dohi, T., Kikinis, R. (eds.) MICCAI 2002. LNCS, vol. 2488, pp. 556–563. Springer, Heidelberg (2002). https://doi.org/10.1007/3-540-45786-0_69
5. Shimizu, A., Ohno, R., Ikegami, T., Kobatake, H., Nawano, S., Smutek, D.: Segmentation of multiple organs in non-contrast 3D abdominal CT images. Int. J. Comput. Assist. Radiol. Surg. 2(3–4), 135–142 (2007)
6. Bradley, C., Pullan, A., Hunter, P.: Geometric modeling of the human torso using cubic hermite elements. Ann. Biomed. Eng. 25(1), 96–111 (1997)
7. Abbena, E., Salamon, S., Gray, A.: Modern Differential Geometry of Curves and Surfaces with Mathematica, 3rd edn. CRC Press, Boca Raton (2017)
8. Fernandez, J.W., Mithraratne, P., Thrupp, S.F., Tawhai, M.H., Hunter, P.J.: Anatomically based geometric modelling of the musculo-skeletal system and other organs. Biomech. Model. Mechanobiol. 2(3), 139–155 (2004)
9. Rueckert, D., Sonoda, L.I., Hayes, C., Hill, D.L.G., Leach, M.O., Hawkes, D.J.: Nonrigid registration using free-form deformations: application to breast MR images. IEEE Trans. Med. Imaging 18(8), 712–721 (1999)

Global Divergences Between Measures: From Hausdorff Distance to Optimal Transport

Jean Feydy[1,2(✉)] and Alain Trouvé[2]

[1] DMA, École Normale Supérieure, Paris, France
`jean.feydy@ens.fr`
[2] CMLA, ENS Paris-Saclay, Cachan, France
`trouve@cmla.ens-cachan.fr`

Abstract. The data fidelity term is a key component of shape registration pipelines: computed at every step, its gradient is the vector field that drives a deformed model towards its target. Unfortunately, most classical formulas are at most semi-local: their gradients saturate and stop being informative above some given distance, with appalling consequences on the robustness of shape analysis pipelines.

In this paper, we build on recent theoretical advances on *Sinkhorn entropies and divergences* [6] to present a unified view of three fidelities between measures that alleviate this problem: the Energy Distance from statistics; the (weighted) Hausdorff distance from computer graphics; the Wasserstein distance from Optimal Transport theory. The ε-Hausdorff and ε-Sinkhorn divergences are *positive* fidelities that interpolate between these three quantities, and we implement them through efficient, freely available GPU routines. They should allow the shape analyst to handle large deformations without hassle.

Keywords: Shape registration · Kernel · Energy Distance
Hausdorff distance · Optimal Transport · GPU

1 Introduction

Shape Registration as a Variational Problem. Given a source shape A and a target B, a key problem in medical image analysis is to register the former onto the latter. That is, to estimate a mapping φ (a change of coordinates) that maps the source A into a model $\varphi(A)$ which is "close enough" to the target.

Most classical registration algorithms strive to minimize an energy

$$\mathrm{E}(\varphi) \;=\; \underbrace{\mathrm{Reg}(\varphi)}_{\text{regularizer}} \;+\; \underbrace{\mathrm{d}\,(\varphi(A), B)}_{\text{fidelity}}$$

which is the sum of a regularization term – encoding a prior on acceptable mappings – and a data attachment term – or *fidelity* – that measures how far the model $\varphi(A)$ is from the target B.

© Springer Nature Switzerland AG 2018
M. Reuter et al. (Eds.): ShapeMI 2018, LNCS 11167, pp. 102–115, 2018.
https://doi.org/10.1007/978-3-030-04747-4_10

The Need for Robust Fidelities and Gradients. Unfortunately, as of today, most fidelities can at best be described as semi-local. Relying on small convolution filters or kernel functions that saturate at long range [8], they stop being informative when parts of the shapes are far away from each other. In recent years, finely crafted formulas have been proposed to alleviate this problem [9]; but they were probably too hard to implement and did not meet widespread adoption. As a result, most users today still rely on finely tuned coarse-to-fine schemes to register shape populations.

Contribution. At MICCAI 2017, we introduced the theory of Optimal Transport to the medical imaging community [5]. Leveraging the ideas and algorithms presented in [11], we showed that using *globally optimal* spring systems to drive a registration routine is tractable, and improves the robustness of pipelines to large deformations. The present paper is about taking advantage of new advances in the field [6] that let us bridge the gap between Optimal Transport and the standard shape analysis toolkit.

In Sect. 1, we review the standard theory of measures and kernel distances (also known as blurred Sums of Squared Distances). We stress the relevance of the scale-invariant kernel $k(x) = -\|x\|$, which induces the global Energy Distance between shapes. We also notice that kernel distances rely on *linear potentials* (influence fields) generated by the shapes.

In Sect. 2, we show how to use and compute *non-linear* potentials. We introduce a family of cheap fidelities between measures, the ε-SoftMin costs, that interpolate between the Energy Distance ($\varepsilon = +\infty$) and the weighted Hausdorff distance ($\varepsilon = 0$) borrowed from computer graphics.

Finally, in Sect. 3, we come back to the optimal transport cost and show that it is nothing but a "Hausdorff" distance under a mass repartition constraint. We interpret the celebrated Sinkhorn algorithm as a *balancing scheme on distance fields* and put an emphasis on two fidelities: the cheap ε-Hausdorff and the high-quality ε-Sinkhorn divergence, with a guarantee of positivity for both (Fig. 10).

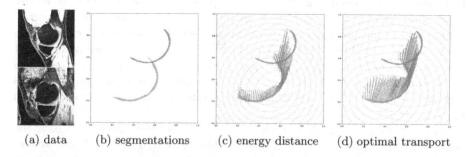

(a) data   (b) segmentations   (c) energy distance   (d) optimal transport

Fig. 1. We focus this paper on the registration of thin segmented volumes (a, from the OsteoArthritis Initiative) encoded as measures on the ambient space (b). We provide efficient GPU routines to compute long-range gradients, from cheap kernel distances (c) to high-quality optimal transport plans (d).

In Practice. Most importantly, we provide efficient CUDA routines – with Matlab, numpy and pytorch bindings – that can be used to implement these new data attachment terms. As shown in Sect. 4, our KeOps library [2] allows users to process curves, surfaces and segmentation maps with up to 100,000 actives vertices on a cheap laptop's GPU. Our code is freely available:

Please visit `github.com/jeanfeydy/global-divergences`.

These new tools fit seamlessly into the standard shape analyst's toolkit; they should help the reader to improve with little to no overhead the robustness to large deformations of its shape analysis pipeline.

1.1 Representing Shapes as Measures on a Space of Features

In This Paper. We choose to focus this paper on a setting that is understood well by all researchers in medical image analysis: the registration of *normalized density maps*. Our source bitmap A (in red) and target B (in blue) will be encoded as measures

$$\alpha = \sum_{i=1}^{N} \alpha_i \delta_{x_i} \quad \text{and} \quad \beta = \sum_{j=1}^{M} \beta_j \delta_{y_j}, \quad \text{with} \quad \sum_{i=1}^{N} \alpha_i = 1 = \sum_{j=1}^{M} \beta_j,$$

where the x_i's (respectively y_j's) are the coordinates of the N (resp. M) nonzero pixels of A (resp. B), with positive weights α_i (resp. β_j) summing up to one.

In most figures, we will display the gradient $\nabla_{x_i} d(\alpha, \beta)$ of a fidelity "d" as a green vector field supported by the x_i's. This descent direction is meant to be used by registration algorithms and is thus the primary information to look at in our pictures. In the background, depending on the section, we also display the level lines of the linear potential "$k \star (\alpha - \beta)$" (in blue) or of the influence fields "a" (in red) and "b" (in blue) – more about that later.

Extensions. The results presented in this paper can be extended to other use cases fairly easily. First, we may wish to use an image-based registration of segmentation maps instead of the mass preserving "Jacobian-free" action. To do so, we should simply compute the gradient $\nabla_{\alpha_i} d(\alpha, \beta)$ of fidelities with respect to the weights of the atomic dirac masses; the presence of long-range interactions is equally important to the robustness of the registration algorithm, with mass contraction (i.e. deletion) replacing the spreading out phenomenon observed in Fig. 3.(a–b).

Most of our results still hold when the source and the target don't have the same mass – the only noticeable changes would be located in Sect. 3, and we recommend [11] as an introduction to the theory of *unbalanced* optimal transport. Going further, these new tools and GPU routines can also be used to handle fiber tracks, curves and surfaces through the *varifold* framework presented in [8].

Notations. In order to let our results be useful to researchers working with curves and surfaces – which are best represented as measures on a product space (position,orientation,curvature) – we will refer to the ambient space $\mathbb{R}^2$ or $\mathbb{R}^3$ as to an abstract *feature space* $\mathcal{X}$. The letters x, y and z will denote points in the feature space, while α, β or μ stand for finitely supported positive measures; finally, a, b and m denote real-valued functions on $\mathcal{X}$ understood as **influence fields generated by their respective measures.**

If $(z_i)_{i \in [\![1,N]\!]}$ is a collection of N points in $\mathcal{X}$ and if $m : \mathcal{X} \to \mathbb{R}$ is a function on the feature space, we will also write "m_{z_i}" to denote the length-N vector $(m(z_i))_{i \in [\![1,N]\!]}$ of values of m sampled on the point cloud z_i.

Finally, if $\mu = \sum_{i=1}^{N} \mu_i \delta_{z_i}$ is a finitely supported measure and if $m : \mathcal{X} \to \mathbb{R}$ is a function on the feature space, we will write

$$\langle \mu, m \rangle = (\mu_i \mid m_{z_i}) = \sum_{i=1}^{N} \mu_i\, m(z_i).$$

Here, $(\mu_i)_{i \in [\![1,N]\!]}$ and $(m_{z_i})_{i \in [\![1,N]\!]}$ are two vectors of $\mathbb{R}^N$: the measure-function duality bracket $\langle \cdot, \cdot \rangle$ is thus understood as a simple scalar product $(\cdot \mid \cdot)$ in $\mathbb{R}^N$.

1.2 Kernel Distances

If α and β represent two shapes in the feature space $\mathcal{X}$, using standard information-theoretic fidelities such as the symmetrised Kullback-Leibler divergence

$$\mathrm{KL}_{\mathrm{sym}}(\alpha, \beta) = \tfrac{1}{2}\mathrm{KL}(\alpha, \beta) + \tfrac{1}{2}\mathrm{KL}(\beta, \alpha) = \tfrac{1}{2}\Big\langle \alpha - \beta, \log\Big(\tfrac{\mathrm{d}\alpha}{\mathrm{d}\beta}\Big) \Big\rangle \geqslant 0 \quad (1)$$

is not recommended: shape analysis routines should take into account the *geometry* of the feature space.

Kernel Norms. A common way of doing so is to endow the feature space $\mathcal{X}$ with a symmetric *kernel function* $k : \mathcal{X} \times \mathcal{X} \to \mathbb{R}$ and to use

$$\mathrm{d}_k(\alpha, \beta) = \tfrac{1}{2}\langle \alpha - \beta, k \star (\alpha - \beta)\rangle = \tfrac{1}{2}\langle \alpha - \beta, b^k - a^k \rangle, \quad (2)$$

$$\text{where} \quad a^k(z) = -(k \star \alpha)(z) = -\sum_{i=1}^{N} \alpha_i\, k(x_i, z) \quad (3)$$

$$\text{and} \quad b^k(z) = -(k \star \beta)(z) = -\sum_{j=1}^{M} \beta_j\, k(y_j, z). \quad (4)$$

In practice, these summations can be implemented as matrix-vector products or, as advocated in Fig. 11, by using the online map-reduce routines of the KeOps library [2]. Popular choices include the Gaussian and Laplacian kernels:

$$\text{Gaussian}_\sigma(x - y) = \exp(-\|x - y\|^2/\sigma^2)$$
$$\text{and} \quad \text{Laplacian}_\sigma(x - y) = \exp(-\|x - y\|/\sigma).$$

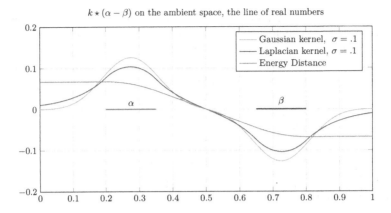

Fig. 2. The linear potential $k \star (\alpha - \beta)$, for standard kernel functions. Here, α and β are sampled from the standard Lebesgue measures on the segments $[.2, .35]$ and $[.65, .8]$, respectively. Out of these three curves, the third is the only one whose (minus) gradient always points from α towards β.

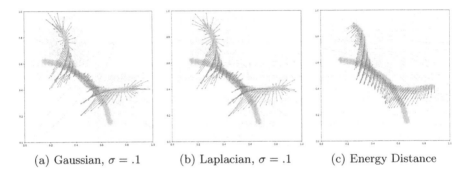

| (a) Gaussian, $\sigma = .1$ | (b) Laplacian, $\sigma = .1$ | (c) Energy Distance |

Fig. 3. The Energy distance is scale-invariant and robust to large deformations. This is the 2D equivalent of Fig. 2, with level lines of $k \star (\alpha - \beta)$ displayed in the background. Notice the spreading out effect in (a–b).

However, as $\nabla_{x_i} d_k(\alpha, \beta)$ is given by the gradient of the linear potential $(b^k - a^k)$ sampled on the x_i's and weighted by the α_i's, we argue in Figs. 2–3 that a more robust baseline could be given by the Energy Distance kernel from statistics [12]:

$$\text{Energy}(x - y) = - \|x - y\|.$$

2   Computing Non-linear Potentials

The Log-sum-exp Trick. In order to build tractable algorithms, restricting ourselves to potentials a and b that depend linearly on the measures α and β seems to be a necessary evil... But we can go further. Indeed, on top of the

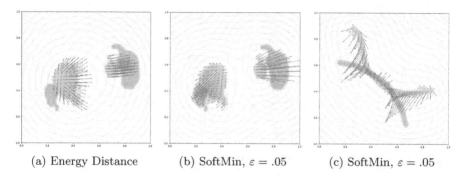

(a) Energy Distance   (b) SoftMin, $\varepsilon = .05$ (c) SoftMin, $\varepsilon = .05$

Fig. 4. Linear potentials can only take you so far. (a) As it faces a mass imbalance, the global gradient of the energy distance tries to split up the largest red mass into pieces. (b–c) The SoftMin fidelity, introduced in Sect. 2, allows us to induce a more "focused" behavior into our algorithms.

$$z \mapsto \min_{x \sim \alpha}{}_\varepsilon |z - x|, \text{ with } \alpha = \tfrac{1}{2}\delta_{.25} + \tfrac{1}{2}\delta_{.75}$$

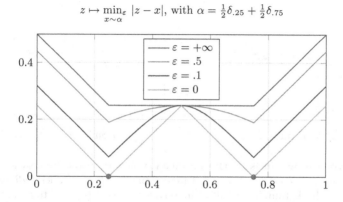

Fig. 5. The SoftMin operator. The log-sum-exp trick allows us to interpolate between two kinds of distance fields to a measure: the "Energy potential" $|\cdot| \star \alpha$ – for $\varepsilon = +\infty$ – and the distance field to the support $\{.25, .75\}$ of α – for $\varepsilon = 0$.

"summation" operation of Eqs. (3–4), we can implement on the GPU another differentiable reduction operator: the log-sum-exp or SoftMax, defined through

$$\log \sum_{i=1}^{N} \exp(v_i) = V + \log \sum_{i=1}^{N} \exp(v_i - V),$$

with $V = \max_i v_i$ taken out of the expression for numerical stability. The KeOps library implements an online variant of this "max-factorization" trick, and lets us scale this operation to large values of N – see Fig. 11.

Definition. Then, we propose to endow the ambient space $\mathcal{X}$ with a symmetric cost function $C : \mathcal{X} \times \mathcal{X} \mapsto C(x, y)$ – say, $\|x - y\|$ – a regularization strength $\varepsilon > 0$ and a kernel function $k_\varepsilon = \exp(-\tfrac{1}{\varepsilon}C(\cdot, \cdot))$ to define

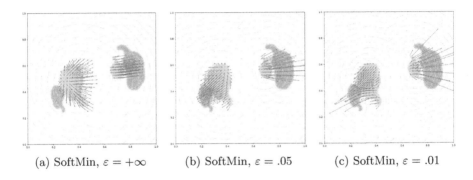

(a) SoftMin, $\varepsilon = +\infty$ (b) SoftMin, $\varepsilon = .05$ (c) SoftMin, $\varepsilon = .01$

Fig. 6. The ε-SoftMin fidelity interpolates between the energy distance and a weighted Hausdorff distance between the supports [1]. Here, we use the simple euclidean cost $C(x, y) = \|x - y\|$.

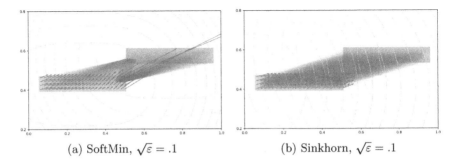

(a) SoftMin, $\sqrt{\varepsilon} = .1$ (b) Sinkhorn, $\sqrt{\varepsilon} = .1$

Fig. 7. Naive projection isn't the panacea. Using an ε-SoftMin cost is equivalent to encoding our shapes through their distance images – the so-called *influence fields*, displayed in the background. (a) Unfortunately, such a cost is prone to giving a disproportionate importance to the extremities of both shapes, as points are only influenced by their *nearest neighbors*. (b) Presented in Sect. 3, the Sinkhorn loop lets us introduce a **mass distribution constraint** to alleviate this problem: we shift the influence fields a (in red) and b (in blue) to retrieve *balanced* gradient fields. Figures computed with $C(x, y) = \|x - y\|^2$.

$$
\begin{aligned}
\min_{x \sim \alpha}{}_{\varepsilon} C(x, z) &= -\varepsilon \log(k_\varepsilon \star \alpha)(z) \\
&= -\varepsilon \log \sum_{i=1}^{N} \exp\left(\log(\alpha_i) - \tfrac{1}{\varepsilon} C(x_i, z) \right).
\end{aligned}
$$

Mimicking Eq. (2), we propose to see the SoftMin functions as non-linear influence fields, analogous to the linear potentials a^k and b^k. Hence, we introduce the ε-SoftMin cost through

$$d_{\varepsilon-\mathrm{SoftMin}}(\alpha,\beta) = \tfrac{1}{2}\langle \alpha - \beta,\, b^\varepsilon - a^\varepsilon\rangle$$
$$= \tfrac{1}{2}(\alpha_i \mid b^\varepsilon_{x_i} - a^\varepsilon_{x_i}) + \tfrac{1}{2}(\beta_j \mid a^\varepsilon_{y_j} - b^\varepsilon_{y_j}),$$
$$\text{where}\quad a^\varepsilon(z) = \min_{x\sim\alpha}{}_\varepsilon\, C(x,z)\quad\text{and}\quad b^\varepsilon(z) = \min_{y\sim\beta}{}_\varepsilon\, C(y,z).$$

Interpretation. Simple calculations show that if $C(x,y) = \|x - y\|$, the ε-SoftMin cost converges towards the Energy distance as ε goes to infinity. At the other end of the spectrum, if $C(x,y) \geqslant 0$ with equality if $x = y$,

$$d_{\varepsilon-\mathrm{SoftMin}}(\alpha,\beta) \xrightarrow{\varepsilon\to 0} \tfrac{1}{2}\sum_{i=1}^{N}\alpha_i \min_j C(x_i,y_j) + \tfrac{1}{2}\sum_{j=1}^{M}\beta_j \min_i C(x_i,y_j)$$

As shown in Figs. 5-6, the SoftMin operators is thus allowing us to interpolate between statistics and computer graphics.

Positivity. Unfortunately, one cannot guarantee the positivity of the ε-SoftMin fidelity: linearizing the cost, we find pairs of measures such that $d_{\varepsilon-\mathrm{SoftMin}}(\alpha + \delta\alpha, \alpha) < 0$. However, if λ is a reference measure on the feature space $\mathcal{X}$ (say, the Lebesgue measure on $\mathbb{R}^D$), then

$$\varepsilon\,\mathrm{KL}_{\mathrm{sym}}((k_\varepsilon \star \alpha)\cdot\lambda, (k_\varepsilon \star \beta)\cdot\lambda) = \tfrac{1}{2}\left\langle \lambda \cdot k_\varepsilon \star (\alpha - \beta),\, \varepsilon\,\log\frac{k_\varepsilon \star \alpha}{k_\varepsilon \star \beta}\right\rangle$$
$$= \tfrac{1}{2}\langle \lambda \cdot k_\varepsilon \star (\alpha - \beta),\, b^\varepsilon - a^\varepsilon\rangle \geqslant 0.$$

In practice, if $(\alpha - \beta)$ is close enough to its ε-blurred image $\lambda \cdot k_\varepsilon \star (\alpha - \beta)$, $d_{\varepsilon-\mathrm{SoftMin}}(\alpha,\beta)$ is thus positive too.

3 Balancing Distance Fields: The Sinkhorn Algorithm

As seen in Fig. 7, adding a **mass distribution constraint** to SoftMin distances can improve the quality of our descent directions. Thankfully, this is now possible thanks to the theory of Optimal Transport, which generalizes the Wasserstein distance – we recommend the recent handbook [11] for reference.

Primal "Monge" Problem. As illustrated in Fig. 8, Optimal Transport is about solving a *convex registration problem*: for $\varepsilon > 0$, we strive to minimize a primal cost OT_ε defined through

$$\mathrm{OT}_\varepsilon(\alpha,\beta) = \min_{\pi_{x_i,y_j}\in\mathbb{R}^{N\times M}_{\geqslant 0}} \underbrace{\sum_{i,j}\pi_{x_i,y_j} C(x_i,y_j)}_{\text{transport cost}\langle\pi,C\rangle} + \varepsilon\underbrace{\sum_{i,j}\pi_{x_i,y_j}\log\frac{\pi_{x_i,y_j}}{\alpha_i\,\beta_j} - \pi_{x_i,y_j} + \alpha_i\beta_j}_{\text{entropic regularization},\,\varepsilon\,\mathrm{KL}(\pi,\alpha\otimes\beta)},$$

under a linear constraint – α should be fully transported onto β:

$$\forall i \in [\![1,N]\!],\ \alpha_i = \sum_{j=1}^{M}\pi_{x_i,y_j}\quad\text{and}\quad \forall j \in [\![1,M]\!],\ \beta_j = \sum_{i=1}^{N}\pi_{x_i,y_j}.$$

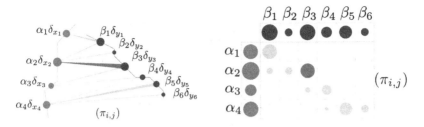

Fig. 8. Looking for a low-cost mapping, from α to β. As we solve the optimal transport problem, we find a *transport plan* π whose marginals are equal to α and β respectively. In practice, we solve a regularized problem whose dual solution is easy to compute on the GPU.

The Sinkhorn Algorithm. Strong duality holds on OT_ε. The major contribution from [3] was to show that the *dual* problem can be solved efficiently on the GPU. In a nutshell, we run the following algorithm:

Algorithm 1.   Sinkhorn Iterative Algorithm: Sink($\alpha_i, x_i, \beta_j, y_j$)

Parameters :   symmetric cost $\mathrm{C} : (x,y) \mapsto \mathrm{C}(x,y)$, regularization $\varepsilon > 0$

Input   :   source $\alpha = \sum_{i=1}^{N} \alpha_i \delta_{x_i}$, target $\beta = \sum_{j=1}^{M} \beta_j \delta_{y_j}$

Output   :   influence fields $a^{\alpha \to \beta}$ and $b^{\beta \to \alpha}$, sampled on the y_j's and x_i's respectively

1: $a_{y_j} \leftarrow \mathrm{zeros}(M)$; $b_{x_i} \leftarrow \mathrm{zeros}(N)$ $\triangleright$ Vectors of size M and N, respectively

2: **for** it $= 1$ **to** n_{its} **do** $\triangleright$ In practice, $n_{\mathrm{its}} = 10$ to 30 is enough

3:      $a_{y_j} \leftarrow \min_{\varepsilon, x \sim \alpha}[\mathrm{C}(x,y_j) - b(x)] = -\varepsilon \log \sum_{i=1}^{N} \exp\left[\log(\alpha_i) - \frac{1}{\varepsilon}(\mathrm{C}(x_i,y_j) - b_{x_i})\right]$

4:      $b_{x_i} \leftarrow \min_{\varepsilon, y \sim \beta}[\mathrm{C}(x_i,y) - a(y)] = -\varepsilon \log \sum_{j=1}^{M} \exp\left[\log(\beta_j) - \frac{1}{\varepsilon}(\mathrm{C}(x_i,y_j) - a_{y_j})\right]$

5: **return** a_{y_j}, b_{x_i} $\triangleright$ Vectors of size M and N, respectively

---

And at convergence, with $(a_{y_j}^{\alpha \to \beta}, b_{x_i}^{\beta \to \alpha}) = \mathrm{Sink}(\alpha_i, x_i, \beta_j, y_j)$, we get

$$\mathrm{OT}_\varepsilon(\alpha,\beta) = \left\langle \alpha, b^{\beta \to \alpha} \right\rangle + \left\langle \beta, a^{\alpha \to \beta} \right\rangle = \left(\alpha_i \mid b_{x_i}^{\beta \to \alpha} \right) + \left(\beta_j \mid a_{y_j}^{\alpha \to \beta} \right).$$

Interpretation. The Sinkhorn algorithm is a block-coordinate ascent on the *dual* variables. Mathematically speaking, these are Lipschitz functions defined on the ambient space $\mathcal{X}$ and sampled on the measures' supports. As illustrated in Fig. 9 and detailed in [6], we propose to understand them as *influence fields* $a^{\alpha \to \beta}$ and $b^{\beta \to \alpha}$ that encode an implicit transport plan $\pi = \exp\left[\frac{1}{\varepsilon}(b \oplus a - \mathrm{C})\right] \cdot \alpha \otimes \beta$.

Towards a Positive Optimal Transport Cost. In [5], we advocated the use of $\mathrm{OT}_\varepsilon(\alpha,\beta)$ as a data attachment term for diffeomorphic registration. Unfortunately though, just as if we used an ε-SoftMin fidelity, the minimum of the loss functional $\alpha \mapsto \mathrm{OT}_\varepsilon(\alpha,\beta)$ is *not* reached when α is exactly equal to β.

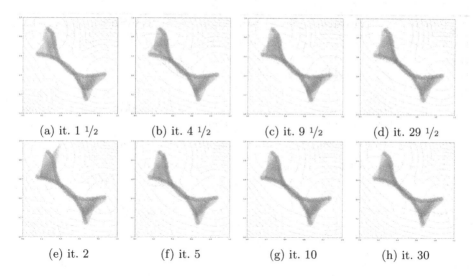

| (a) it. 1 ½ | (b) it. 4 ½ | (c) it. 9 ½ | (d) it. 29 ½ |

| (e) it. 2 | (f) it. 5 | (g) it. 10 | (h) it. 30 |

Fig. 9. The (standard) Sinkhorn algorithm brings balance to the force. On top of α, β, $a^{\alpha\to\beta}$ (in red) and $b^{\beta\to\alpha}$ (in blue), we display the mean "springs" linking the x_i's to β (in red) and the y_j's to α (in blue). Algorithm 1 is all about normalizing the blue (line 3) and red (line 4) springs until reaching equilibrium. (Color figure online)

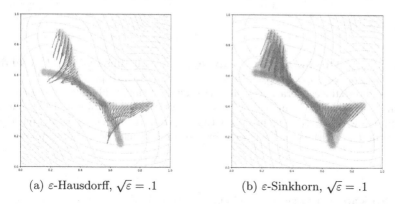

| (a) ε-Hausdorff, $\sqrt{\varepsilon} = .1$ | (b) ε-Sinkhorn, $\sqrt{\varepsilon} = .1$ |

Fig. 10. Computing ε-Hausdorff and ε-Sinkhorn divergences. On this page, we use a quadratic cost $C(x, y) = \|x - y\|^2$ so that ε is homogeneous to a squared distance. As evidenced in (b), the gradient of the ε-Sinkhorn divergence is good enough for one-shot registration in simple cases.

With collaborators [6], we thus decided to shift our attention towards a new *geometric* entropy:

$$F_\varepsilon(\alpha) \;=\; -\tfrac{1}{2}\mathrm{OT}_\varepsilon(\alpha, \alpha) \;=\; \varepsilon \min_{\mu_i \in \mathbb{R}_{\geq 0}^N} \left\langle \alpha,\, \log \tfrac{d\alpha}{d\mu} \right\rangle + \tfrac{1}{2}\langle \mu,\, k_\varepsilon \star \mu \rangle - \tfrac{1}{2}, \quad (5)$$

with $\mu = \sum_{i=1}^N \mu_i \delta_{x_i}$ – this identity stands thanks to a change of variable "$\mu_i = \exp(a_{x_i}/\varepsilon)\,\alpha_i$". We let SymSink denotes the *symmetrized* Sinkhorn algorithm:

Algorithm 2. Symmetric Sinkhorn Algorithm: SymSink(α_i, x_i, y_j)

Parameters : symmetric cost $\mathrm{C} : (x,y) \mapsto \mathrm{C}(x,y)$, regularization $\varepsilon > 0$
Input   : source $\alpha = \sum_{i=1}^N \alpha_i \delta_{x_i}$, target point cloud $(y_j)_{j \in [\![1,M]\!]}$
Output : influence field $a^{\alpha \leftrightarrow \alpha}$ sampled on the x_i's and the y_j's

1: $a_{x_i} \leftarrow$ zeros(N) $\triangleright$ Vector of size N
2: **for** it = 1 to $n_{\mathrm{its}} - 1$ **do** $\triangleright$ In practice, $n_{\mathrm{its}} = 3$ is enough
3:     $a_{x_i} \leftarrow \frac{1}{2}(a_{x_i} + \min_{\varepsilon, x \sim \alpha}[\mathrm{C}(x_i, x) - a(x)])$
$\qquad = \frac{1}{2}\Big(a_{x_i} - \varepsilon \log \sum_{k=1}^N \exp\big[\log(\alpha_k) - \frac{1}{\varepsilon}(\mathrm{C}(x_i, x_k) - a_{x_k})\big]\Big)$
4: $a'_{x_i} \leftarrow \min_{\varepsilon, x \sim \alpha}[\mathrm{C}(x_i, x) - a(x)] = -\varepsilon \log \sum_{k=1}^N \exp\big[\log(\alpha_k) - \frac{1}{\varepsilon}(\mathrm{C}(x_i, x_k) - a_{x_k})\big]$
5: $a''_{y_j} \leftarrow \min_{\varepsilon, x \sim \alpha}[\mathrm{C}(y_j, x) - a(x)] = -\varepsilon \log \sum_{k=1}^N \exp\big[\log(\alpha_k) - \frac{1}{\varepsilon}(\mathrm{C}(y_j, x_k) - a_{x_k})\big]$

6: **return** a''_{y_j}, a'_{x_i} $\triangleright$ Vectors of size M and N, respectively

---

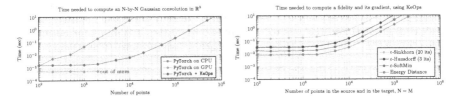

Fig. 11. The KeOps library lets shape analysis routines scale up to real data.
Performances on a cheap laptop's GPU (GTX 960M). (a) As it provides CUDA routines
for online map-reduce operations, our "KErnelOPerationS" library – developed with
Benjamin Charlier and Joan A. Glaunès – allows Matlab, numpy and pytorch users
to compute huge N-by-N convolutions without having to store large kernel matrices in
the GPU memory. (b) Experiments performed on point clouds in $\mathbb{R}^3$, endowed with a
euclidean cost $C(x,y) = \|x - y\|$.

The ε-Sinkhorn divergence. Then, we can define

$$
\begin{aligned}
\mathrm{d}_{\varepsilon\text{-Hausdorff}}(\alpha, \beta) &= \tfrac{1}{2}\langle \alpha - \beta, \nabla \mathrm{F}_\varepsilon(\alpha) - \nabla \mathrm{F}_\varepsilon(\beta) \rangle \\
&= \tfrac{1}{2}\big(\alpha_i \mid b_{x_i}^{\beta \leftrightarrow \beta} - a_{x_i}^{\alpha \leftrightarrow \alpha}\big) + \tfrac{1}{2}\big(\beta_j \mid a_{y_j}^{\alpha \leftrightarrow \alpha} - b_{y_j}^{\beta \leftrightarrow \beta}\big), \\
\mathrm{d}_{\varepsilon\text{-Sinkhorn}}(\alpha, \beta) &= \mathrm{OT}_\varepsilon(\alpha, \beta) - \tfrac{1}{2}\mathrm{OT}_\varepsilon(\alpha, \alpha) - \tfrac{1}{2}\mathrm{OT}_\varepsilon(\beta, \beta) \\
&= \big(\alpha_i \mid b_{x_i}^{\beta \to \alpha} - a_{x_i}^{\alpha \leftrightarrow \alpha}\big) + \big(\beta_j \mid a_{y_j}^{\alpha \to \beta} - b_{y_j}^{\beta \to \beta}\big),
\end{aligned}
$$

with $(a_{y_j}^{\alpha \leftrightarrow \alpha}, a_{x_i}^{\alpha \leftrightarrow \alpha}) = $ SymSink(α_i, x_i, y_j), $(b_{x_i}^{\beta \leftrightarrow \beta}, b_{y_j}^{\beta \leftrightarrow \beta}) = $ SymSink
(β_j, y_j, x_i) and $(a_{y_j}^{\alpha \to \beta}, b_{x_i}^{\beta \to \alpha}) = $ Sink$(\alpha_i, x_i, \beta_j, y_j)$.

The ε-Hausdorff divergence is the symmetrized Bregman divergence associated to F_ε on the space of probability measures on $\mathcal{X}$, and can be shown to
behave like the ε-SoftMin cost at the small and large ε limits. Meanwhile, the

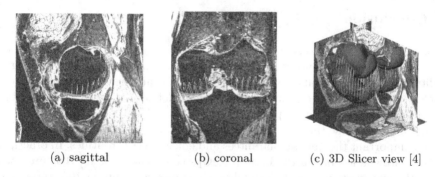

(a) sagittal   (b) coronal   (c) 3D Slicer view [4]

Fig. 12. On real data. Our routines could be used to registrate thin structures such as these knee caps from the OsteoArthritis Initiative – special thanks to Zhenlin Xu and Marc Niethammer for letting us know about this dataset. Here, the source and target volumes are respectively made up of 52,319 and 34,966 voxels – out of a 192-192-160 volume. As advertised in Fig. 11, this Energy Distance's gradient was computed in half a second on the author's laptop.

ε-Sinkhorn divergence is an "unbiased" Optimal Transport cost that has been recently introduced in the Machine Learning community [7].

The intuition here is that since $\mathrm{OT}_\varepsilon(\alpha, \beta)$ converges towards a kernel scalar product $\langle \alpha, \mathrm{C} \star \beta \rangle$ when ε goes to infinity, adding the self-correlation corrective terms lets us converge towards a genuine kernel squared norm $\frac{1}{2}\|\alpha - \beta\|^2_{-\mathrm{C}}$ – say, the Energy Distance if $\mathrm{C}(x, y) = \|x - y\|$. Most importantly, we are able to prove that both formulas define *positive* divergences for $\varepsilon > 0$:

Theorem 1 (Positivity). *Let* α *and* β *be two positive measures with finite support and same total mass on a feature space* $\mathcal{X}$. *Let us choose a smoothing scale* $\varepsilon > 0$ *and a cost function* C *on* $\mathcal{X} \times \mathcal{X}$ *such that*

$$k_\varepsilon(x, y) \;=\; \exp(-\mathrm{C}(x, y)/\varepsilon)$$

defines a **positive kernel** *function on* $\mathcal{X}$. *Then, one can show that*

$$0 \;\leqslant\; d_{\varepsilon\text{-}Hausdorff}(\alpha, \beta) \;\leqslant\; d_{\varepsilon\text{-}Sinkhorn}(\alpha, \beta),$$

with a null value if and only if $\alpha = \beta$.

Proof. The proof of this result is given in [6].
In a nutshell: the first inequality relies on the positivity of the kernel k_ε, as it ensures the convexity of the potential F_ε – Eq. (5) – and the positivity of the associated Bregman divergence. The second inequality derives from the convexity of $\mathrm{OT}_\varepsilon(\alpha, \beta)$ with respect to α and β varying independently.

4   Conclusion

Overview. All things considered, we introduced three positive divergences to the shape analysis community: the cheap and global Energy Distance; the high-quality ε-Sinkhorn cost; and, sitting in-between, a brand new ε-Hausdorff divergence inspired by computer graphics. All of them define well-posed, differentiable loss functions for registration problems.

As we linked these theories with each other in Sects. 2 and 3, we were able to provide important theoretical guarantees and efficient GPU routines. In practice, we advocate the use of the PyTorch + KeOps combination [2,10] that provides *automatic differentiation* and scalability to shapes with up to 100,000 active vertices.

Going Further. Now, which one of these formulas should we use in practice? As seen in Fig. 10, using an ε-Sinkhorn divergence is equivalent to performing a full convex registration – with no guarantee of topology preservation – every time we need a descent direction... Do we really need to go that far?

The answer to this question is highly dependent on the remainder of the registration pipeline. In months to come, we thus plan to test our new fidelities in a wide range of settings – from standard LDDMM to Deep Learning based methods – as we strive to provide our colleagues with reliable tools.

References

1. Aspert, N., Santa-Cruz, D., Ebrahimi, T.: Mesh: measuring errors between surfaces using the hausdorff distance. In: Proceedings 2002 IEEE International Conference on Multimedia and Expo, 2002 ICME 2002, vol. 1, pp. 705–708. IEEE (2002)
2. Charlier, B., Feydy, J., Glaunès, J.: Kernel operations on the GPU, with autodiff, without memory overflows. www.kernel-operations.io, Accessed 15 Oct 2018
3. Cuturi, M.: Sinkhorn distances: lightspeed computation of optimal transport. In: Advances in neural information processing systems, pp. 2292–2300 (2013)
4. Fedorov, A., Beichel, R., Kalpathy-Cramer, J., Finet, J., et al.: 3D slicer as an image computing platform for the quantitative imaging network. Magn. Reson. Imaging **30**(9), 1323–1341 (2012)
5. Feydy, J., Charlier, B., Vialard, F.-X., Peyré, G.: Optimal transport for diffeo-morphic registration. In: Descoteaux, M., Maier-Hein, L., Franz, A., Jannin, P., Collins, D.L., Duchesne, S. (eds.) MICCAI 2017. LNCS, vol. 10433, pp. 291–299. Springer, Cham (2017). https://doi.org/10.1007/978-3-319-66182-7_34
6. Feydy, J., Séjourné, T., Vialard, F.X., Amari, S.i., Trouvé, A., Peyré, G.: Interpolating between Optimal Transport and MMD using Sinkhorn Divergences. arXiv preprint arXiv:1810.08278
7. Genevay, A., Peyré, G., Cuturi, M.: Learning generative models with sinkhorn divergences. In: Storkey, A., Perez-Cruz, F. (eds.) Proceedings of the Twenty-First International Conference on Artificial Intelligence and Statistics, PMLR, vol. 84, pp. 1608–1617. 09–11 April 2018. Proceedings of Machine Learning Research
8. Kaltenmark, I., Charlier, B., Charon, N.: A general framework for curve and surface comparison and registration with oriented varifolds. In: Computer Vision and Pattern Recognition (CVPR) (2017)

9. Lombaert, H., Grady, L., Pennec, X., Ayache, N., Cheriet, F.: Spectral log-demons: diffeomorphic image registration with very large deformations. Int. J. Comput. Vis. **107**(3), 254–271 (2014)
10. Paszke, A., et al.: Automatic differentiation in PyTorch (2017)
11. Peyré, G., Cuturi, M.: Computational optimal transport. arXiv preprint arXiv:1803.00567 (2018)
12. Székely, G.J., Rizzo, M.L.: Energy statistics: a class of statistics based on distances. J. Stat. Plann. Infer. **143**(8), 1249–1272 (2013)

Parallel Transport of Surface Deformations from Pole Ladder to Symmetrical Extension

Shuman Jia[1]([⊠]), Nicolas Duchateau[2], Pamela Moceri[1,3], Maxime Sermesant[1], and Xavier Pennec[1]

[1] Université Côte d'Azur, Epione Project, Inria, Sophia Antipolis, France
shuman.jia@inria.fr
[2] Creatis, CNRS UMR5220, INSERM U1206, Université Lyon 1, Lyon, France
[3] Hôpital Pasteur, CHU de Nice, Nice, France

Abstract. Cardiac motion contains information underlying disease development, and complements the anatomical information extracted for each subject. However, normalization of temporal trajectories is necessary due to anatomical differences between subjects. In this study, we encode inter-subject shape variations and temporal deformations in a common space of diffeomorphic registration. They are parameterized by stationary velocity fields. Previous normalization algorithms applied in medical imaging were first order approximations of parallel transport. In contrast, pole ladder was recently shown to be a third order scheme in general affine connection spaces and exact in one step in affine symmetric spaces. We further improve this procedure with a more symmetric mapping scheme, which relies on geodesic symmetries around mid-points. We apply the method to analyze cardiac motion among pulmonary hypertension populations. Evaluation is performed on a 4D cardiac database, with meshes of the right-ventricle obtained by commercial speckle-tracking from echo-cardiogram. We assess the stability of the algorithms by computing their numerical inverse error. Our method turns out to be very accurate and efficient in terms of compactness for subspace representation.

1 Introduction

Analyzing cardiac function, notably myocardial deformation along cardiac cycle, can reveal subtle changes underlying disease development, and therefore improve risk stratification for patients. However, temporal deformations (cyclical or longitudinal) are complex due to subject-specific anatomy. Normalization of these trajectories into a common reference frame is an essential prerequisite in statistical analysis [1,4].

Nevertheless, it is a challenging task to construct a robust method for the normalization of temporal deformations, both theoretically and numerically. In cardiac imaging, the first step often includes segmenting the region of interest

© Springer Nature Switzerland AG 2018
M. Reuter et al. (Eds.): ShapeMI 2018, LNCS 11167, pp. 116–124, 2018.
https://doi.org/10.1007/978-3-030-04747-4_11

from the images, which generates its surface or volume as results. Then, to model the deformation between two shapes, depending on properties of the shapes, different non-rigid registration algorithms may be suitable in specific scenario. We choose to place our method in a space of diffeomorphic transformations. In particular, diffeomorphism provides invertible and folding-free registration results, which enables a symmetric encoding of deformation trajectories.

Given that diffeomorphisms are parameterized via flow of velocity fields, here stationary velocity field (SVF) [13], their normalization requires vector-based transport. In differential geometry, parallel transport specifies how to realize an infinitesimal transformation (a tangent vector) along a curve from one point to another of a manifold, as illustrated in Fig. 1(a). The concept was introduced in medical imaging by [14] and used for neuroimaging studies in [11]. To apply it to cardiac sequences, we need to:

- Parameterize the temporal deformations Φ_{t_i} from the subject-specific shape S at baseline to its shape S'_{t_i} at time t_i by SVF v_{t_i}; this step amounts to computing the logarithm of the deformations such that $\Phi_{t_i} = \exp(v_{t_i})$, or to register S to S'_{t_i}.
- Transfer these SVFs along the inter-subject deformation geodesic Φ_S from the space of S to a common geometry T, often called a template.

These steps lead to a representation of all the subject-specific deformations as infinitesimal deformations of the same anatomy. We can thus perform proper population comparison in terms of shape evolution along the cardiac cycle, as shown in Fig. 1(b).

Despite the fact that the definition of logarithm may be well developed in theory, implementations of its computation could be unstable due to numerical inconsistency. While computing registration/geodesics, the logarithms of surface deformations are only sparsely defined in the space (on the shape), which differs from image deformations. Careful numerical implementation of parallel transport algorithm is also needed.

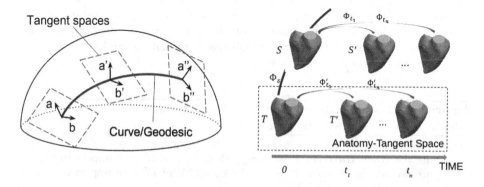

Fig. 1. Illustration of parallel transport of vectors a and b along a curve (left) and its application to cardiac imaging (right) with a focus on surfaces.

Algorithm 1. Pole ladder transport of the vector u along the geodesic $[S, T]$

- Compute the midpoint $M = \exp_S(\frac{1}{2}\log_S(T))$ on the intersubject geodesic;
- Compute the geodesic form the endpoint $S' = \exp_S(u)$ of the temporal geodesic segment to the midpoint M, and shoot twice to get the inverse endpoint: $T'' = \exp_{S'}(2\log_{S'}(M))$;
- Return the vector $trans(u) = -\log_T(T'')$ and then apply it to T: $T' = \exp_T(trans(u))$.

Parallel transport methods in medical image analysis are currently based on ladders (like Schild's and pole ladders [6,7]) or on variations of Jacobi Fields [8,14]. These methods are first order approximation schemes which need to be iterated along the curve. In contrast, pole ladder was recently discovered to be of third order in general affine connection spaces [10], which makes it a very attractive method to implement. In order to further improve the symmetry and thus the numerical stability with respect to the implementation of [7], our method relies on the definition of middle point and geodesic symmetry.

2   Methodology

2.1   Pole Ladder

Pole ladder is based on using the curve as the diagonal of the geodesic parallelogram to realize parallel transport (see Fig. 2 and Algorithm 1). Let u be the initial tangent vector to the geodesic segment that encodes the temporal deformation $\exp_S(tu)$ ($t \in [0, 1]$). Originally, pole ladder computes a midpoint on the geodesic $[S, T]$ and expands twice the geodesic form the endpoint S' to the midpoint to obtain the point T''. In this paper, we propose to reformulate the doubling of the geodesics with a mid-point geodesic symmetry (Algorithm 2). The mid-point M of a geodesic segment $[S, T]$ is defined as $M = \gamma_{[S,T]}(\frac{1}{2})$. The mappings from M towards the two sides meet the definition of a geodesic symmetry: $\gamma_{[M,S]}(t) = -\gamma_{[M,T]}(t)$. Although this novel version of pole ladder is theoretically equivalent to the previous one, it is numerically more stable in our experiments. This may be emphasized by the fact that in medical imaging we are encoding tangent vectors with infinitesimal deformations and that changing the object which is deformed may have a drastic numerical impact.

Algorithm 2. Mid-point symmetric pole ladder transport of the geodesic segment $[S, S']$ along the geodesic $[S, T]$

- Compute the midpoint $M = \gamma_{[S,T]}(\frac{1}{2})$ on the intersubject geodesic;
- Compute the symmetric point $T'' = \exp_M(-\log_M(S'))$ of S' with respect to M;
- Compute the symmetric point $T' = \exp_T(-\log_T(T''))$ of T'' with respect to T, and return the geodesic segment $[T, T']$.

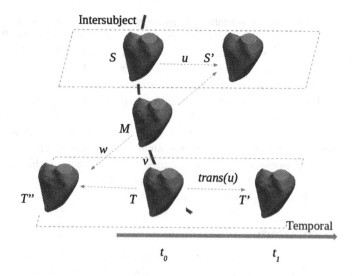

Fig. 2. The symmetry-based pole ladder structure.

2.2 Numerical Accuracy

Recent mathematical developments have enabled the numerical analysis of pole ladder in affine connection spaces with symmetric connections [10]. In Lie groups, the Baker-Campbell-Hausdorff (BCH) formula provides an expansion of the composition of two group exponentials in the Lie algebra: $BCH(v, u) = \log(\exp(v) \circ \exp(u))$. This formula has been thoroughly used in registration algorithms [2]. In general affine connection manifolds, a somewhat similar formula can be established based on the curvature instead of the Lie bracket [5]. The double exponential $\exp_x(v, u) = \exp_y(\Pi_x^y u)$ corresponds to a first geodesic shooting from the point x along the vector v, followed by a second geodesic shooting from $y = \exp_x(v)$ along the parallel transport $\Pi_x^y u$ of the vector u. [5] has shown that the Taylor expansion of the log of this endpoint $h_x(v, u) = \log_x(\exp_x(v, u))$ is:

$$h_x(v, u) = v + u + \frac{1}{6}R(u, v)v + \frac{1}{3}R(v, u)u + \frac{1}{12}\nabla_v R(u, v)v + \frac{1}{24}(\nabla_u R)(u, v)v$$
$$+ \frac{5}{24}(\nabla_v R)(u, v)u + \frac{1}{12}(\nabla_u R)(u, v)u + O(\|u + v\|^5).$$

When applied to our reformulation of pole ladder using geodesic symmetry, we find that the error on one step of pole ladder to transport the vector u along a geodesic segment of tangent vector $[S, T] = [\exp_M(-v), \exp_M(v)]$ (all quantities being parallel translated at the mid-point M) is:

$$\Pi_T^M trans(u) - \Pi_S^M u = \frac{1}{12}\left((\nabla_v R)(u, v)(5u - 2v) + (\nabla_u R)(u, v)(v - 2u)\right) + O(\|v + u\|^5).$$

We see here that one single step of pole ladder is of order three, thus much more accurate than the other first order parallel transport schemes. Moreover, the fourth order error term vanishes in affine symmetric spaces since the curvature is covariantly constant in these spaces. In fact, one can actually prove that all error terms vanish in a convex normal neighborhood of an affine connection space: one step of pole ladder realizes an exact parallel transport (provided that geodesics and mid-points are computed exactly of course) [10]. This result makes pole ladder a very attractive scheme. In particular, Lie groups have a canonical symmetric space structure thanks to the symmetry $s_g(h) = gh^{-1}g$ for any elements g, h of the Lie group. This is an affine structure which is generally not metric. The symmetry generates a canonical connection which is exactly the symmetric Cartan-Schouten connection. Since the geodesics of this connection going through identity are parameterized the flow of SVFs, we can conclude that pole ladder on SVFs is exact, at least theoretically.

2.3   SVF-Based Transport

In practice, we consider sparse point-to-point correspondences between two shapes (established here with the commercial speckle-tracking software) to compute diffeomorphic transformation. Thus, here the solution for the log is not unique and needs to be spatially regularized. Following [12], the sparse displacement field on the mesh vertices is interpolated to a dense image grid using with a standard thin-plate spline (TPS) kernel (stiffness of zero) [3]. The TPS fits the smooth surfaces and resistance in myocardial contraction. Then, a symmetric iterative procedure computes explicitly a SVF from the displacement field using BCH formula. The result gives a smooth SVF that linearly extends outside the grid borders.

The SVFs for temporal and intrasubject transformations are then used to compute the transported SVF to the template space using our symmetric pole ladder transport. In this context, we hypothesize that cardiac shape variations and temporal deformations can be efficiently modeled in a space of diffeomorphic transformations. The detailed shape variability that is lost during registration process will be transported. That is the reason why we report fiducial localisation error due to shape registration in Sect. 3.

2.4   Benchmark Transport Algorithm

Simple transport, conjugate action, which has been tested for cardiac motion analysis [1,4], serves as a benchmark. The conjugate action of two transformations is defined as $Conj_{\Phi_s}(\Phi_t) = \Phi_s\Phi_t\Phi_s^{-1}$. Numerically, it can be computed as the solution of $\exp(trans(v_t)) = \exp(v_s)\exp(v_t)\exp(-v_s)$ in the SVF setting using iterated BCH formulas.

3   Experiments

3.1   Materials

We assess our methods on a 4D cardiac database of right-ventricular (RV) meshes. The population includes 34 healthy subjects, and 104 subjects with pulmonary hypertension, which are divided into three classes according to the severity of the disease (New York Heart Association - NYHA, classes II, III and IV). The motion of the myocardium was given by point-to-point correspondences from commercial speckle-tracking of the RV from 3D trans-thoracic echocardiography (by 4D RV Function 2.0 software, TomTec Imaging Systems GmbH, Germany). For the acquisition of images, please refer to [9].

3.2   Template Estimation and Registration

The meshes were spatially aligned at baseline time, end-diastole (ED), using rigid deformations with the iterative closest point algorithm. Then for meshes of different instants but belonging to one subject, we preserved their relative position between cardiac sequences by applying to them the same rigid deformation. A template was built at baseline time ED as a mean shape in the healthy group using point distribution model.

Then we compute the deformation from each subject's shape at ED towards the template. The middle point on this geodesic serves as the midpoint for the two symmetric mappings in pole ladder to transport temporal deformations, $[M, S']$, $[M, T'']$ and $[T, T'']$, $[T, T']$, as shown in Fig. 2. The computation of SVFs is implemented in C++.

3.3   Consistency

Inverse consistency was tested by transporting the velocity field corresponding to the end-diastole-end-systole (ED-ES) deformation forward along the geodesic encoding the subject-specific RV shape changes with respect to the template at ED, and then backward along the reverse geodesic. If the numerical implementation is accurate, the result of the inverse transport should be exactly the original vector.

Consistency was quantified by the error between the final warped end-systole (ES) shape and the original subject's ES shape (Table 1). The errors should be compared to the mismatch of each registration method (fiducial localisation error of vertices). We can see that SVF pole ladder transport was very consistent.

Table 1. Numerical consistency of parallel transports. Fiducial localisation error due to shape registration (left) and to forward/backward transport (right) ($\mu \pm \sigma$ in mm).

Registration error (FLE)	Inverse Transport	
SVF	Pole ladder SVF	Conjugate SVF
0.15 ± 0.15	0.12 ± 0.10	0.22 ± 0.12

3.4   Application to the Statistical Modeling of Cardiac Deformation

In this subsection, we model ED-ES deformation in the whole subgroup of healthy subjects using parallel transports. Similar to the first step described in the previous experiments, we transported the velocity fields associated to each subject's ED-ES changes to the template at ED. Then, we applied principal component analysis (PCA) on the transported velocity fields, and warped the template with resulting principal components to show the main modes of deformation among this subgroup. We also compared this with the PCA modes obtained from the point-to-point ED-ES displacement.

The first mode from point-to-point displacement accounts for the elongation (no relative displacement of the two valves), the second accounts for the vertical displacement and a slight orientation of the tricuspid valve. The first two modes from the pole ladder with SVF are mainly related to the orientation and the relative position of the tricuspid valve and the pulmonary valve. Figure 3 summarizes these results for the point-to-point displacement and pole ladder with SVF. We compared the compactness of the representations (Table 2) and found pole ladder with SVF a very good explanation.

Table 2. Compactness of the representations

Explained variations	85%	95%	98%
Displacement	6	11	16
Pole ladder SVF	7	10	14

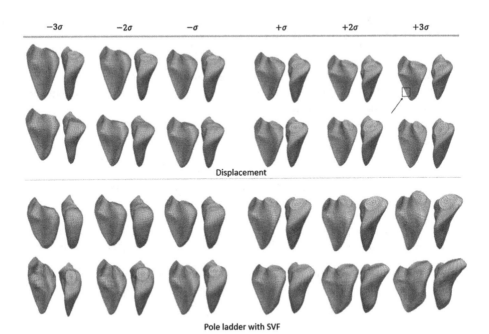

Fig. 3. Fist two modes of variation after applying PCA on the transported ED-ES changes, for the healthy subgroup. Comparison of point-to-point (top) and pole ladder with SVF (bottom). Surface folds appear at the arrow.

3.5   Limitations

Cardiac motion tracking establishes point-to-point correspondences between mesh vertices, available here to benchmark our method. For databases that do not have such correspondence, one option is to register the segmented surfaces to the template, with the framework of currents or varifold-based deformation, which provide elegant mathematical approaches to match surfaces and establish point-to-point correspondence. The limitation of the method notably lays in registration accuracy, but this is compensated by the stability and one-step transport structure of the algorithm.

4   Conclusion

We proposed a general scheme to perform statistical modeling of the temporal deformation of the heart, directly based on meshes. The extensions of the pole ladder for parallel transport to mesh deformations were stable and accurate, of importance for the assessment of pathological changes. They also provided a more compact and interpretable representation that is useful for statistical modeling, and prevented surface folds in the range of population variability.

The method is adaptable to other anatomies with temporal or longitudinal data. Perspectives notably include synthetic experiments; the possibility to simulate physiologically-realistic motion on a given subject's anatomy, of relevance to better understand shape and motion interactions, or inversely to generate template sequences derived from populations, to be used for physiological modeling.

Acknowledgments. Part of the research was funded by the Agence Nationale de la Recherche (ANR)/ERA CoSysMed SysAFib project. The authors would like to thank fellows from Hôpital Pasteur, CHU de Nice, France for preparing the data.

References

1. Bai, W., et al.: A bi-ventricular cardiac atlas built from 1000+ high resolution mr images of healthy subjects and an analysis of shape and motion. Med. Image Anal. **26**(1), 133–145 (2015)
2. Bossa, M., Hernandez, M., Olmos, S.: Contributions to 3D diffeomorphic atlas estimation: application to brain images. In: Ayache, N., Ourselin, S., Maeder, A. (eds.) MICCAI 2007. LNCS, vol. 4791, pp. 667–674. Springer, Heidelberg (2007). https://doi.org/10.1007/978-3-540-75757-3_81
3. Davis, M.H., Khotanzad, A., Flamig, D.P., Harms, S.E.: A physics-based coordinate transformation for 3-D image matching. IEEE Trans. Med. Imaging **16**(3), 317–328 (1997)
4. Duchateau, N., et al.: A spatiotemporal statistical atlas of motion for the quantification of abnormal myocardial tissue velocities. Med. Image Anal. **15**(3), 316–328 (2011)
5. Gavrilov, A.V.: Algebraic properties of covariant derivative and composition of exponential maps. Matematicheskie Trudy **9**(1), 3–20 (2006)

6. Lorenzi, M., Ayache, N., Pennec, X.: Schild's ladder for the parallel transport of deformations in time series of images. In: Székely, G., Hahn, H.K. (eds.) IPMI 2011. LNCS, vol. 6801, pp. 463–474. Springer, Heidelberg (2011). https://doi.org/10.1007/978-3-642-22092-0_38

7. Lorenzi, M., Pennec, X.: Efficient parallel transport of deformations in time series of images: from Schild's to pole ladder. J. Math. Imaging Vis. **50**(1–2), 5–17 (2014)

8. Louis, M., Bône, A., Charlier, B., Durrleman, S.: Parallel transport in shape analysis: a scalable numerical scheme. In: Nielsen, F., Barbaresco, F. (eds.) GSI 2017. LNCS, vol. 10589, pp. 29–37. Springer, Cham (2017). https://doi.org/10.1007/978-3-319-68445-1_4

9. Moceri, P., et al.: Three-dimensional right-ventricular regional deformation and survival in pulmonary hypertension. Eur. Heart J. Cardiovasc. Imaging **19**, 450–458 (2017)

10. Pennec, X.: Parallel transport with pole ladder: a third order scheme in affine connection spaces which is exact in affine symmetric spaces. arXiv preprint arXiv:1805.11436 (2018)

11. Qiu, A., Younes, L., Miller, M.I., Csernansky, J.G.: Parallel transport in diffeomorphisms distinguishes the time-dependent pattern of hippocampal surface deformation due to healthy aging and the dementia of the Alzheimer's type. NeuroImage **40**(1), 68–76 (2008)

12. Rohé, M.-M., Datar, M., Heimann, T., Sermesant, M., Pennec, X.: SVF-Net: learning deformable image registration using shape matching. In: Descoteaux, M., Maier-Hein, L., Franz, A., Jannin, P., Collins, D.L., Duchesne, S. (eds.) MICCAI 2017. LNCS, vol. 10433, pp. 266–274. Springer, Cham (2017). https://doi.org/10.1007/978-3-319-66182-7_31

13. Vercauteren, T., Pennec, X., Perchant, A., Ayache, N.: Symmetric log-domain diffeomorphic registration: a demons-based approach. In: Metaxas, D., Axel, L., Fichtinger, G., Székely, G. (eds.) MICCAI 2008. LNCS, vol. 5241, pp. 754–761. Springer, Heidelberg (2008). https://doi.org/10.1007/978-3-540-85988-8_90

14. Younes, L.: Jacobi fields in groups of diffeomorphisms and applications. Q. Appl. Math. **65**, 113–134 (2007)

4D Continuous Medial Representation Trajectory Estimation for Longitudinal Shape Analysis

Sungmin Hong[✉], James Fishbaugh, and Guido Gerig

Department of Computer Science,
Tandon School of Engineering, New York University, Brooklyn, USA
sungmin.hong@nyu.edu

Abstract. Morphological change of anatomy over time has been of great interest for tracking disease progression, aging, and growth. Shape regression methods have shown great success to model the shape changes over time to create a smooth and representative shape trajectory of sparsely scanned medical images. Shape changes modeled by shape regression methods can be affected by pose changes of shapes caused by neighboring anatomies. Such pose changes can cause informative local shape changes to be obscured and neglected in longitudinal shape analysis. In this paper, we propose a method that estimates a continuous trajectory of medial surfaces with correspondence over time to track longitudinal pose changes and local thickness changes separately. A spatiotemporally continuous medial surface trajectory is estimated by integrating velocity fields from a series of continuous medial representations individually estimated for each shape in a continuous 3D shape trajectory. The proposed method enables straightforward analysis on continuous local thickness changes and pose changes of a continuous multi-object shape trajectory. Longitudinal shape analysis which makes use of correspondence and temporal coherence of the estimated continuous medial surface trajectory is demonstrated with experiments on synthetic examples and real anatomical shape complexes.

1 Introduction

Analysis of disease progression and anatomical growth or degeneration over time is critical for diagnosis of neurodegenerative diseases and tracking post-treatment improvement of patients. Longitudinal shape analysis reveals morphological changes of anatomy over time which can provide crucial information for such analysis [3].

Conventional shape analysis methods are often performed with an assumption that shapes are initially aligned. The methods are heavily influenced by such alignment, as local direction and speed of growth may be dramatically different due only to different initial alignment. The challenge is more obvious for multi-object shape complexes where individual alignment of each shape eliminates important interactions between shapes in a complex [4]. To address the

© Springer Nature Switzerland AG 2018
M. Reuter et al. (Eds.): ShapeMI 2018, LNCS 11167, pp. 125–136, 2018.
https://doi.org/10.1007/978-3-030-04747-4_12

importance of including multiple sources of geometry for longitudinal analysis, ambient space regression methods based have been proposed [1,2].

Although the shape regression methods successfully estimate a continuous shape changes over time which can be represented by a 4D function (3D shape + time), it is not straightforward to interpret the relationship between the estimated shape trajectories and disease progression because of high dimensionality of shapes and deformation fields. Statistical analysis of shape change estimated by these methods is challenging since pose changes caused by adjacent objects influence deformation vectors of the ambient space. Deformation vectors encode both local geometric changes and pose changes, and it is precisely this ambiguity which hinders statistical analysis and interpretation. It is possible that informative shape changes independent from pose changes are obscured in deformation vectors which reflect an unknown combination of both types of change. For example, consider the multi-object shape complex of the basal ganglia, where all anatomy in the shape complex are pushed outward over time by the expansion of the adjacent lateral ventricles. The deformation vectors of each object are estimated to be large due to the external effect, even if a shape itself does not deform much except for translation. Therefore, it is important to decompose pose changes from coupled shape changes while not eliminating them since pose changes also reflect valuable information about interaction between shapes within a shape complex.

Skeletonization methods are widely used to reveal symmetry and local thickness of shapes [10–12]. Because of the inherent symmetry of a shape to its medial surface, the methods decompose a shape property to a nonlinear pose of a shape by medial positions in a medial surface and local thickness property. Medial representations (M-Rep) in [10, 12] were suggested to aid the statistical analysis on a medial manifold by forcing correspondence between medial surfaces with a topologically fixed M-Rep graph. Skeletonization methods have great potential to decompose the coupled longitudinal shape changes to pose changes by deformation of a medial surface and local thickness changes. However, only a handful of studies have been suggested to explore the ability and potential of 4D skeletonization. In [6], we proposed a 4D skeleton method by applying Hamilton-Jacobi skeletonization [11] to a geodesic shape regression [2]. Statistical analysis on medial surfaces was not obvious because of a noisy boundary of each medial surface and the lack of correspondence between medial surfaces of a trajectory. 4D continuous medial representation (CM-Rep) estimated by geodesic shape regression on medial surfaces and linear regression on local thickness fields was suggested in [5]. The method showed a promising result on decomposed thickness fields linear trends could reveal the difference between clinical risk groups by making use of correspondence between medial surfaces.

In this paper, we propose a novel method that estimates a continuous trajectory of medial surfaces with correspondence over time to track longitudinal pose changes and local thickness changes. The proposed method is integrated with ambient space shape regression methods [1,2] which estimate a representative continuous trajectory of 3D shapes from a set of shape complexes over time. Our method generates a continuous trajectory of medial surfaces by adapting CM-Rep [12] and inducing temporal coherence between medial surfaces by integrating a flow of velocity vectors for CM-Rep surface deformations and thickness field changes. While we take into account of interactions between shapes in a shape complex, the proposed method decomposes a 4D function that represents a 3D shape changes over time to 4D functions of pose changes and local thickness changes with more flexibility than the previous methods. Also, correspondence between medial surfaces and also reconstructed shape boundaries are well-established by making use of CM-Rep inverse skeletonization with a fixed graph medial surface template. As a consequence, the proposed method enables statistical analysis on continuous local thickness changes and pose changes of a continuous multi-object shape trajectory which can uncover local structure changes related with disease progression and anatomical structure change which cannot be shown in the ambient space regression methods. The proposed method was experimented on synthetic examples and real anatomical multi-object shape complexes sampled from a large cohort study on Huntington's disease (PREDICT-HD) [9] to show its ability on decomposing shape changes and correspondence on medial surfaces within a CM-Rep trajectory and 3D shape trajectories.

2   Methods

2.1   Continuous Shape Trajectory and CM-Rep

Continuous Shape Trajectory Estimation. The proposed method requires a continuous 3D shape trajectory to estimate a continuous CM-Rep trajectory. A continuous 3D shape trajectory is a continuous trajectory of shapes with volume which are typically surface boundaries of anatomical structures. The proposed medial surface trajectory estimation method can be applied to any continuous 3D shape trajectory. In this paper, we use a geodesic shape regression method [1,2] to create a continuous 3D shape trajectory which represent the development of anatomical structures over time of a given set of shapes.

The set of sparsely observed shape complexes $\mathbf{O} = \{O_{t_0}, ..., O_{t_N}\}$, where t_is are time points which are ages or disease progression parameters of subjects at observation. We assume that all shapes in $\mathbf{O}$ are diffeomorphic to 2-sphere (genus 0) for inverse skeletonization using CM-Rep.

The representative 3D shape trajectory can be considered as a trend of shape changes over time of the given set of sparsely distributed shapes over time. Let $\phi(\mathbf{X}, t)$ be an estimated continuous 3D shape trajectory of $\mathbf{O}$. We discretize the continuous trajectory $\phi(\mathbf{X}, t)$ with any fixed time interval δ, $t_s = s\delta$, $s = 0, ..., S$. The discretization can be done with any intervals or any number of time points since we assume the trajectory to be continuous as long as it is dense enough to represent the continuous trajectory. For each shape in the discretized shape trajectory $[\phi(\mathbf{X}, t_0), \phi(\mathbf{X}, t_1), ..., \phi(\mathbf{X}, t_S)]$, a medial surface and a local thickness field are estimated by CM-Rep inverse skeletonization [12] to decompose pose and local thickness of each shape in the 3D shape trajectory.

Continuous Medial Representation. For each shape $\phi(\mathbf{X}, t_s)$ at t_s in a 3D shape trajectory, we estimate a medial surface and a local thickness field by CM-Rep [12]. A CM-Rep surface $\mathbf{m}$ is a parameterized continuous surface with thickness field $\mathbf{R}$ encoded on the surface. A CM-Rep surface $\mathbf{m}$ is a surface without a hole, 1-sphere (genus 0) which is located at the middle of $\phi(\mathbf{X}, t_s)$. $\mathbf{m}$ is represented by a triangle mesh for implementation. Local thickness field $\mathbf{R}$ is attached to vertices of $\mathbf{m}$. At each vertex, the position of the vertex and the radius encoded at the vertex forms a medial atom.

Inverse skeletonization of shape surface starts with initial template CM-Rep medial surface $\mathbf{m}_0$ and a local thickness fields $\mathbf{R}_0$ attached to atoms of $\mathbf{m}_0$. We used an ellipsoid with a thickness field from an ellipse as $\mathbf{m}_0$ for 2-sphere shapes. The inverse skeletonization minimizes the difference between $\phi(\mathbf{X}, t)$ and $\mathbf{B}$ by deforming the geometry of medial surface $\mathbf{m}$ and updating a local thickness field $\mathbf{R}$. The geometry of a CM-Rep surface is deformed to match an input shape by minimizing the negative log of a Bayesian posterior probability of a shape matching likelihood with regularity on smoothness and validity on medial geometry. With the regularization on deformation, the surface property of a CM-Rep surface $\mathbf{m}$ remains consistent, e.g. the number of vertices and edge indices do not change, after deformation from the template CM-Rep surface $\mathbf{m}_0$. $\mathbf{R}$ is solved by bi-harmonic PDE with a potential function and boundary condition defined on a fixed $\mathbf{m}$. For more details, see [12].

A shape boundary $\mathbf{B}$ of $\mathbf{m}$ is reconstructed by maximum inscribed ball (MIB) with thickness $\mathbf{R}$.

$$\mathbf{B}(u) = \mathbf{m}(u) + \mathbf{R}(u)\mathbf{U}^{\pm}(u) \tag{1}$$

where u represents a surface parameter of $\mathbf{m}$ and $\mathbf{U}^{\pm}$ is the unit outward normal vectors on both hemispheres of $\mathbf{B}$. $\mathbf{U}^{\pm}$ is defined by the normal of $\mathbf{m}$ and the gradient of $\mathbf{R}$ on $\mathbf{m}$. The CM-Rep $\mathbf{m}$ is represented as a surface triangular mesh with a fixed number of vertices. The edge information of the reconstructed shape $\mathbf{B}$ is copied from $\mathbf{m}$ on both sides of $\mathbf{B}$ to create a surface mesh of $\mathbf{B}$. This will guarantee that the surface mesh of $\mathbf{B}$ is well-defined.

By individual CM-Rep estimation of each shape $\phi(\mathbf{X}, t_i)$ in a series of 3D shapes from a continuous 3D shape trajectory, the series of CM-Re surface $[\mathbf{m}(t_0), \mathbf{m}(t_1), ..., \mathbf{m}(t_S)]$ and thickness fields $[\mathbf{R}(t_0), \mathbf{R}(t_1), ..., \mathbf{R}(t_S)]$ are estimated. Although the CM-Rep estimation is done individually, correspondence between CM-Rep surfaces $\mathbf{m}(t_i)$ are well-established by fixing the topology of $\mathbf{m}(t_i)$ with a fixed CM-Rep surface template. Correspondence on the reconstructed shape surfaces $\mathbf{B}$ is propagated from $\mathbf{m}$ since the vertex and the edge information is copied from $\mathbf{m}$ on each hemisphere of $\mathbf{B}$.

2.2 Continuous CM-Rep Trajectory

The series of $[\mathbf{m}(t_0), \mathbf{m}(t_1), ..., \mathbf{m}(t_S)]$ and $[\mathbf{R}(t_0), \mathbf{R}(t_1), ..., \mathbf{R}(t_S)]$ are not continuous over time because the inverse skeletonization was processed without considering temporal correlation between CM-Reps. To estimate a continuous trajectory of $\mathbf{m}(t)$, $\mathbf{R}(t)$ with temporal coherence and, as a result, reconstructed surface boundaries $\mathbf{B}(t)$, the proposed method adapt the integration of velocity vectors in [7] to integrate deformation of CM-Reps $\mathbf{m}(t)$ and local thickness change $\mathbf{R}(t)$ over time from an individually estimated series of CM-Rep surfaces. At each time point, we use a temporal gradient by the derivative of Gaussian, $\dot{\mathbf{m}}(t) = \frac{d}{dt}G(\mathbf{m}(t), \sigma_t)$ on a temporal axis and a spatial covariance matrix $\mathbf{K}_{\mathbf{m}}(t)$, as a spatial kernel, to calculate a velocity vector $v_{\mathbf{m}}(t)$ at each corresponding vertex of shapes in a series.

The spatial covariance matrix $\mathbf{K}_{\mathbf{m}}(t)$ is defined as,

$$\mathbf{K}_{\mathbf{m}}(\mathbf{m}(t)) = \begin{pmatrix} K(\mathbf{m}(m_1,t), \mathbf{m}(m_1,t)) & \cdots & K(\mathbf{m}(m_1,t), \mathbf{m}(m_P,t)) \\ \vdots & \ddots & \vdots \\ K(\mathbf{m}(m_P,t), \mathbf{m}(m_1,t)) & \cdots & K(\mathbf{m}(m_P,t), \mathbf{m}(m_P,t)) \end{pmatrix}, \quad (2)$$

where $K(\cdot, \cdot) \in \Re^3$ is a 3×3 diagonal Gaussian kernel matrix of the positions of $\mathbf{m}(m_i,t)$ and $\mathbf{m}(m_j,t)$. Then a velocity field at t is calculated by convoluting $\mathbf{K}_{\mathbf{m}}$ to $\dot{\mathbf{m}}(t)$,

$$\hat{v}_{\mathbf{m}}(\mathbf{m}, t) = \sum_{p=1}^{P} \mathbf{K}_{\mathbf{m}}(\mathbf{m}(m_p,t), \mathbf{m}) \sum_{q=1}^{P} (\mathbf{K}^{-1}(\mathbf{m}(t)))_{pq} \dot{\mathbf{m}}(m_q,t), \quad (3)$$

where P is the number of vertices in $\mathbf{m}$. A continuous trajectory of $\mathbf{m}$, $\mathbf{m}(t)$ as a flow of velocity fields can be integrated as follows,

$$\hat{\mathbf{m}}(m, t_S) = \int_{t_0}^{t_S} \hat{v}_{\mathbf{m}}(m, t)dt + \mathbf{m}_0, \quad (4)$$

where $\mathbf{m}_0$ is a CM-Rep surface at the initial time point.

A trajectory of local thickness fields $\mathbf{R}(t)$ is calculated analogous to $\mathbf{m}(t)$ with a kernel matrix $\mathbf{K}_{\mathbf{R}} \in \Re$, which is a matrix of a Gaussian kernel of thickness fields $K(\mathbf{R}(m_i,t), \mathbf{R}(m_j,t))$, where $i, j = 1, ..., P$.

$$\mathbf{K}_{\mathbf{R}}(\mathbf{R}(t)) = \begin{pmatrix} K(\mathbf{R}(m_1,t), \mathbf{R}(m_1,t)) & \cdots & K(\mathbf{R}(m_1,t), \mathbf{R}(m_P,t)) \\ \vdots & \ddots & \vdots \\ K(\mathbf{R}(m_P,t), \mathbf{R}(m_1,t)) & \cdots & K(\mathbf{R}(m_P,t), \mathbf{R}(m_P,t)) \end{pmatrix}. \quad (5)$$

Then a velocity field at t is calculated by convoluting $\mathbf{K}_{\mathbf{R}}$ to $\dot{\mathbf{R}}(t)$ and then integrated to calculate a trajectory of thickness field change over time,

$$\hat{v}_{\mathbf{R}}(\mathbf{R}, t) = \sum_{p=1}^{P} \mathbf{K}_{\mathbf{R}}(\mathbf{R}(m_p,t), \mathbf{R}) \sum_{q=1}^{P} (\mathbf{K}^{-1}(\mathbf{R}(t)))_{pq} \dot{\mathbf{R}}(m_q,t), \quad (6)$$

$$\hat{\mathbf{R}}(m, t_S) = \int_{t_0}^{t_S} \hat{v}_{\mathbf{R}}(m, t)dt + \mathbf{R}_0, \quad (7)$$

where $\mathbf{R}_0$ is a thickness field at the initial time point. As final output, we have continuous trajectories of CM-Rep surfaces $\hat{\mathbf{m}}(t)$, local thickness fields $\hat{\mathbf{R}}(t)$, and reconstructed shape boundaries $\hat{\mathbf{B}}(t)$ for $t \in [t_0, t_S]$.

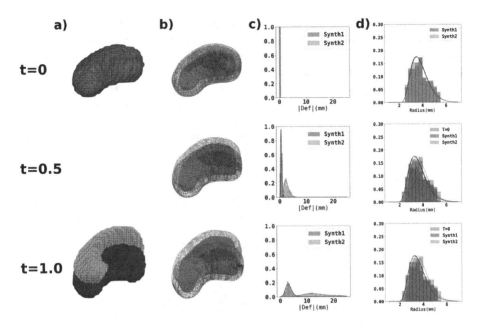

Fig. 1. Example of synthetic shape data. (a) Two sets of synthetic shapes, one with only nonlinear deformation (Set 1, blue) and one with induced translation and rotation (Set 2, green). (b) The estimated CM-Rep trajectories. (c) Deformation based analysis quantified by distributions of deformation magnitude in the ambient space model imply significant shape differences between two sets. (d) Thickness changes measured by our proposed method shows clearly that only a change in pose is present between the two sets, rather than a change in shape itself. (Color figure online)

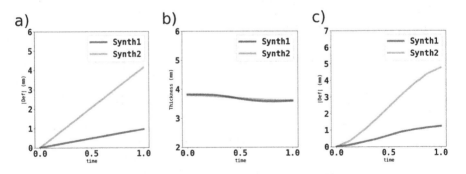

Fig. 2. Comparison between average deformation magnitude over time of 3D shape trajectories and local thickness changes. (a) Average deformation magnitude from an initial baseline shape ($t = 0$) of synthetic examples from ambient space regression methods only shows that there is dramatic difference between shape changes of set 1 and 2 which is caused by pose difference. (b) Average local thickness change over time reveals that two sets' local shape properties are similar while the difference caused by pose difference is encoded by the deformation of CM-Rep surfaces shown in (c) average deformation magnitude of CM-Rep surfaces of set 1 and 2.

3   Results

The proposed method is evaluated with a synthetic example and real anatomical data from the population study of Huntington's disease (HD) PREDICT-HD [9]. The synthetic experiment demonstrate the ability of the proposed method to decompose pose and intrinsic shape changes. 4D atlases of control group (normative spatiotemporal atlas) and high risk group (high risk spatiotemporal atlas) are estimated by the proposed method and statistically compared.

3.1   Synthetic Data

Two synthetic examples are constructed to show how the proposed method decomposes a 3D shape change to unveil a local shape change represented by a thickness field while it does not lose information about pose change. Each example consists of a shape set: an ellipsoid as the source and a putamen shape as the target. In the second set (green), we induce a pose change with translation and rotation to the target putamen shape, so the two synthetic shape sets differ only in pose (Fig. 1a). We applied the shape matching method suggested in [1] to estimate a continuous 3D shape trajectory for each set. A CM-Rep trajectory of each set with a reconstructed shape boundary is visualized in Fig. 1(b). Please note that input shapes are only initial baseline shapes at $t = 0$ and target shapes at $t = 1$. 3D Shapes and medial surfaces at $t = 0.5$ are captured from estimated continuous reconstructed shape boundary trajectories and continuous CM-Rep surface trajectories, respectively, by the proposed method which are not given as input. The average deformation changes over time in Fig. 1(c) captured by the deformation vectors of the ambient space model [1] show significant differences between the two sets. An analysis based on such deformation statistics would not reveal that the two sets differ only in pose. However, local thickness distributions which are extracted from the proposed method visualized as histograms in Fig. 1(d) properly reveal that shapes at corresponding time points in the two shape sets have the same geometry. Local thickness changes are thus decomposed from pose changes and reveal a slight atrophy over time. At $t = 0$, median thickness of an initial baseline shape was 3.7562 mm. At $t = 1.0$, median thickness of a final shape of set 1 and 2 were measured to 3.5284 mm and 3.5525 mm, respectively. Such a subtle local shape changes over time to match an ellipsoid to a putamen shape is completely hidden in the ambient space model, due to the larger effect of translation and rotation. The average deformation magnitude estimated by the ambient space model of set 1 at $t = 1$ from $t = 0$ is 4.2510 mm while 18.5419 mm for set 2, also displayed in Fig. 2. Pose changes are separately encoded as deformations of CM-Rep surfaces, demonstrating that our method does not lose this potentially valuable information. The average deformation magnitude of a CM-Rep surface trajectory at $t = 1$ from $t = 0$ is 5.6872 mm while 21.3158 mm for set 2. Figure 2 shows the average deformation magnitude from an initial baseline shape at $t = 0$ estimated by the ambient space model and the average thickness changes estimated by the proposed method. It shows that, while ambient space models overestimates shape changes in the presence of pose changes, our proposed method estimates consistent thickness between two sets which differ only in pose. The proposed method separates subtle local shape changes from changes of pose.

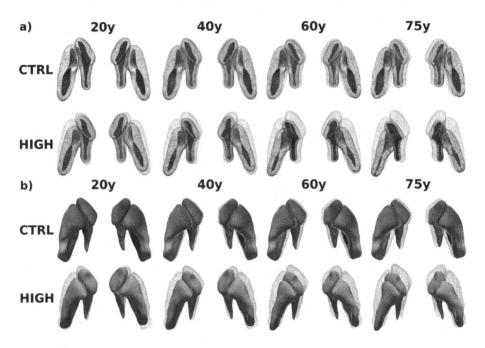

Fig. 3. Estimated continuous shape trajectories. From the continuous shape trajectories, each shape complex at age 20, 40, 60, and 75 years old were captured for visualization. (a) CM-Rep trajectories estimated by the proposed method from a control group and a high risk HD group. Reconstructed surface trajectories are visualized as gray wireframes. A shape complex at age 20 of a control group (green) is overlaid as a reference. Thickness fields are visualized on CM-Rep surfaces by a blue-red color map from thin (blue) to thick (red). (b) Continuous 3D shape trajectories estimated by the geodesic shape regression method. Blue-red color maps display the magnitude of velocity at each time point from less (blue) to more deformation (red). The bottom tips of caudate nuclei and putamina show more deformation caused by an adjacent ventricle expansion. (Color figure online)

3.2   HD Risk Group Regression

We apply the proposed method to analyze the shape changes of caudate nuclei and putamina of the basal ganglia complex of a control and a high risk group in PREDICT-HD Huntington's disease (HD) database [9] as a comparative analysis. The shapes were segmented by an automatic segmentation method and manually cleaned by experts [8]. We make use of sparsely observed 243 scans of

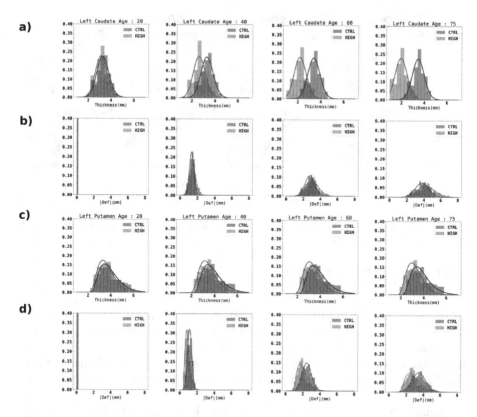

Fig. 4. Histograms of thickness distribution extracted by the proposed method and deformation magnitude distribution by the ambient space regression method captured at age 20, 40, 60, and 75 of (a, b) left caudate and (c, d) left putamen. The deformation magnitude is measured from an initial baseline shape at age 20, therefore zero deformation for both groups. For a control group, thickness distribution does not change much while a high risk group clearly shows the shift to thinner structures.

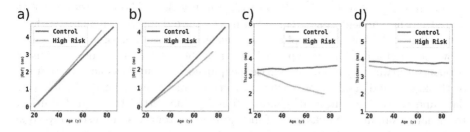

Fig. 5. Mean deformation magnitude change over time estimated by the ambient space regression method for (a) left caudate and (b) putamen. Left caudate show more deformation for a control group than a high risk group and vice versa for left putamen. Mean thickness change over time estimated by the proposed method for (c) left caudate and (d) putamen. Both caudate and putamen show significant atrophy over time for a high risk group.

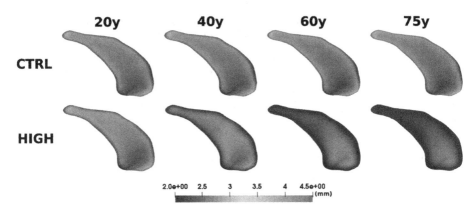

Fig. 6. Estimated thickness of left caudates over time from a control group and a high risk group (HD) are visualized on a fixed CM-Rep surface. Along all ages, local thickness shows that the high risk group's putamen is thinner and atrophies significantly faster when compared to a control group.

107 subjects over time 20 to 85 years old and 319 scans of 114 subjects from 20 to 75 years old for a control group and a high risk group, respectively. Then a continuous 3D shape trajectory for each group was estimated by geodesic shape regression method [2] cross-sectionally. The continuous 3D shape trajectory is sampled with one year interval to have a series of shapes for the proposed method.

Figure 3 visualizes (a) the continuous CM-Rep surface trajectory and the reconstructed shape boundary trajectory of each group and (b) the continuous 3D shape trajectory estimated by the geodesic shape regression method [2]. Shape complexes of the continuous trajectories at age 20, 40, 60 and 75 were captured for the visualization to show the changes over ages for each group. A shape complex of a control group at age 20 is overlaid as a reference. Local thickness fields estimated by the proposed method are displayed as a blue-red color map from thin to thick on CM-Rep surfaces in Fig. 3(a). The velocity fields estimated by the ambient space regression method are displayed on shape surfaces in Fig. 3(b). The bottom tips of caudate nuclei and putamina of a control group show more deformation on shape surfaces than the heads of structures because it is pushed outward by adjacent ventricle expansion. Figure 4 displays histograms of thickness fields and deformation magnitudes distribution of (a, b) left caudate and (c, d) left putamen. Gamma functions are fitted to the distributions to visualize summarized changes of histograms. Histograms are also sampled at same time points, 20, 40, 60, and 75 years old. Thickness distribution of left caudate shows left shift to a thinner structure which indicates significant atrophy over ages in Fig. 4(a). For example, at age 20, 40, 60, and 75 years old, mean thickness of left putamen were estimated as 3.9491 mm, 3.9084 mm, 3.8697 mm and 3.8490 mm for a control group and 3.6694 mm, 3.4897 mm, 3.3953 mm and 3.2943 mm for a high risk group, respectively.

Figure 5(a, b) shows average deformation magnitude of left caudate and putamen in the shape complex estimated by the ambient space method. A high risk group shows more deformation for a left caudate than a control group. However, it is opposite for a left putamen that a control group's putamen deformed more. It is because putamina are placed further away from a center of a shape complex and pushed further away by ventricle expansion. Average thickness changes of left putamen in Fig. 5(c, d) shows that there is significant difference between a control group and a high risk group over ages which are separated from pose changes caused by neighborhood structures. It is worthwhile to note that pose changes over time of a shape trajectory are preserved by deformations of CM-Rep surfaces.

Figure 3(b) shows thickness distribution changes of left caudate over ages. It shows that the difference in local thickness distributions becomes more significant over time as the left caudate of high risk group (red) atrophies faster compared to the control group (blue).

A trajectory of a control group shows almost mere pose changes over ages without any atrophy while a high risk group's trajectory shows significant atrophy. Also, a high risk group's left putamen and caudate have thinner structures than a control group's at an initial baseline time point, age 20. Comparison of shape characteristics at the initial baseline time point is not available with the ambient space regression method because deformation at an initial baseline time point is all zero as shown in Fig. 4(b, d) and Fig. 5(a, b).

To show local shape changes of anatomy estimated by the proposed method, we display thickness fields of left caudates on a fixed CM-Rep surface in Fig. 6. Correspondence between any CM-Rep surfaces among shape trajectories enables local analysis of shape property changes. Local thickness fields over ages in each group reveals which part of anatomy atrophies over ages, for example, a left caudate of a high risk group in Fig. 6 shows more significant atrophy at the center area of the anatomy. We suggest readers to see the supplementary video as it fully visualizes the longitudinal shape changes estimated by the proposed method.

4   Conclusions

In this paper, we proposed a method to estimate a continuous CM-Rep trajectory derived from a continuous 3D shape trajectory estimated by shape regression methods from a set of multi-object shape complexes distributed over time. A continuous CM-Rep surface trajectory avails intuitive analysis on continuous pose changes and local thickness changes of shape complexes separately over time. For future work, we will focus on theoretical derivation of temporally smooth CM-Rep trajectory that guarantees not to violate valid medial properties over temporal changes of CM-Reps. To draw more valid clinical results, regression methods that account for individual differences of a subject will be explored for Huntington's disease risk group analysis. We will also investigate to increase matching accuracy of CM-Rep estimation by exploring other medial models as well to capture more details of 3D shapes by medial models.

Acknowledgement. This research was supported by NIH NIBIB RO1EB021391 and New York Center for Advanced Technology in Telecommunications (CATT).

References

1. Durrleman, S., Pennec, X., Trouvé, A., Braga, J., Gerig, G., Ayache, N.: Toward a comprehensive framework for the spatiotemporal statistical analysis of longitudinal shape data. Int. J. Comput. Vis. **103**(1), 22–59 (2013)
2. Fishbaugh, J., Prastawa, M., Gerig, G., Durrleman, S.: Geodesic shape regression in the framework of currents. In: Gee, J.C., Joshi, S., Pohl, K.M., Wells, W.M., Zöllei, L. (eds.) IPMI 2013. LNCS, vol. 7917, pp. 718–729. Springer, Heidelberg (2013). https://doi.org/10.1007/978-3-642-38868-2_60
3. Gerig, G., Fishbaugh, J., Sadeghi, N.: Longitudinal modeling of appearance and shape and its potential for clinical use. Med. Image Anal. **33**, 114–121 (2016)
4. Gorczowski, K., et al.: Statistical shape analysis of multi-object complexes. In: Computer Vision and Pattern Recognition, pp. 1–8. IEEE (2007)
5. Hong, S., Fishbaugh, J., Gerig, G.: 4D continuous medial representation by geodesic shape regression. In: ISBI 2018. IEEE EMBS (2018)
6. Hong, S., et al.: Subject-specific longitudinal shape analysis by coupling spatiotemporal shape modeling with medial analysis. In: Medical Imaging. SPIE (2017)
7. Joshi, S.C., Miller, M.I., Grenander, U.: On the geometry and shape of brain submanifolds. IJPRAI **11**(8), 1317–1343 (1997)
8. Kim, E.Y., Johnson, H.J.: Robust multi-site MR data processing: iterative optimization of bias correction, tissue classification, and registration. Front. Neuroinform. **7**, 29 (2013)
9. Paulsen, J.S., et al.: Clinical and biomarker changes in premanifest Huntington disease show trial feasibility: a decade of the PREDICT-HD study. Front. Aging Neurosci. **6**, 78 (2014)
10. Pizer, S.M., Gerig, G., Joshi, S., Aylward, S.R.: Multiscale medial shape-based analysis of image objects. Proc. IEEE **91**(10), 1670–1679 (2003)
11. Siddiqi, K., Bouix, S., Tannenbaum, A., Zucker, S.W.: Hamilton-Jacobi skeletons. Int. J. Comput. Vis. **48**(3), 215–231 (2002)
12. Yushkevich, P.A.: Continuous medial representation of brain structures using the biharmonic PDE. NeuroImage **45**(1), S99–S110 (2009)

Probabilistic Fitting of Active Shape Models

Andreas Morel-Forster[(⊠)], Thomas Gerig, Marcel Lüthi, and Thomas Vetter

University of Basel, 4051 Basel, Switzerland
{andreas.forster,thomas.gerig,marcel.luethi,thomas.vetter}@unibas.ch
http://gravis.dmi.unibas.ch

Abstract. Active Shape Models (ASMs) are a classical and widely used approach for fitting shape models to images. In this paper, we propose a fully probabilistic interpretation of ASM fitting as Bayesian inference. To infer the posterior, we use the Metropolis-Hastings algorithm. We then use the maximum a posteriori sample as the segmentation result. Our approach has several advantages compared to classical ASM fitting: (1) We are left with fewer parameters that we need to choose. (2) It is less prone to get trapped in local minima. (3) It becomes straightforward to extend the approach to include additional information, such as expert annotations. (4) It is even simpler to implement than the classical ASM fitting method.

We apply our algorithm to the SLIVER dataset and show that it achieves a higher segmentation accuracy than the standard ASM approach. We further demonstrate the flexibility and expressivity of the framework by integrating experts annotations along parts of the outline to further increase the accuracy. The code used for fitting is based on open-source software and made available to the community.

Keywords: Active shape model · Statistical shape model
Gaussian process · MCMC · Sampling · Metropolis Hastings
Bayesian · Liver

1 Introduction

To automate medical diagnosis, treatments or the planning of interventions, a segmentation of an organ is a useful preprocessing step. However, analyzing volumetric computed tomography (CT) images is a difficult task, because human organs are highly variable in terms of shape and appearance. Possible shifts from neighboring organs can change the visual appearance of the boundary. An often used approach to organ segmentation is the Active Shape Model (ASM) [2] algorithm.

An ASM consists of two main parts. A point distribution model (PDM) is used to summarize prior knowledge about the shapes of the organs. An instance of an organ's shape is fully described using a set of parameters. In addition, the

© Springer Nature Switzerland AG 2018
M. Reuter et al. (Eds.): ShapeMI 2018, LNCS 11167, pp. 137–146, 2018.
https://doi.org/10.1007/978-3-030-04747-4_13

ASM has a built-in prior for the appearance of the volume around the organ boundary. The appearance is modeled at a sparse set, of so-called profile points. Visual features are extracted in the normal direction and approximated using a Gaussian distribution. When adapting the shape, better locations for the profile points are searched. To increase robustness while fitting, new points are removed when the point or appearance distance is larger than a given threshold. The shape is updated using the remaining points. To keep the segmented shapes plausible the model parameters are restricted to a certain interval.

In this paper, we propose a probabilistic interpretation of this model. The probabilistic formulation has several advantages: (1) It makes many of the implicit assumptions taken in the ASM explicit. (2) It does not rely on seemingly arbitrary parameters. (3) We can apply standard inference procedures developed in the statistics community for fitting the model. (4) It provides a principled way of extending the algorithm with additional information such as expert annotations.

We propose to use a sampling-based strategy for model fitting based on the Metropolis-Hastings (MH) algorithm. This leads to a simple, stochastic algorithm, which is less prone to get stuck in local optima and provides an estimate of the posterior distribution. In this approach, the only parameter to choose is a proposal distribution for the MH algorithm. While in theory, the exact choice of this distribution has no influence on the result, in practice, this can change the efficiency of the algorithm. Our experiments on the SLIVER dataset [5] show that our method is more robust and leads to better segmentation performance compared to the standard, deterministic search-based approach. Finally, we demonstrate how we can incorporate expert annotations, and that such additional information significantly improves on the segmentation performance.

Prior Work: The ASM approach, as introduced by Cootes and Taylor [1,2], is a generic approach to model-based image segmentation. It has many components and parameters, which affect its performance. An overview of different possibilities to tune the algorithm is given by van Ginneken et al. [12]. Consequently, a lot of work has been done. In the following, we concentrate on reviewing some work addressing specific limitations of the standard ASM: Wimmer et al. [13] replaces the Gaussian assumption with a probabilistic likelihood of the boundary profile based on a k-nearest-neighbor estimate using positive and negative boundary profiles. Norajitra et al. replaced the search for better boundary locations in [10] with random forests, which, when compared to the line profiles, take information of a larger volume into account. Kirschner et al. [7] use a non-linear shape prior based on a kernel PCA. They showed the superior performance of the non-linear model for vertebra, which we think holds also for livers. Note, that our proposed method for model adaptation is orthogonal to all formerly mentioned changes and can make use of improved shape or appearance models.

There is also work on advanced fitting strategies in the recent literature about ASMs. In [3], Esfandiarkhani et al. propose a non-linear fitting scheme. Zhan et al. present a method related to the inverse gradient descent optimization used for active appearance models [14]. In contrast to those, our proposed method is simple to implement, fully probabilistic and provides a principled mechanism for integrating additional information.

Van Ginneken et al. proposed an extension of ASM to allow for interactive fitting [4]. In contrast to our method, their method requires the use of corresponding landmarks, while we can incorporate information, which is given as line to surface correspondence only. Furthermore, in our approach, the constraint is formulated probabilistically, which allows us to add the user annotation as uncertain observation, in a principled way.

The most closely related work to ours is the one of Schönborn et al. [11]. They propose to use sampling to adapt a 3D face model to 2D photographs using computer graphics.

2   Background : Active Shape Models

An Active Shape Model consists of two main components: (1) A *Point Distribution Model (PDM)*, which represents the normal shape variation of the modeled anatomical structure and (2) an intensity model, which models the intensities in a neighborhood around dedicated points of the PDM. Before discussing the main fitting algorithm, we discuss these two main components in more detail.[1]

Point Distribution Models: The main idea behind a PDM is that given a set of $i = 1, \ldots, N$ typical example surfaces $\{\Gamma_i\}$ of a certain shape, it becomes possible to learn the mean shape and the normal variability of this shape. For this to be possible, it is necessary that the example surfaces are in correspondence. This means that each surface is defined using the same number of boundary points, $\Gamma_i = (x_1^i, \ldots, x_n^i)$, and that the points $\{x_k^i\}$ on each of the surfaces $\{\Gamma_i\}$ are at the same anatomical location. Assuming that all the surfaces $\{\Gamma_i\}$ are rigidly aligned to each other, we can define the mean of a boundary point as $\overline{x}_k = \frac{1}{N} \sum_{i=1}^{N} x_k^i$. The corresponding mean shape is given as $\overline{\Gamma} := (\overline{x}_1, \ldots, \overline{x}_n)$. Furthermore, we can compute from the example surfaces $\{\Gamma_i\}$ a set of $N-1$ principal components, which represent the directions of main variation in the data. In our model, the possible locations of a point x_k is defined as a linear combination of the principal components with coefficient vector $\alpha = (\alpha_1, \ldots, \alpha_{N-1})$ as follows:

$$x_k(\alpha) := \overline{x}_k + \sum_{i=1}^{N-1} \alpha_i u_k^i$$

where $u_k^i \in \mathbb{R}^3$ denotes a displacement direction for the k-th point given by the i-th principal component. The corresponding shape $\Gamma(\alpha)$ with coefficients α is in turn defined as $\Gamma(\alpha) := (x_1(\alpha), \ldots, x_N(\alpha))$.

---

[1] Note that, while the mathematically concepts are equivalent to the classical ASM papers [1,2], our exposition of PDMs is based on the notation and interpretation of Point Distribution Models as Discrete Gaussian processes, as presented by Lüthi et al. [9].

A probabilistic model of shape variation is obtained by assuming that the coefficients α_i are independent and normally distributed, $\alpha_i \sim N(0,1)$. For this to hold, the eigenvectors forming the basis are scaled by the square root of the corresponding eigenvalue. The model can then be seen as a multivariate normal distribution of shapes centered around $\overline{\Gamma}$, the mean shape.

For explaining an organ's shape in a new image, it is not sufficient to model shape variation, but also the pose needs to be modeled. Thus we define a translation parameter $t \in \mathbb{R}^3$ and a rotation matrix $R(\phi, \psi, \rho)$, which itself is parametrized by the three Euler angles (ϕ, ψ, ρ). For notational convenience, we summarize all parameters in a single vector $\theta = (t, R, \alpha)$. Using this full parametrization, the $k-$th model point becomes

$$x_k(\theta) := R\left(\overline{x}_k + \sum_{i=1}^{N-1} \alpha_i u_k^i\right) + t$$

and the notation $\Gamma(\theta)$ is used again to refer to the full surface induced by θ.

Intensity Models: On top of the PDM, an Active Shape Model describes an intensity model. The intensity model summarizes the intensity distribution around a subset of the N points that define the model. We refer to these points as profile points. For every such profile point x_k, an ASM models the variation of some intensity feature $\rho_k \in \mathbb{R}^d$. Usually, it is assumed that ρ_k follows a normal distribution $\rho_k \sim N(\mu_k, \Sigma_k)$, with a mean μ_k and covariance matrix Σ_k. The parameters are estimated during training time from a set of example images. For a given point x and image I, we can extract the corresponding feature vector $\rho(x, I)$ and use the model to evaluate how likely this point is to correspond to the boundary point x_k:

$$p(\rho(x, I)) = \frac{1}{Z} \exp\left((\rho(x, I) - \mu_k)^T \Sigma_k^{-1} (\rho(x, I) - \mu_k)\right) \tag{1}$$

Hence we can use this intensity model to select the most likely boundary point during model fitting.

Active Shape Model Fitting: With these concepts defined, we now formulate the ASM algorithm in Algorithm 1. Note that once we have found the best matching points, the optimal rotation and shape parameters on line 10, can be computed in closed form (see e.g. [1] for details). The seemingly arbitrary constraint on line 12 involving the threshold κ_α is usually motivated by assuming that α_i follow a standard normal distribution, which implies that values of α_i which are more than three standard deviations away from the mean are very unlikely. New point locations are dropped if they are unlikely under the shape model using κ_S, or if they are unlikely under the appearance model using κ_T.

3 Method

In this section, we introduce our fully probabilistic interpretation of the ASM fitting. We use the ASM in a Bayesian setting, where our goal is to compute the

---

Algorithm 1. Active Shape Model fitting

1: $\theta_0 \leftarrow$ intialization
2: **for** $i = 1$ **to** *max-iterations* **or** *converged* **do**
3:     **for** $x_k \in \{x_1, \ldots, x_K\}$ **do**
4:         generate candidate locations $x_c, c = 1, \ldots, C$
5:         find best new candidate x'_k as $\arg\max_{x_c} p(\rho_k(x_c, I))$
6:         **if** $\| \arg\min_{\alpha} R x_k(\alpha) + t - x'_k \| > \kappa_S$ **or**
$$\sqrt{(\rho_k(x'_k, I) - \mu_k)^T \Sigma_k^{-1} (\rho_k(x'_k, I) - \mu_k)} > \kappa_T \text{ then}$$
7:             drop the correspondence pair (x_k, x'_k)
8:         **end if**
9:     **end for**
10:     calculate rigid alignment R, t of remaining sets $\{x_k\}$ and $\{x'_k\}$
11:     find best α given R, t and remaining sets $\{x_k\}$ and $\{x'_k\}$
12:     $\alpha_i \leftarrow \max(\min(\alpha_i, \kappa_\alpha), -\kappa_\alpha)$
13: **end for**

---

posterior distribution over the parameters θ given the observed image I, which we would like to segment. The posterior is defined as:

$$p(\theta|I) = \frac{p(\theta)p(I|\theta)}{\int p(\theta)p(I|\theta)d\theta} \propto p(\theta)p(I|\theta). \tag{2}$$

As we will see later, our inference procedure makes it possible to work with the unnormalized posterior, hence we only have to specify the prior $p(\theta)$ and likelihood function $p(I|\theta)$.

Prior Distributions: The prior distribution defines our assumptions about the value of the parameters, before we have seen any data. We assume independence between components of the prior, i.e.

$$p(\theta) = p(t, R, \alpha) = p(t)p(R)p(\alpha). \tag{3}$$

For the pose parameters t and R we assume that every possible value is equally likely, so $p(\phi) = p(\psi) = p(\rho) = p(t_1) = p(t_2) = p(t_3) = \mathcal{U}(-\infty, \infty)$. For the shape prior, we use the PDM distribution, which states that the coefficients α_i are independent and follow a standard normal distribution $\alpha_i \sim N(0, 1)$.

Likelihood Functions: Let $x_k \in \Gamma_R$ denote the k-th point of the model, which has an associated intensity distribution $N(\mu_k, \Sigma_k)$ (Cf. Eq. 1). The likelihood for a fixed point x_k of the model is then given by

$$p(I|\theta, x_k) = \frac{1}{Z} \exp(-(\rho(x_k(\theta), I)) - \mu_k)^T \Sigma_k(\rho(x_k(\theta), I)) - \mu_k)$$

where Z is a normalization constant. Assuming independence between the observed values, we can define the shape likelihood as

$$p(I|\theta) = \prod_{k=1}^{N} p(I|\theta, x_k) \tag{4}$$

We can integrate additional constraints in the posterior formulating them as an additional likelihood. We demonstrate this in terms of a few strokes drawn by an expert along the perceived boundary of the liver. We integrate the lines as a discrete set of points $\{x_l\}, l = 1, \ldots, L$ using the likelihood

$$p(\{x_l\}|\theta) = \prod_{l=1}^{L} \mathcal{N}(x_l|CP(x_l, \Gamma(\theta)), \sigma_l). \tag{5}$$

Here, the function CP returns the point from the surface $\Gamma(\theta)$ which is closest to the point x_l.

Approximating the Posterior Distribution: The posterior distribution from Eq. (2) cannot be expressed in closed form. However, it is possible to draw samples from it, which we can use to find shapes that are likely under the posterior distribution. For this, our method uses the Metropolis-Hastings algorithm. The main idea is, that instead of sampling from the posterior $p(\theta|I)$ directly, we sample from a proposal distribution $Q(\theta'|\theta)$, which proposes a new sample θ' given the current sample θ. This generated proposal is then accepted or rejected using an acceptance criterion based on the unnormalized posterior probability $p(\theta|I)$.

The MH algorithm we propose to use for ASM fitting is shown in Algorithm 2. The individual terms in the ratio a, are given by the shape prior and the appearance model of the ASM. Note that we do not need to choose any parameter. The only part we have to provide is the proposal distribution Q. Also note that the denominator in (2), the normalization constant which is usually intractable, is equal for all θ and hence cancels in the ratio on line 4.

Algorithm 2. Metropolis Hastings sampling

1: $\theta_0 \leftarrow$ arbitrary initialization
2: **for** $i = 1$ to S **do**
3:    $\theta' \leftarrow$ sample from $Q(\theta'|\theta)$
4:    $a \leftarrow \frac{q(\theta|\theta')p(\theta'|I)}{q(\theta'|\theta)p(\theta|I)} = \frac{q(\theta|\theta')p(\theta')p(I|\theta)}{q(\theta'|\theta)p(\theta)p(I|\theta)}$. {acceptance threshold}
5:    $r \leftarrow$ sample from $\mathcal{N}(0, 1)$
6:    **if** $a > r$ **then**
7:       $\theta_i \leftarrow \theta'$
8:    **else**
9:       $\theta_i \leftarrow \theta_{i-1}$
10:   **end if**
11: **end for**

The most commonly used proposal distribution is a random walk proposal, defined as $Q(\theta'|\theta) \sim N(\theta, \sigma^2 I)$. We change this to a block-wise proposal distribution, meaning that we update only either, α, ϕ, ψ, ρ or t at a time. Further, we use for each block a mixture of Gaussians with three different σ to account for the initial phase of convergence before we get the samples from the true posterior. When we generate a proposal, a part of the mixture is selected with a predefined probability ω.

4   Experimental Setup

In this section, we experimentally compare our proposed fitting method to the standard ASM method. For both methods, we use the same basic ASM. The methods are compared on the SLIVER dataset. In order to retain reproducibility, we use only the 20 livers from the training set with the provided ground-truth. We report the errors for the results of the model using all examples, also including the test item, as well as for all the leave-one-out setups.

We rigidly align the provided data using eight manually-clicked landmarks. The landmarks are shown in Fig. 1a on the surface of the handcrafted reference. We register the livers using the model-based registration presented by Lüthi et al. [9].

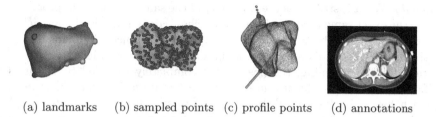

(a) landmarks   (b) sampled points   (c) profile points   (d) annotations

Fig. 1. We show the reference liver with the annoated 8 landmarks in (a), the 1k sampled profile anchor points in (b), the locations for the appearance feature extraction (blue) and the sampled search points (green) for different profile anchor points (red) in (c) and the expert annotations in (d). (Color figure online)

We model the appearance at 1000 evenly sampled points (see Fig. 1b). The values of the image gradient are taken at seven points with a spacing of 8 mm to from the appearance feature (see Fig. 1c). The full appearance model consists of all 1000 individual local Gaussian appearance models[2].

As we aligned the SLIVER dataset initially before we built the models, we do not have to align the model to the data at test time. For the standard ASM fitting, we sample 61 search points over a distance of 60 mm around the current profile point location (see Fig. 1c). We choose $\kappa_T = 6$, $\kappa_S = 3$ and $\kappa_\alpha = 3$ to prevent unlikely updates.

For the sampling-based approach, we use the PDM prior from Eq. 3 and the appearance likelihood from Eq. 4. In the experiment including the expert annotated lines, we additionally include the line likelihood from Eq. 5 in the posterior. The expert annotations depicted in Fig. 1d mark parts of the organ boundary on three axis-aligned slices. We use the introduced multiscale, block-wise Gaussian distribution for generating the proposals (See footnote 2). As

---

[2] The code for the model adaptation is available online at github.com/unibas-gravis/probabilistic-fitting-ASM.

this proposal distribution is symmetric the correction term of the transition probability ratio cancels on line 4 in the Algorithm 2.

For the standard ASM fitting, we take the last state after a maximum of 1000 iterations or convergence. When sampling, we draw 10k samples and use the one with the highest posterior value as result. We use a higher number of samples compared to the standard fitting steps. This is motivated by the fact that the standard approach looks at the appearance of 61 locations per iteration while for one sample we evaluate only one. We report the dice coefficient, the bi-directional average surface distance, and the Hausdorff distance to compare the results.

5   Results

Simplicity: What is striking is the simplicity of the sampling-based approach. We can use the exact same model in both approaches. For the standard approach, we need to define a search strategy, choose the search distance, the point distance threshold, the feature distance threshold and the model coefficient threshold. In contrast, for the sampling, the posterior is completely specified by the model itself. We need only to define the proposal distribution. Further, the standard approach has a fixed search distance. In contrast, when we generate samples from the proposal distribution, the model deformations depends on the local variance of the PDM and hence is locally adaptive.

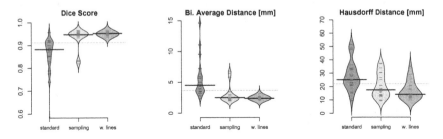

Fig. 2. Segmentation accuracy using the model including the test item. This figure shows that sampling finds a better segmentation compared to the standard ASM fitting. The sampling has the higher dice score as well as the lower bi-directional average distance value and Hausdorff distance. Including expert annotations further improves the result.

Full Model: In the Fig. 2, we show the evaluation of the results for the first experiment, where the target shape is contained in the model. For the Dice coefficient, the bi-directional average surface distance and the Hausdorff-distance one can observe that the sampling outperforms the standard fitting. Including also the expert annotations further improves the result.

Leave-One-Out: The leave-one-out experiments in Fig. 3 show the same trends. Comparing the values to the last experiment we can observe that the Hausdorff distance drops much more than the other measures. This was to be expected, as in this experiment the test item is excluded from the model, but often has a very specific local shape compared to the training items. The expert annotations have a stronger impact on the leave-one-out experiment. Note, also for this experiment, the used model for a specific test case is the same for all methods.

We conclude from the experiments that sampling is a better strategy to adapt an ASM to data. In addition, integrating additional constraints in a straightforward manner, we showed the example of expert annotations along the boundary, helps to improve the accuracy further.

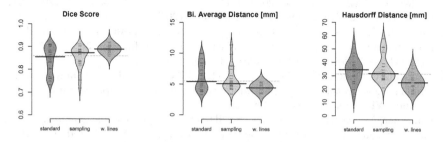

Fig. 3. Segmentation accuracy of the leave-one-out experiment. The sampling outperforms the standard ASM fitting approach. Again, the result further improves when expert annotations are provided.

6 Conclusion

We presented a fully probabilistic interpretation of ASM based segmentation as Bayesian inference. Using a Metropolis-Hastings sampling approach, we determine the maximum a posteriori segmentation. Our method is simple to implement and leads to better results compared to the standard ASM algorithm. As all the terms in our posterior formulation are motivated by the model, no arbitrary thresholds are needed. Furthermore, the probabilistic formulation provides a principled way of integrating additional information, such as expert annotations. For future work, additional constraints, such as regions in the image, which the fitting result should not enter could be integrated. The crucial component for the performance of our method is the proposal distribution. The better it reflects the (unknown) target distribution, the more efficient the sampling is while convergence is always guaranteed asymptotically. Smarter choices of the proposal distribution than the used random walk proposals, which take the image intensities into account, could improve the convergence rate. Such proposals could be based on random forest regression steps [8], on a global estimated parameter distribution [6] or even include deep learning.

Acknowledgment. This work was supported by the Innosuisse project 25622.1 PFLS-LS.

References

1. Cootes, T., Baldock, E., Graham, J.: An introduction to active shape models. In: Image Processing and Analysis, pp. 223–248 (2000)
2. Cootes, T.F., Taylor, C.J., Cooper, D.H., Graham, J.: Active shape models-their training and application. Comput. Vis. Image Underst. **61**(1), 38–59 (1995)
3. Esfandiarkhani, M., Foruzan, A.H.: A generalized active shape model for segmentation of liver in low-contrast CT volumes. Comput. Biol. Med. **82**, 59–70 (2017)
4. van Ginneken, B., de Bruijne, M., Loog, M., Viergever, M.A.: Interactive shape models. In: Medical Imaging 2003: Image Processing, vol. 5032, pp. 1206–1217. International Society for Optics and Photonics (2003)
5. Heimann, T., van Ginneken, B., et al.: Comparison and evaluation of methods for liver segmentation from CT datasets. IEEE Trans. Med. Imaging **28**(8), 1251–1265 (2009). https://doi.org/10.1109/TMI.2009.2013851
6. Jampani, V., Nowozin, S., Loper, M., Gehler, P.V.: The informed sampler: a discriminative approach to Bayesian inference in generative computer vision models. Comput. Vis. Image Underst. **136**, 32–44 (2015)
7. Kirschner, M., Becker, M., Wesarg, S.: 3D active shape model segmentation with nonlinear shape priors. In: Fichtinger, G., Martel, A., Peters, T. (eds.) MICCAI 2011. LNCS, vol. 6892, pp. 492–499. Springer, Heidelberg (2011). https://doi.org/10.1007/978-3-642-23629-7_60
8. Lindner, C., Thiagarajah, S., Wilkinson, J., Consortium, T., Wallis, G., Cootes, T.: Fully automatic segmentation of the proximal femur using random forest regression voting. IEEE Trans. Med. Imaging **32**(8), 1462–1472 (2013)
9. Lüthi, M., Gerig, T., Jud, C., Vetter, T.: Gaussian process morphable models. IEEE Trans. Pattern Anal. Mach. Intell. **40**, 1860–1873 (2017)
10. Norajitra, T., Maier-Hein, K.H.: 3D statistical shape models incorporating landmark-wise random regression forests for omni-directional landmark detection. IEEE Trans. Med. Imaging **36**(1), 155–168 (2017)
11. Schönborn, S., Egger, B., Morel-Forster, A., Vetter, T.: Markov chain Monte Carlo for automated face image analysis. Int. J. Comput. Vis. **123**(2), 160–183 (2017). https://doi.org/10.1007/s11263-016-0967-5
12. Van Ginneken, B., Frangi, A.F., Staal, J.J., ter Haar Romeny, B.M., Viergever, M.A.: Active shape model segmentation with optimal features. IEEE Trans. Med. Imaging **21**(8), 924–933 (2002)
13. Wimmer, A., Soza, G., Hornegger, J.: A generic probabilistic active shape model for organ segmentation. In: Yang, G.-Z., Hawkes, D., Rueckert, D., Noble, A., Taylor, C. (eds.) MICCAI 2009. LNCS, vol. 5762, pp. 26–33. Springer, Heidelberg (2009). https://doi.org/10.1007/978-3-642-04271-3_4
14. Zhang, Q., Bhalerao, A., Helm, E., Hutchinson, C.: Active shape model unleashed with multi-scale local appearance. In: 2015 IEEE International Conference on Image Processing (ICIP), pp. 4664–4668. IEEE (2015)

Automatic Extraction of a Piecewise Symmetry Surface of a 3D Mesh: Application to Scoliosis

Marion Morand[1,2(✉)], Olivier Comas[2], Gérard Subsol[1], and Christophe Fiorio[1]

[1] Research-Team ICAR, LIRMM, University of Montpellier/CNRS,
Montpellier, France
{gerard.subsol,christophe.fiorio}@lirmm.fr
[2] DMS Imaging, Nîmes, France
{mmorand,ocomas}@dms-imaging.com

Abstract. Symmetry analysis of the surface of anatomical structures offers good promise for diagnosis, follow-up and therapy planning of pathologies causing abnormal deformities. This paper addresses the problem of detecting and modelling symmetry of bilateral structures, even in cases where the transformation between the two lateral parts is not a simple planar reflection but a symmetry with respect to a curved symmetry surface. We describe a new method to compute a piecewise curved symmetry surface for 3D objects. The algorithm is based on the computation of a 3D symmetry line, which defines strips by orthogonal slicing. A local symmetry plane is computed for each strip by an ICP-like method. The set of all local symmetry planes forms a piecewise symmetry surface. The method is first validated on parametric objects. Then, we show its potential as a non-invasive technique for the study of patients affected by scoliosis. Finally, our approach is generic enough that it could be extended to other medical applications such as facial dysplasia.

Keywords: Symmetry analysis · Curved reflection · Scoliosis

1 Introduction

Reflection is one of the main characteristics of many human anatomical structures. Its loss is often linked to pathologies causing abnormal deformities. Analysis of the 3D symmetry of the anatomical structure surface gives very useful information for diagnosis, follow-up or therapy planning. With the development of 3D medical imaging, quantifying automatically the symmetry in 3D data of anatomical structures (either as 3D image or 3D mesh) has become an important research topic in medicine, especially for brain [17], face [7] or back pathologies [9]. For example, some recent work [17] on the brain proposed an algorithm to extract a 3D symmetry surface, which results in a better left/right hemisphere segmentation. Moreover, the deviation of this symmetry surface with respect to the anatomical sagittal plane allows one to characterise brain torque [11].

© Springer Nature Switzerland AG 2018
M. Reuter et al. (Eds.): ShapeMI 2018, LNCS 11167, pp. 147–159, 2018.
https://doi.org/10.1007/978-3-030-04747-4_14

Nevertheless, most of the work dealing with algorithms to detect automatically 3D symmetry in anatomical structures focuses on planar symmetry [15]. Symmetry is then quantified by finding a symmetry plane Π, aligning the original structure with its corresponding reflection with respect to this plane and by analysing point-to-point distances [10]. For a straight bilateral structure, there exists a unique reflected point y that corresponds to a point x with respect to Π and conversely. However, it is well-known that most of bilateral anatomical structures do not present a planar symmetry but a "curved" symmetry [13]. In this case, we may not have a unique correspondence between x and y but several reflected points y_i for a unique original point x (see Fig. 1).

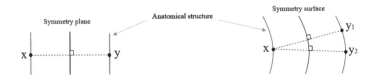

Fig. 1. Differences between a planar and a curved symmetry

Related Work. Methods to compute curved symmetry surfaces can be separated into three groups.

The first group of methods is based on 2D slicing. Lee *et al.* [12] cut the 3D structure along parallel planes and get a set of 2D slices. They then propose an algorithm to obtain a 2D curved glide-reflection symmetry for each slice. By interpolating all the 2D symmetry curves, they obtain a parametric 3D symmetry surface. However, their method depends heavily on the chosen orientation for the 2D slicing procedure.

The second group is based on a refinement of a global symmetry plane. Sato et al. [16] use the Hough transform to estimate an initial symmetry plane. Two refinement processes to obtain a symmetry surface are then proposed. The first one uses a quadratic fitting function instead of a plane. The second process consists in applying the planar symmetry detection method only to the contour points within a local window and extracting the curved symmetry by linking local planar symmetries detected at each point along the occluding contour. In his Ph.D. thesis, Combès [3] computes an initial symmetry plane by an ICP-based method and divides the 3D mesh orthogonally to this plane. For each submesh, a new symmetry plane is estimated and the surface of symmetry is globally parametrised with a Leclerc function. It is then assumed that the curved symmetry can be seen locally as a planar symmetry. However, the results of this group of methods are limited to anatomical structures which are not too curved due to the global smoothness of the fitting functions.

A third group can be defined by the approaches that are specific to brain applications. They are based on 3D MR images of the brain and use the variation of intensities of the cerebral structures. For example, Kuijf *et al.* [11] segment the brain in the MR image and detect automatically the interhemispheric fissure that gives an initial symmetry plane. Then, control points are defined to deform this initial symmetry plane into an optimised surface, modelled by a bicubic spline. After the approximation of a symmetry plane of the brain, Davarpanah et al. [5] propose a refinement process that is applied on 2D slices of the 3D MR images based on fractal dimension and specific intensity values of the cerebral structures. A symmetry surface is eventually constructed as a stack of resulting curves in different slices. Stegman et al. [17] suggest to compute symmetry pixels in 2D slices of the 3D MR brain image maximising a local symmetry measure based on a correlation coefficient and the image intensity at the slice centre voxel. All these methods cannot be directly generalised to other anatomical structures, especially if the latter are given as 3D meshes.

Contributions. Due to the 2D character of the first class of methods and the specific application of the third class, we choose to focus on the second class and propose to generalise their application to large bending.

In this paper, we introduce a new method for automatically assessing the curved reflection of a 3D mesh by extraction of a piecewise symmetry surface. We present this algorithm in detail in Sect. 2: a set of local symmetry planes is computed and forms a piecewise symmetry surface. In Sect. 3, we assess our approach on parametrical 3D meshes. In Sect. 4, we study its application to 3D meshes of the back of patients affected by scoliosis.

2   Piecewise Symmetry Surface Extraction

Our method is designed to automatically detect a piecewise symmetry surface of a 3D mesh even in the case of a very curved structure. In practice, we choose to decompose the 3D mesh into a set of strips S_i which are defined orthogonally to a free-form 3D curve L which we call "symmetry line" and then compute their planes of symmetry Π_i. The method is iterative and begins with an initial symmetry line and strips. At each step n, we get a new set of Π_i^n. At the end of the iterative process, when the symmetry line is stable, we obtain an optimised set of local symmetry planes that we fuse to form the piecewise symmetry surface of the 3D mesh. The overview of the iterative method is illustrated Fig. 2 and we describe each step in the following.

2.1   Determination of the Initial Symmetry Line and Strips

To initialise the symmetry line and the strips, we decompose roughly the 3D mesh into submeshes that we call regions where the symmetry is consistent. For this, the user manually defines two points on the 3D mesh that describe a straight line. Between this couple of points and perpendicularly to the direction of the line, we define N_R regions delimited by $(N_R + 1)$ equidistant and parallel planes. N_R is defined by the user.

The Principal Component Analysis (PCA) method is applied to every submesh to compute their principal axis for a coarse estimate of the direction of the

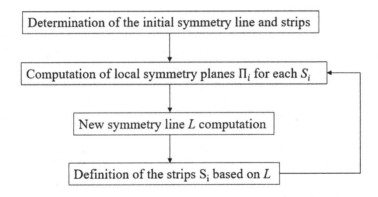

Fig. 2. Piecewise symmetry extraction method

regions. We then subdivide each region orthogonally to its axis into N_S equidistant surface strips S_i. This step is illustrated Fig. 3. In fact, the N_R axes define the initial symmetry line.

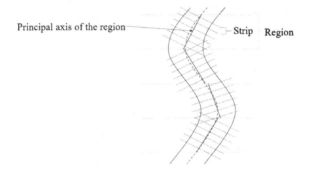

Fig. 3. 2D illustration of the computation of the initial symmetry line and strips

In practice, for general objects, the two seed points are chosen at the extremities of the structure and belonging to the symmetry surface.

2.2   Computation of Local Symmetry Planes

Initialisation. If a surface is perfectly symmetrical, it is well-known that its symmetry plane is orthogonal to a PCA axis [18]. So PCA is used to initialise the symmetry plane Π_i^0 for each strip S_i. We roughly define the direction of the symmetry and the PCA axis that has the closest orientation is selected to act as the normal unit vector $\mathbf{u_i^0}$ of Π_i^0. We assume that Π_i^0 goes through the centroid of S_i which defines the distance d_i^0 to the origin. The couple $(\mathbf{u_i^0}, d_i^0)$ gives an initial symmetry plane Π_i^0 for each strip S_i.

Optimisation. For each strip S_i, we launch the Iterative Closest Point (ICP)-like algorithm described in [4]. This method directly computes the parameters of the optimal symmetry plane for bilateral objects presenting a perfect or imperfect reflection symmetry. To make the method more robust, we integrate the TrimmedICP (trICP) algorithm proposed by Chetverikov $et\ al.$ [2]. While the standard ICP algorithm assumes that all data points can be paired, trICP rejects outliers points. The optimisation of the symmetry plane localisation follows an iterative scheme. At iteration n of the algorithm, we have the 3 following steps:

(1) The points of the strip S_i are reflected with respect to the current estimated symmetry plane Π_i^n. Using the k-d tree method, each point $\mathbf{x_k}$ of S_i is paired with the closest reflected point of S_i. From the set of registered point couples $(\mathbf{x_k}; \mathbf{y_k^n})$ obtained, the individual squared distances are computed and sorted in increasing order. We only select the first $q_i N_i$ couples of points, with q_i the overlap rate from the trICP and N_i the number of points included in the strip S_i. The optimal value of q_i is searched in a range of $[0.4; 1.0]$ by minimising the Mean Squared Error of distance $(\mathbf{x_k}, \mathbf{y_k^n})$ while trying to use as many points as possible [2]. Notice that $(\mathbf{x_k}, \mathbf{y_k^n})$ is different at each step as it depends on Π_i^n.

(2) The parameters $(\mathbf{u_i^{n+1}}, d_i^{n+1})$ of the new estimation of the symmetry plane of S_i are computed by the two following formulas given in [4]:

   - $\mathbf{u_i^{n+1}}$ is collinear with the eigenvector corresponding to the smallest eigenvalue of the 3×3 matrix U_{n+1} defined as:

$$U_{n+1} = \sum_{(\mathbf{x_k}:\mathbf{y_k^n})} (\mathbf{x_k} - \mathbf{g_1} + \mathbf{y_k^n} - \mathbf{g_2})(\mathbf{x_k} - \mathbf{g_1} + \mathbf{y_k^n} - \mathbf{g_2})^T - (\mathbf{x_k} - \mathbf{y_k^n})(\mathbf{x_k} - \mathbf{y_k^n})^T$$

   with $\mathbf{g_1} = \frac{1}{N} \sum \mathbf{x_k}$ and $\mathbf{g_2} = \frac{1}{N} \sum \mathbf{y_k^n}$.
   - $d_i^{n+1} = \frac{1}{2}(\mathbf{g_1} + \mathbf{g_2})^T \mathbf{u_i^{n+1}}$

(3) Go back to step 1 if the mean distance between $(\mathbf{x_k}, \mathbf{y_k^n})$ has changed between the iterations and if a maximal number of iterations has not been reached.

Finally, we obtained a local symmetry plane Π_i for each strip S_i and therefore a set of local symmetry planes which forms the piecewise symmetry surface.

2.3   New Symmetry Line Computation

For each Π_i, we note $\mathbf{P_i^{inf}}$ and $\mathbf{P_i^{sup}}$ the 2 points that are defined at the intersection between the surface, Π_i and respectively the inferior and superior plane of the strip. We compute the $(N_S + 1)$ symmetry points $\mathbf{P_i^{sym}}$ as the middle between $\mathbf{P_i^{sup}}$ and $\mathbf{P_{i+1}^{inf}}$ (see Fig. 4). The new symmetry line L is formed by the interpolation of the set of symmetry points $\mathbf{P_i^{sym}}$ by a third order parametric spline curve.

2.4   Definition of the Strips Based on the Symmetry Line

This symmetry line L acts as a base for creating new adaptive strips S_i^a (see Fig. 5). Each new adaptive strip S_i^a is defined as the intersection between the object surface and two planes:

- The superior plane of the strip is characterised by the vector defined by $\mathbf{P}_{i+1}^{sym}$ and $\mathbf{P}_{i+2}^{sym}$ and passing through $\mathbf{P}_{i+1}^{sym}$.
- The inferior plane of the strip is characterised by the vector defined by $\mathbf{P}_i^{sym}$ and $\mathbf{P}_{i-1}^{sym}$ and passing through $\mathbf{P}_i^{sym}$.

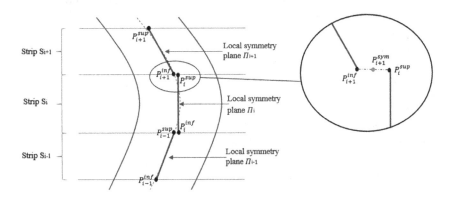

Fig. 4. 2D illustration of the computation of the symmetry points

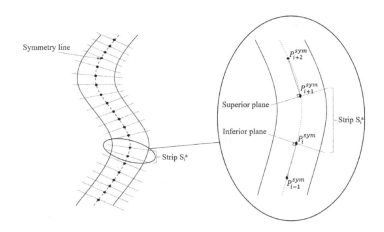

Fig. 5. 2D illustration of the strip refinement

3   Validation on Parametrical 3D Meshes

3.1   Method

To validate our method on objects presenting curved reflection, we generate mathematically different swept 3D meshes which are curved and we assess the method accuracy with respect to bending. We define a half-ellipse in the plane (Oxy) centered in $(0, 0, 0)$, with a semi-major axis of 20 mm along Ox and a semi-minor axis of 10 mm along Oy. The symmetry point of this half-ellipse is then located at $(0, 5.0, 0)$. We extrude this curve along a 3D parametric curve involving cosine and sine. Each model is sampled into a 3D mesh made of 75 000 vertices. The set of meshes is shown in the Table 1. The extrusion of the symmetry points of the half-ellipse gives the symmetry line. For a height z, the theoretical local symmetry plane is given by the binormal of the Frenet-Serret frame along this symmetry line.

We can then compare our piecewise symmetry surface to this theoretical plane both in localisation and orientation. For the localisation we compute the depth and lateral Root Mean Square Deviations, defined as the quadratic mean of the distances projected along an axis: Oy for RMSD$_{depth}$ and Ox for RMSD$_{lat}$. We assess the orientation of each local symmetry plane by calculating the angle θ defined as $\theta = arccos(\mathbf{n}.\mathbf{u})$, where $\mathbf{n}$ is the normal unit vector of the theoretical symmetry plane and $\mathbf{u}$ is the normal unit vector of the symmetry plane obtained by our method.

3.2   Results

Our method was implemented in Matlab (R2015a). We have chosen 4 regions ($N_R = 4$) and 5 strips have been created in each of them ($N_s = 5$). The number of iterations is arbitrarily fixed at 100 for each strip. Table 1 shows the comparison of our piecewise symmetry surface (in red) with the theoretical one.

Table 1. Evaluation of the proposed method on geometrical swept models

Model	1	2	3	4	5	6	7
RMSD$_{lat}$ (mm)	0.16	0.50	0.64	0.80	0.62	1.10	1.75
RMSD$_{depth}$ (mm)	0.00	0.01	0.02	0.02	0.01	0.03	0.09
Mean value θ (°)	0.5	1.3	1.9	2.2	1.8	2.8	4.0
Maximum value θ (°)	2.1	2.37	4.5	5.9	3.9	6.4	11.1

The maximums for both the distance and the orientation θ are always observed at the apex section of the curve. This can be explained by the definition of the local symmetry plane. We assume that for a planar symmetry and by extension for small bending surface, we have $\mathbf{x_k} = \mathbf{S_\Pi}(\mathbf{y_k^n})$ and $\mathbf{y_k^n} = \mathbf{S_\Pi}(\mathbf{x_k})$. However, for large bending $\mathbf{y_k^n} = \mathbf{S_\Pi}(\mathbf{x_k})$ is not guaranteed. This is why the orientation of our plane does not perfectly match the orientation of the Frenet-Serret frame, which is only an approximate solution along the translated 3D curve used as trajectory during the mesh generation. We observe that one iteration of the refinement is enough to obtain stable symmetry lines and good results, but it may be necessary to carry out additional iterations for more complex structures.

Comparing to other existing methods, our method promises good results. The method proposed by Sato et al. [16] seems to fail for surfaces with a single bending which is smaller than ours. In the same way, the methods proposed by Combès [3] and Lee et al. [12] are limited for detecting symmetry of structures with large or multiple curvatures, due to their initialisations. In particular, the initial slicing process of the 3D mesh proposed by [12] is only parallel and so will negatively affect the results in case of curved structures.

4   Application to Scoliosis

Scoliosis is characterised by a lateral deviation of the spine, associated to a local axial rotation of vertebrae in the horizontal plane. This 3D spinal deformity may lead to severe impairment of the outer appearance of the back surface. To limit hazardous X-ray examinations prescribed during the treatment, there is a growing interest for non-invasive methods based on 3D measurements of the back mesh [1,9].

The aim of these methods is to find 3D parameters that yield better quantification of the back deformation. In particular, one of the interesting parameters to assess scoliosis is the left/right asymmetry in order to determine the number, direction and location of deformed parts for classifying the scoliosis [1]. We apply our method to the 3D meshes of the backs of patients affected by scoliosis with the following parameters:

- The initial direction of the subdivision of the back into regions is computed from the straight line defined by the prominent vertebra and the middle of the posterior superior iliac spine. In order to fully automate the method, the detection of these anatomical landmarks may be based only on the surface curvature as proposed in [8].
- We used 3 regions and 6 strips per regions to represent the 18 vertebrae localised between the two seed points. An adaptation of the height of each strip to the height of each vertebra is statistically computed from the height of the spine.

The result on one example of a scoliotic patient can be seen in Fig. 6.

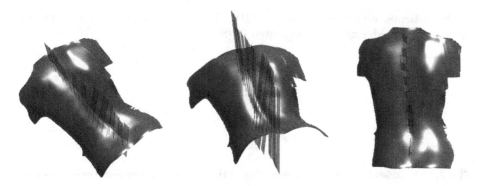

Fig. 6. 3D piecewise symmetry surface of the back of a scoliotic patient. Notice how the orientations of the local planes (in green and red) follow the back deformations. (Color figure online)

4.1 Symmetry Line of the Back Mesh

The lateral deviation and the anteroposterior curvature are measured with respect to the spinal midline, which is the line that passes over the centre point of the vertebral bodies. The midline can be estimated by the symmetry line of the back shape [9]. We have already showed the potential of a simpler version of our method to compute the symmetry line for 3D objects [14]. The comparison between the line manually determined by landmarks placed by clinician and this symmetry line assesses the mean error deviation to 5.8 mm, the $RMSD_{lat}$ to 4.82 mm and the $RMSD_{depth}$ to 0.69 mm. These indicators remain constant with the variations of the disease severity and patient morphology. These results demonstrate that the method is consistent with the reference method and robust with respect to the disease severity and the patient morphology.

4.2 Vertebral Rotation

We propose to use our new method to evaluate the local back surface rotation that can be correlated to the axial rotations of vertebrae [9]. 51 scoliotic patients were acquired with the $BIOMOD^{TM}$ system[1]. This device provides bi-planar radiographic 3D reconstructions of the spines coupled with optical acquisitions of back surfaces. They are both expressed in a patient-specific reference system. For each vertebra, we have the 3D coordinates of the spinous process, noted S, and the centre of the vertebra C. We compute the direction SC and we recover its projection in the horizontal plane. In the same way, we compute the horizontal component of the direction provided by the local symmetry plane corresponding to the same vertebra. We compute α the angle between these two directions, as illustrated Figs. 7 and 8, for each vertebra for every patient. On the set of

---

[1] Acquisition device developed by AXS Medical (DMS Imaging): http://www.dms.com/biomod-3s/.

the 51 patients, we get: $\alpha = 3.81° \pm 2.93°$. This preliminary result seems to be promising, considering those presented in [8].

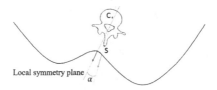

Fig. 7. Comparison between the orientation of the local symmetry plane and the actual vertebral rotation

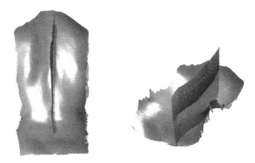

Fig. 8. Example of a piecewise symmetry surface on the back of a scoliotic patient. Note that red crosses correspond to spinous processes on the back surface and green crosses to the centre of vertebrae. (Color figure online)

4.3   Adaptation to the Lateral Bending Posture

Patients are often examined in lateral bending as this position is optimal to evaluate the spine flexibility for surgery planning. However most of the proposed methods to analyse this pathology fail for asymmetric postures [6]. We apply our method on a patient in bending posture (Fig. 9). Notice how the spine curve is well emphasised by the piecewise symmetry surface.

5   Future Work

We have described a method for computing out a piecewise symmetry surface on 3D meshes. Future work will focus on interpolating the piecewise surface to obtain a continuous curved symmetry surface. To provide reproducible and objective results, a fully automatic calculation of the method parameters (N_R

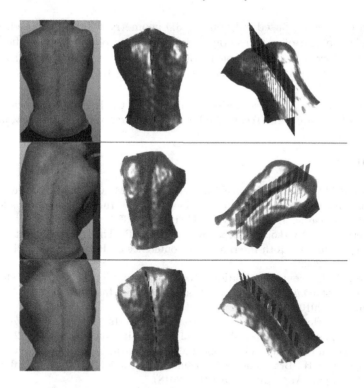

Fig. 9. Piecewise symmetry surface on the 3D meshes of the back of a patient in bending (∼180 000 vertices and ∼360 000 faces).

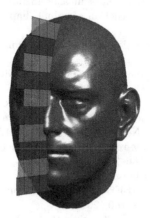

Fig. 10. Computation of a piece wise symmetry surface of a 3D face mesh (∼41 000 vertices and ∼81 500 faces)

and N_s in particular) based only on the 3D geometry will be proposed. On the clinical side, we also plan to use our local symmetry planes for classification of scoliosis [1]. Moreover, our approach could be extended to other medical applications such as facial dysplasia (see for example Fig. 10).

Acknowledgements. This work was supported by a CIFRE grant (French National Association of Research and Technology) for the doctoral work of Marion Morand.

References

1. Aroeira, R.M.C., de Las Casas, E.B., Pertence, A.E.M., Greco, M., Tavares, J.M.R.: Non-invasive methods of computer vision in the posture evaluation of adolescent idiopathic scoliosis. J. Bodyw. Mov. Ther. **20**(4), 832–843 (2016)
2. Chetverikov, D., Svirko, D., Stepanov, D., Krsek, P.: The trimmed iterative closest point algorithm. In: 16th International Conference on Pattern Recognition, vol. 3, pp. 545–548 (2002)
3. Combès, B.: Efficient computational tools for the statistical analysis of shape and asymmetry of 3D point sets. Ph.D. thesis. Signal and Image Processing, University of Rennes 1 (2010)
4. Combès, B., Hennessy, R., Waddington, J., Roberts, N., Prima, S.: Automatic symmetry plane estimation of bilateral objects in point clouds. In: 26th IEEE Conference on Computer Vision and Pattern Recognition, Anchorage, US (2008)
5. Davarpanah, S.H.: Brain mid-sagittal surface extraction based on fractal analysis. Neural Comput. Appl. **30**(1), 153–162 (2018)
6. Di Angelo, L., Di Stefano, P., Spezzaneve, A.: Symmetry line detection for non-erected postures. Int. J. Interact. Des. Manuf. **7**(4), 271–276 (2013)
7. Di Angelo, L., Di Stefano, P.: Bilateral symmetry estimation of human face. Int. J. Interact. Des. Manuf. **7**(4), 217–225 (2013)
8. Drerup, B., Hierholzer, E.: Back shape measurement using video rasterstereography and three-dimensional reconstruction of spinal shape. Clin. Biomech. **9**(1), 28–36 (1994)
9. Drerup, B.: Rasterstereographic measurement of scoliotic deformity. Scoliosis **9**(1), 22 (2014)
10. Krajíček, V., Dupej, J., Veleminská, J., Pelikán, J.: Morphometric analysis of mesh asymmetry. J. WSCG **20**(1), 65–72 (2012)
11. Kuijf, H.J., Veluw, S.J.V., Geerlings, M.I., Viergever, M.A., Jan, G., Koen, B.: Automatic extraction of the midsagittal surface from brain MR images using the Kullback–Leibler measure. Neuroinformatics **12** (2013)
12. Lee, S., Liu, Y.: Curved glide-reflection symmetry detection. IEEE Trans. Pattern Anal. Mach. Intell. **34**(2), 266–278 (2012)
13. Lee, T.S.H., Fidler, S., Dickinson, S.: Detecting curved symmetric parts using a deformable disc model. In: IEEE International Conference on Computer Vision, Sydney, Australia, pp. 1753–1760 (2013)
14. Morand, M., Comas, O., Fiorio, C., Subsol, G.: Automatic extraction of the 3D symmetry line of back surface: application on scoliotic adolescents. In: 40th International IEEE Conference on Engineering in Medicine and Biology Society, EMBS, Honolulu, US (2018)
15. Quan, L., Zhang, Y., Tang, K.: Curved reflection symmetric axes on free-form surfaces and their extraction. IEEE Trans. Autom. Sci. Eng. **15**(1), 111–126 (2018)

16. Sato, Y., Tamura, S.: Detecting planar and curved symmetries of 3D shapes from a range image. Comput. Vis. Image Underst. **64**(1), 175–187 (1996)
17. Stegmann, M.B., Skoglund, K., Ryberg, C., Plads, R.P., Lyngby, D.K.: Mid-sagittal plane and mid-sagittal surface optimization in brain MRI using a local symmetry measure. In: Medical Imaging 2005: Image Processing, vol. 5747, pp. 568–579 (2005)
18. Sun, C., Sherrah, J.: 3D symmetry detection using the extended Gaussian image. IEEE Trans. Pattern Anal. Mach. Intell. **19**(2), 164–169 (1997)

Image Registration and Predictive Modeling: Learning the Metric on the Space of Diffeomorphisms

Ayagoz Mussabayeva[1,3]([⊠]), Alexey Kroshnin[1,3], Anvar Kurmukov[1,3],
Yulia Denisova[1], Li Shen[4], Shan Cong[5], Lei Wang[6], and Boris A. Gutman[1,2]

[1] The Institute for Information Transmission Problems, Moscow, Russia
ayagoz.muss@gmail.com
[2] Department of Biomedical Engineering, Illinois Institute of Technology,
Chicago, IL, USA
[3] Higher School of Economics, Moscow, Russia
[4] Department of Biostatistics, Epidemiology and Informatics,
University of Pennsylvania, Philadelphia, PA, USA
[5] Indiana University, Indianapolis, IN, USA
[6] Department of Psychiatry and Behavioral Sciences,
Northwestern University Feinberg School of Medicine, Chicago, IL, USA

Abstract. We present a method for metric optimization in the Large Deformation Diffeomorphic Metric Mapping (LDDMM) framework, by treating the induced Riemannian metric on the space of diffeomorphisms as a kernel in a machine learning context. For simplicity, we choose the kernel Fischer Linear Discriminant Analysis (KLDA) as the framework. Optimizing the kernel parameters in an Expectation-Maximization framework, we define model fidelity via the hinge loss of the decision function. The resulting algorithm optimizes the parameters of the LDDMM norm-inducing differential operator as a solution to a group-wise registration and classification problem. In practice, this may lead to a biology-aware registration, focusing its attention on the predictive task at hand such as identifying the effects of disease. We first tested our algorithm on a synthetic dataset, showing that our parameter selection improves registration quality and classification accuracy. We then tested the algorithm on 3D subcortical shapes from the Schizophrenia cohort Schizconnect. Our Schizophrenia-Control predictive model showed significant improvement in ROC AUC compared to baseline parameters.

Keywords: Image registration · Machine learning · Subcortical shape
Expectation Maximization · Metric learning · LDDMM

1 Introduction

Image registration, and more generally geometric alignment underlies a large number of analyses in medical imaging, particularly neuroimaging. As one of the

© Springer Nature Switzerland AG 2018
M. Reuter et al. (Eds.): ShapeMI 2018, LNCS 11167, pp. 160–168, 2018.
https://doi.org/10.1007/978-3-030-04747-4_15

mainstays of medical image analysis, the problem has been addressed extensively over the last 2+ decades, with several flavors of robust algorithms [1]. A number of registration approaches develop an explicit metric space comprised of the geometric objects of interest—anatomical shapes, diffusion tensors, images, etc. Prominent among these is the Large Deformation Diffeomorphic Metric Mapping (LDDMM) framework [2]. Instead of treating images as objects of interest directly, LDDMM builds a space of image-matching diffeomorphisms using a Riemannian metric on velocity fields. This metric is induced by a differential operator which at once controls the nature of the metric space and regularizes the registration.

The structure of such a space—a manifold of smooth mappings with well-defined geodesics—enables generalizations of several standard statistical analysis methods. These methods adapted to the Riemannian setting has been repeatedly shown to improve their sensitivity and ability to discern population dynamics when compared to projecting the data onto Euclidean domains. Works in this area include computation of the geometric median and metric optimization for robust atlas estimation [3,4], time series geodesic regression [5], and principal geodesic analysis [6].

With the exception of [4], in the works above the metric is assumed to be fixed. Further, the metricity and Riemannian inner product with which the LDDMM space is endowed has not been used explicitly in predictive modeling up to now. In this work, we strive for two complementary aims: (1) to exploit the Riemannian metric on registration-defining velocities as a kernel in a classification task and (2) to optimize the metric to improve classification. We follow an Expectation-Maximization (EM) approach similar to [4], alternating between minimizing image misalignment for kernel estimation, and optimizing model quality over the kernel parameters. In this work, we choose the kernel Fischer linear discriminant classifier for simplicity, though other predictive models are admissible in our framework as well. It is our hope that by explicit tuning the diffeomorphism metric to questions of biological interest, the carefully crafted manifold properties of LDDMM will gain greater practical utility.

Our experiments consist of synthetic 2-dimensional shape classification, as well as classifying hippocampal shapes extracted from brain MRI of the Schizconnect schizophrenia study. In both cases, the classification accuracy and ROC area under the curve (AUC) improved significantly compared to default baseline kernel parameters.

2 Methods

2.1 Metric on Diffeomorphisms

The Large Deformation Diffeomorphic Metric Mapping (LDDMM) was first introduced in [2]. The goal of the registration is to compute a diffeomorphism $\phi \colon \Omega \to \Omega$, where the Ω is the image domain. The diffeomorphism ϕ is generated by the flow of a time-dependent velocity vector field v, defined as follows:

$$\frac{\partial\phi(t,x)}{\partial t} = v(t, \phi(t,x)),$$

$$\phi(0,x) = id,$$

(1)

where id is the identity transformation: $id(x) = x$, $\forall x \in \Omega$. This equation gives a path $\phi_t \colon \Omega \to \Omega$, $t \in [0,1]$, in the space of diffeomorphisms. Estimation of the optimal diffeomorphism via the basic variational problem in the space of smooth velocity fields V on Ω takes the following form, constrained by 1:

$$v^* = \underset{v}{\operatorname{argmin}} \left(\int_0^1 \|v_t\|_L^2 \, dt + \frac{1}{\sigma^2} \|I_0 \circ \phi - I_1\|^2 \right).$$

(2)

The required smoothness is enforced by defining the norm $\|\cdot\|_L$ on the space V of smooth velocity vector fields through a Riemannian metric L.

The Riemannian metric L should be naturally defined by the geometric structure of the domain. The inner product $\|v\|_L^2 = \langle Lv, v \rangle$ can also be thought of as a metric between images, i.e. the minimal diffeomorphism required to transform the appearance of I_0 to be as similar as possible to I_1. Since the diffeomorphism space is a Lie Group with respect to Eq. 1, the Riemannian metric defined suggests a right-invariance property. The original LDDMM work [2] defines L as a smooth differential self-adjoint operator $L = (\alpha\Delta + \beta E)$, where E is identity operator. Here, we choose to use an L based on the biharmonic operator $L = (\alpha\Delta + \beta E)^2$, as e.g. in [7]. The parameters (α, β) correspond to convexity and normalization terms, respectively. These parameters significantly affect the quality of the registration. It is not obvious how to select α and β, though they effectively define the geometric structure of the primal domain. Indeed, these are the parameters we optimize in our EM scheme below.

2.2   Predictive Model

Consider a standard binary classification problem: given a sample $\left(x_i, y(x_i)\right)_{i=1}^n$, where $y(x_i) \in \{1, -1\}$ is a class label, find a classification function $\hat{y}$ approximating the true one y. One of the standard linear techniques in statistical data analysis is the Fisher's linear discriminant analysis (LDA). The kernel Fisher Discriminant Analysis (KLDA) introduced in [8] is a generalization of the classical LDA. There are several approaches to derive more general class separability criteria. KLDA derives a linear classification in the embedding feature space (RKHS [9]) induced by a kernel k, what corresponds to a non-linear decision function in the original, or "input" space. The main idea of LDA is to find a one-dimensional projection w in the feature space that maximizes the between-class variance while minimizing the within-class variance. KLDA seeks an analogous projection in the embedding space, where means (M_z) and covariance matrices (Σ_z) for each class $z \in \{-1, 1\}$ are computed. The (K)LDA cost function takes the following quadratic rational form:

$$J(w) = \frac{w^T(M_1 - M_{-1})(M_1 - M_{-1})^T w}{w^T(\Sigma_{-1} + \Sigma_1)w} = \frac{w^T M w}{w^T N w}, \tag{3}$$

where

$$(M_z)_i = \frac{1}{n_z} \sum_{x_\ell : y(x_\ell) = z} k(x_i, x_\ell),$$

$$(\Sigma_z)_{i,j} = \frac{1}{n_z} \sum_{x_\ell : y(x_\ell) = z} k(x_i, x_\ell)k(x_j, x_\ell) - (M_z)_i(M_z)_j.$$

Here n_z is a number of objects from class z in the sample.

The solution of the problem $J(w) \to \min$ is known to be $\hat{w} = N^{-1}(M_1 - M_{-1})$. The decision function for a new observation x is based on the projected distance to the training sample means, $w^T(M_z - x)$. The M-step in an EM formulation requires a differentiable measure of model quality which in our case is the accuracy of classification. The more common approach is to formulate a probabilistic model which leads to a log-likelihood optimization. Such an approach is used e.g. in [4]. In our case, this can be done by modeling the classifier's output with a parametric distribution.

However, we found that such a formulation using the sigmoid distribution function leads to an unstable solution. Instead, we propose to use the hinge loss defined for KLDA as

$$h(x', z) = \max\{0, 1 - z\,y(x')\}$$

$$y(x') = \sum_{i=1}^{n} w_i \left(k(x_i, x') - \frac{(M_1)_i + (M_{-1})_i}{2} \right), \tag{4}$$

where $z \in \{-1, 1\}$ is a true label for the new observation x' and $k(x_i, x')$ is the inner product (i.e. the kernel) between x' and the training observation x_i. While both hinge loss and log-likelihood formulations eventually lead to some locally optimal solutions on simple problems, such as our synthetic dataset, the former exhibits greater stability. For the hippocampal data, only hinge loss minimization leads to a stable solution.

2.3   Learning the Diffeomorphic Metric

The main goal of this work is to use the registration-derived metric to classify images. Let us denote the Riemannian metric by $K_L(\alpha, \beta) = \langle Lv, v \rangle$. In practice, β plays an insignificant role and can be fixed, as multiplication of the velocity by a constant does not change the optimization problem in LDDMM. We focus on optimizing α, fixing $\beta = 1$ as a normalization term.

We optimize α in the EM framework as follows.

- E-step:

Register each pair of images in our training sample optimizing Eq. 2 to derive $K_L(x_i, x_j)$. Define $K(x_i, x_j) = \exp\{-\gamma K_L(x_i, x_j)\}$ and apply KLDA using $K(x_i, x_j)$. The parameter gamma is estimated by grid search to make a computation easier, but it can be also estimated by gradient descent. Estimate the hinge loss 4 given a fixed α.

- M-step:

Minimize the hinge loss 4 with respect to α.

The primary computational challenge above is in the M-step. Though the decision function is non-convex with respect to α, we seek a local minimum via gradient descent. We give the gradient direction with respect to $\theta = (\alpha, \beta)$ below, keeping in mind that β is fixed.

$$\frac{dh(x', z)}{d\theta} = \begin{cases} -z\frac{dy(x')}{d\theta}, & \text{if } zy(x') < 1, \\ 0, & \text{otherwise.} \end{cases} \tag{5}$$

Using the matrix notation $y(x') = w^T\big(k(x') - (M_1 + M_{-1})/2\big)$ with $k_i(x') = K(x_i, x')$ one can obtain

$$\frac{dy(x')}{d\theta} = \left(k(x') - \frac{M_1 + M_{-1}}{2}\right)^T \frac{dw}{d\theta} + w^T\left(\frac{dk(x')}{d\theta} - \frac{1}{2}\frac{d(M_1 + M_{-1})}{d\theta}\right),$$

$$dw = -N^{-1}(dN)N^{-1}(M_1 - M_{-1}) + N^{-1}(dM_1 - dM_{-1}),$$

$$\frac{dK(x_i, x')}{d\theta} = -\gamma K(x_i, x')\frac{dK_L(x_i, x')}{d\theta}$$

$$\frac{dK_L(x_i, x')}{d\theta} = \begin{pmatrix} 2\langle(\alpha\Delta^2 + \beta\Delta)v_{x,x'}, v_{x,x'}\rangle, \\ 2\langle(\alpha\Delta + \beta E)v_{x,x'}, v_{x,x'}\rangle. \end{pmatrix} \tag{6}$$

The resulting algorithm requires $n \times (n - 1)$ registrations at each EM step to train, and n registrations to a new image from each of n images in training sample to apply.

3 Experiments

To derive a baseline set of metrics between pairs of images, we selected α to maximize mutual information between registered images. This metric was then used to define the kernel in the KLDA classifier, the results of which we used as a baseline accuracy for our proposed method.

Our initial experiments were based on 100 images of rectangles, and 100 images of ellipses, each generated with a random locally affine deformation sufficiently noisy to obscure the original class of the image to the naked eye (Fig. 1). Using 50 deformed ellipses and 50 deformed rectangles as a training dataset, we optimized α until hinge loss convergence. Figure 2 (left) shows that EM converges stably after several iterations based on ROC AUC. The final model, chosen based on the best training ROC AUC, performed nearly as well on the synthetic test dataset: ROC AUC = 0.84.

Original Images   Locally Affine Transformation

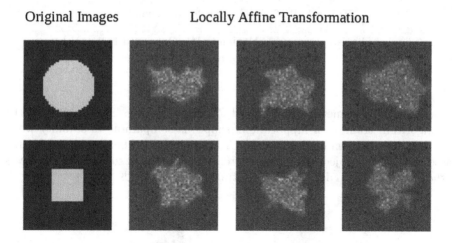

Fig. 1. Synthetic data generation

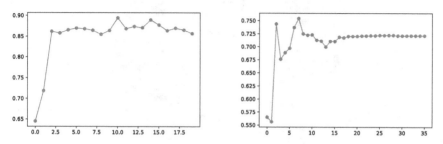

Fig. 2. ROC area under the curve vs. EM iterations on (left) synthetic data and (right) hippocampal shape

Our 3D hippocampal shape sample was derived from the SchizConnect brain MRI dataset [10]. We used right hippocampal segmentations extracted with FreeSurfer [11] from 227 Schizophrenia (SCZ) patients and 496 controls (CTL). All shapes were affinely registered to the ENIGMA hippocampal shape atlas [12], and their binary mask was computed from the transformed mesh model.

We again used 100 training examples (50 CTL, 50 SCZ) in all our experiments below, using the remaining sample as a test dataset. To derive baseline results to compare with our algorithm's performance on hippocampal shapes, we constructed two additional discriminative models.

(1) A logistic regression model simply using the vectorized binary mask. No spatial information is used in this model.
(2) A KLDA model constructed using LDDMM metrics optimized for registration quality.

ROC AUC scores for the three models are shown in Table 1.

As expected, ignoring spatial information leads to significant drop in performance. It is also encouraging to see improvement in the classification accuracy

Table 1. ROC AUC scores for three models

	Logistic regression	Maximum MI	Optimized LDDMM-kernel
ROC AUC	0.36 ± 0.02	0.72 ± 0.06	0.75 ± 0.06

when the LDDMM metric is optimized for this explicitly. The stability of the EM algorithm trained on hippocampal shapes is comparable to stability when synthetic data, as seen in Fig. 2 (right). To visualize the difference in the kernel-based models, we project the mean difference between SCZ subjects and controls in the scalar momenta defining the registration velocity fields [7], as seen in Fig. 3.

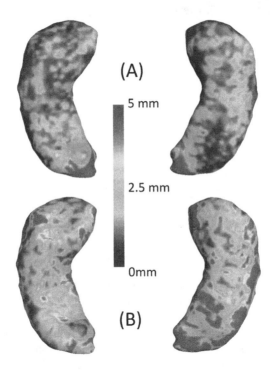

Fig. 3. Mean momentum difference between Schizophrenics and healthy subjects, using (A) a classification-optimized metric and (B) a metric optimized for pairwise mutual information. The effect in the latter is diffuse, while the classification-aware metric focuses on the hippocampal tail.

4   Conclusion

We have presented a method to optimize registration parameters for improved classification performance. Method exploits the geodesic distance on the space of diffeomorphisms as an image similarity measure to be learned in the fashion of traditional metric learning [13]. Our aim in this work was twofold: (1) to show that the metricity of a high dimensional space of geometric objects can be successfully used to improve predictive modeling, and (2) to suggest a means of making the sophisticated mathematical machinery of constructions such a LDDMM more useful in medical imaging practice. As a first attempt, we believe this work shows progress towards both goals. A stable LDDMM metric optimization is devised, and classification accuracy in our real-world application is indeed improved. The main drawback is the significant computational burden, as $N \times N$ training registrations are required. One approach to alleviate this problem is to lift the classification problem onto the tangent space at identity, thus requiring only N training registrations to an atlas, similar to [4]. Other generalizations of the idea presented here are possible both in LDDMM and other metric frameworks. We hope our work will inspire these generalizations to be developed.

Acknowledgements. This work was funded in part by the Russian Science Foundation grant 17-11-01390.

References

1. Klein, A., et al.: Evaluation of 14 nonlinear deformation algorithms applied to human brain MRI registration. Neuroimage **46**(3), 786–802 (2009)
2. Beg, M.F., Miller, M.I., Trouvé, A., Younes, L.: Computing large deformation metric mappings via geodesic flows of diffeomorphisms. Int. J. Comput. Vis. **61**(2), 139–157 (2005)
3. Fletcher, P.T., Venkatasubramanian, S., Joshi, S.C.: The geometric median on Riemannian manifolds with application to robust atlas estimation. NeuroImage **45**(1 Suppl), S143–52 (2009)
4. Zhang, M., Singh, N., Fletcher, P.T.: Bayesian estimation of regularization and atlas building in diffeomorphic image registration. In: Gee, J.C., Joshi, S., Pohl, K.M., Wells, W.M., Zöllei, L. (eds.) IPMI 2013. LNCS, vol. 7917, pp. 37–48. Springer, Heidelberg (2013). https://doi.org/10.1007/978-3-642-38868-2_4
5. Hong, Y., Golland, P., Zhang, M.: Fast geodesic regression for population-based image analysis. In: Descoteaux, M., Maier-Hein, L., Franz, A., Jannin, P., Collins, D.L., Duchesne, S. (eds.) MICCAI 2017. LNCS, vol. 10433, pp. 317–325. Springer, Cham (2017). https://doi.org/10.1007/978-3-319-66182-7_37
6. Zhang, M., Fletcher, P.T.: Probabilistic principal geodesic analysis. In: Proceedings of the 26th International Conference on Neural Information Processing Systems, NIPS 2013, USA, vol. 1, pp. 1178–1186. Curran Associates Inc. (2013)
7. Mang, A., Gholami, A., Biros, G.: Distributed-memory large deformation diffeomorphic 3D image registration. In: International Conference for High Performance Computing, Networking, Storage and Analysis, SC 2016, pp. 842–853 (2016)
8. Mika, S., Ratsch, G., Weston, J., Scholkopf, B., Mullers, K.R.: Fisher discriminant analysis with kernels. In: Proceedings of the 1999 IEEE Signal Processing Society Workshop on Neural Networks for Signal Processing IX, pp. 41–48. IEEE (1999)
9. Aronszajn, N.: Theory of reproducing kernels. Trans. Am. Math. Soc. **68**(3), 337–404 (1950)

10. Wang, L., et al.: SchizConnect: mediating neuroimaging databases on schizophrenia and related disorders for large-scale integration. NeuroImage **124**, 1155–1167 (2016). Sharing the wealth: Brain Imaging Repositories in 2015
11. Fischl, B.: FreeSurfer. Neuroimage **62**(2), 774–781 (2012)
12. Roshchupkin, G.V., et al.: Heritability of the shape of subcortical brain structures in the general population. Nat. Commun. **7**, 13738 (2016)
13. Bellet, A., Habrard, A., Sebban, M.: A survey on metric learning for feature vectors and structured data. ArXiv e-prints, June 2013

Joint Registration of Multiple Generalized Point Sets

Zhe Min[✉], Jiaole Wang, and Max Q.-H. Meng

Robotics, Perception and Artificial Intelligence Lab,
The Chinese University of Hong Kong, Shatin, N.T., Hong Kong, China
{zmin,max}@ee.cuhk.edu.hk

Abstract. To align different views or representations of anatomy is an essential task in computer-assisted surgery (CAS). In this paper, we propose a probabilistic approach to the joint rigid registration problem of multiple generalized point sets. A generalized point set consist of high-dimensional points which include both positional and orientational information (normal vector). A hybrid mixture model (HMM) combining Gaussian and Von-Mises-Fisher distributions is used to model the positional and orientational components of the generalized point sets, respectively. All generalized point sets are jointly registered under the expectation maximization framework. In E-step, the posterior probabilities representing point correspondence confidences are computed. In M-step, the transformation matrices, positional variances and orientational concentration parameters are updated for each point set. We validate the proposed algorithm using the human femur bone surface points extracted from the CT data. The experimental results show that the proposed algorithm outperforms the state-of-the-art ones in terms of the registration accuracy, the robustness to noise and outliers, and the convergence speed.

1 Introduction

The registration problem is commonly used to align (a) pre-operative with intra-operative spaces [9–12,14]; (b) different imaging modalities in image-guided surgery (IGS) [5]. When the *surface registration* technique is used, the correspondences between points in two spaces to be registered are not known. In this situation, generally, an iterative framework is utilized to seek the best rigid transformation matrice. Iterative closest point (ICP) is a classical two-step framework to solve such registrations where the first step finds the best correspondences between points in two sets and the second step computes the best transformation matrice that aligns the two sets given the current correspondences. The two steps are repeated until convergence. On the other hand, an alternative way to conduct such registrations is to reformulate the registration into a maximum likelihood (ML) problem and solve the problem under the expectation maximization (EM) framework. In the *E-step*, the posterior probability of one point in the observed set corresponding to one point in the model set is computed.

© Springer Nature Switzerland AG 2018
M. Reuter et al. (Eds.): ShapeMI 2018, LNCS 11167, pp. 169–177, 2018.
https://doi.org/10.1007/978-3-030-04747-4_16

In the *M-step*, the best rigid transformation matrice is updated given the current posterior probabilities. The EM steps will terminate until convergence. The advantage of the EM-based method is that it does not impose a one-to-one correspondence between two point sets. There exists a large amount of work using EM technique to solve the registration problem.

There is few work attempting to utilize the normal vector associated with a point for pair-wise registrations. Under the ICP framework, the authors utilize the Gaussian and Von-Mises-Fisher distribution to model the positional and orientation localization uncertainties [3,4]. The same authors also extend their work to 2d/3d case for video-CT registration [1,5]. More recently, in [13], the authors utilize Student's t distribution and Von-Mises-Fisher distribution to tackle the group-wise 3d/3d registration problem. One disadvantage of the pair-wise registration is that it assumes one point set to be the noise-free model set. In other words, points in the model set are assumed to be perfect without noise. This will cause an imbalance between two point sets to be registered.

The most relevant registration algorithm with ours is the JRMPC method [7]. In the JRMPC, multiple point sets to be registered are assumed to be one specific realization of *Gaussian Mixture Models (GMMs)*. JRMPC algorithm was verified to outperform the state-of-the-art registration methods in terms of the robustness and accuracy. However, only the positional information is used in JRMPC. In this work, we utilize the hybrid mixture models and further formulate the EM-based approach to jointly register multiple *generalized point sets*. By jointly registering multiple point sets, the noise and outliers existing in all point sets can be dealt with more properly. With the orientational information incorporated at into each point, we demonstrate with extensive experiments that the proposed algorithm is more accurate, more robust and converges faster than the state-of-the-art algorithms.

2   Methods

Let $\mathbf{D}_j = [\mathbf{d}_{j1}...\mathbf{d}_{ji}...\mathbf{d}_{jN_j}] \in \mathbb{R}^{6 \times N_j}$ be N_j *generalized points* that belong to the j-th point set, and let N be the number of point sets. We denote $\mathbf{D} = \{\mathbf{D}_j\}_{j=1}^N$ be the union of all these sets. The aim of the registration problem is to find the best rotation matrix set $\{\mathbf{R}_j\}_{j=1}^N$ and translation vector set $\{\mathbf{t}_j\}_{j=1}^N$ which align the observed point sets to an *unknown model* point set. The joint registration problem is formally formulated into a maximum likelihood (ML) problem. Under the assumption that all the observed generalized points are generated from the same hybrid mixture models (HMMs):

$$p(\mathbf{d}_{ji}) = w\frac{1}{N_j} + (1-w)\sum_{m=1}^M \frac{1}{M}p(\mathbf{d}_{ji}|m) \qquad (1)$$

where $\mathbf{d}_{ji} = (\mathbf{x}_{ji}; \widehat{\mathbf{x}}_{ji})$, $\mathbf{x}_{ji}; \widehat{\mathbf{x}}_{ji}$ represent the positional and orientational vectors, and one additional uniform distribution $p(\mathbf{x}_{ji}, \widehat{\mathbf{x}}_{ji}|M+1) = \frac{1}{N_j}$ is added to account for noise and outliers, w denotes the weight of the uniform distribution.

We now introduce the hidden variables $\mathcal{Z} = \{z_{ji}|j \in [1...N], i \in [1...N_j]\}$ such that $z_{ji} = k$ indicates that one observation $\mathbf{d}_{ji}$ is assigned to the k-th component of the HMMs. Gaussian and Von-Mises-Fisher distributions are utilized to model the positional and orientational error, respectively. Assuming that the positional and orientational error vectors are independent, the probability that the i-th observed six-dimensional point $\mathbf{d}_{ji}$ in the j-th point set is generated by the m-th hybrid mixture model point $\mu_m = (\mathbf{y}_m, \widehat{\mathbf{y}}_m)$ is defined as the following:

$$p(\mathbf{d}_{ji}|z_{ji} = m) = \underbrace{\frac{1}{(2\pi\sigma_j^2)^{\frac{3}{2}}} e^{-\frac{1}{2\sigma_j^2}\|\mathbf{x}_{ji} - (\mathbf{R}_j\mathbf{y}_m + \mathbf{t}_j)\|^2}}_{\text{Position}} \underbrace{\frac{\kappa_j}{2\pi(e^{\kappa_j} - e^{-\kappa_j})} e^{\kappa_j(\mathbf{R}_j\widehat{\mathbf{y}}_m)^\top \widehat{\mathbf{x}}_{ji}}}_{\text{Orientation}}$$

(2)

where σ_j^2 and κ_j represent the positional variance and the concentration parameter corresponding to the j-th point set.

Assuming that the observed data vectors in $\mathbf{D}$ are in independent and identically distributed (i.i.d.), the expectation of the complete *negative log-likelihood function* is the following,

$$E(\Theta) = -\sum_{j=1}^{N}\sum_{i=1}^{N_j}\sum_{m=1}^{M} \alpha_{jim}\log p(\mathbf{x}_{ji}, \widehat{\mathbf{x}}_{ji}|m; \Theta)$$

(3)

where $\Theta = (\{\mathbf{y}_m, \widehat{\mathbf{y}}_m\}_{m=1}^{M}, \{\kappa_j, \sigma_j^2, \mathbf{R}_j, \mathbf{t}_j\}_{j=1}^{N})$ are the model parameters, $\alpha_{jim} = p(\mathbf{x}_{ji}, \widehat{\mathbf{x}}_{ji}|z_{ji} = m)$ are the posterior probabilities. By ignoring the constants and utilizing the standard expressions of the likelihoods [6], we can rewrite Eq. (3) as the following:

$$E(\Theta) = -\sum_{j=1}^{N} N_{\mathbf{P}j}\log\kappa_j + \sum_{j=1}^{N} N_{\mathbf{P}j}\log(e^{\kappa_j} - e^{-\kappa_j}) - \sum_{jim} \kappa_j\alpha_{jim}(\mathbf{R}_j\widehat{\mathbf{y}}_m)^\top\widehat{\mathbf{x}}_{ji}$$
$$+ \frac{3}{2}\sum_{j=1}^{N} N_{\mathbf{P}j}\log\sigma_j^2 + \sum_{jim} \frac{1}{2\sigma_j^2}\alpha_{jim}\|(\mathbf{x}_{ji} - \mathbf{R}_j\mathbf{y}_m - \mathbf{t}_j)\|^2$$

(4)

where $N_{\mathbf{P}j} = \sum_{i=1}^{N_j}\sum_{m=1}^{M} \alpha_{jim}$ for $j = 1, \ldots, N$.

2.1 Expectation-Maximization Framework

Expectation-Maximization framework is used to solve the above ML problem. The EM steps iterates until convergence or some certain termination criteria is satisfied. Note that like the case in [7], the standard M-step of the standard Gaussian parameters are replaced with two M steps. In the two M steps, the model parameters Θ is updated.

E-Step. In *E-step*, the posterior probabilities $\alpha_{jim} = P(\mathbf{z}_{ji} = m|\mathbf{d}_{ji})$ are computed:

$$P(\mathbf{z}_{ji} = m|\mathbf{d}_{ji}) = \frac{P(\mathbf{z}_{ji} = m)p(\mathbf{d}_{ji}|\mathbf{z}_{ji} = m)}{p(\mathbf{d}_{ji})}$$

(5)

where $P(m) = \frac{1}{M}$ and $p(\mathbf{x}_{ji}, \widehat{\mathbf{x}}_{ji}|\mathbf{z}_{ji} = m)$ and are computed using Eq. (2).

M-Rigid Step. In this section, we update the rotation matrice set $\{\mathbf{R}_j\}_{j=1}^N$ by minimizing the value of the expression in Eq. (4) with respect to $\mathbf{R}_j$ for $j = 1, \ldots, N$:

$$\mathbf{R}_j^\star = \mathrm{argmin}_{\mathbf{R}_j} -\left(\underbrace{\sum_{i=1}^{N_j} \sum_{m=1}^M \frac{1}{\sigma_j^2} \alpha_{jim} (\mathbf{x}'_{ji})^\mathsf{T} \mathbf{R}_j \mathbf{y}'_{m,j}}_{\mathbf{H}_{1j}} + \underbrace{\sum_{i=1}^{N_j} \sum_{m=1}^M \kappa_j \alpha_{jim} (\mathbf{R}_j \widehat{\mathbf{y}}_m)^\mathsf{T} \widehat{\mathbf{x}}_{ji}}_{\mathbf{H}_{2j}} \right)$$

(6)

$\mathbf{x}'_{ji} = \mathbf{x}_{ji} - \boldsymbol{\mu}_{x,j}$ and $\mathbf{y}'_{m,j} = \mathbf{y}_m - \boldsymbol{\mu}_{y,j}$, wherein $\boldsymbol{\mu}_{x,j}$ and $\boldsymbol{\mu}_{y,j}$ are defined as follows:

$$\boldsymbol{\mu}_{x,j} = \frac{\sum_{i=1}^{N_j} \sum_{m=1}^M \alpha_{jim} \mathbf{x}_{ji}}{N_{\mathbf{P}j}}$$

(7)

$$\boldsymbol{\mu}_{y,j} = \frac{\sum_{i=1}^{N_j} \sum_{m=1}^M \alpha_{jim} \mathbf{y}_m}{N_{\mathbf{P}j}}$$

(8)

We can reformulate the objective function in Eq. (6) as the following: $\mathbf{R}_j = \mathrm{argmax}\left(\overbrace{\mathbf{H}_{1j} + \mathbf{H}_{2j}}^{\mathbf{H}_j} \right)$. After doing the singular value decomposition (SVD) of $\mathbf{H}_j$ as $\mathbf{H}_j = \mathbf{U}_j \mathbf{S}_j \mathbf{V}_j^\mathsf{T}$, we can now get the updated rotation matrice set $\{\mathbf{R}_j^\star\}_{j=1}^N, \forall j \in [1...N]$ as:

$$\mathbf{R}_j^\star = \mathbf{V}_j \, \mathrm{diag}\left([1, 1, \det(\mathbf{V}_j \mathbf{U}_j^\mathsf{T})] \right) \, \mathbf{U}_j^\mathsf{T}$$

(9)

Next, by computing the partial derivative of $E(\Theta)$ in Eq. (4) with respect to $\{\mathbf{t}_j\}$ and equaling the result to zero, we can get the updated translation vectors $\{\mathbf{t}_j^\star\}_{j=1}^N, \forall j \in [1...N]$ as

$$\mathbf{t}_j^\star = \frac{\sum_{i=1}^{N_j} \sum_{m=1}^M \alpha_{jim} \mathbf{x}_{ji} - \sum_{i=1}^{N_j} \sum_{m=1}^M \alpha_{jim} \mathbf{R}_j^\star \mathbf{y}_m}{N_{\mathbf{P}j}}$$

(10)

We should note the updated translation vector $\mathbf{t}_j^\star$ is only up to the positional information associated with each point.

M-Var Step. The positional variances $\{\sigma_j^2\}_{j=1}^N$ are updated by $\partial E(\Theta)/\partial \sigma_j^2 = 0, \forall j \in [1...N]$:

$$(\sigma_j^2)^\star = \frac{\sum_{i=1}^{N_j} \sum_{m=1}^M ||\mathbf{x}_{ji} - (\mathbf{R}_j^\star \mathbf{y}_m + \mathbf{t}_j^\star)||^2}{3N_{\mathbf{P}j}}$$

(11)

We again notice that the updated variance $(\sigma_j^2)^\star$ is only up to the positional information associated with each point. The concentration parameters $\{\kappa_j\}_{j=1}^N$

are updated by solving $\partial E(\Theta)/\partial \kappa_j = 0, \forall j \in [1...N]$:

$$\frac{1}{\kappa_j} = \frac{e^{\kappa_j} + e^{-\kappa_j}}{e^{\kappa_j} - e^{-\kappa_j}} - \frac{1}{N_{\mathbf{P}j}} \sum_{i}^{N_j} \sum_{m=1}^{M} \alpha_{jim} (\mathbf{R}_j^\star \widehat{\mathbf{y}}_m)^\mathsf{T} \widehat{\mathbf{x}}_{ji} \tag{12}$$

where fixed point iteration method is used to solve the above nonlinear equation.

M-Model Step. Now we update the GMMs' means by solving $\partial E(\Theta)/\partial \mathbf{y}_m = 0, \forall m \in [1...M]$, which yields

$$\mathbf{y}_m^\star = \frac{\sum_{i=1}^{N_j} \sum_{j=1}^{N} \alpha_{jim} (\mathbf{R}_j^{\star\mathsf{T}} \mathbf{x}_{ji} - \mathbf{R}_j^{\star\mathsf{T}} \mathbf{t}_j^\star)}{N_{\mathbf{P}j}} \tag{13}$$

We update the FMM means $\{\widehat{\mathbf{y}}_m\}_{m=1}^M$ by maximizing $\mathbf{H}_{2j}$ in Eq. (4) with respect to $\widehat{\mathbf{y}}_m$ subject to the constraints $||\widehat{\mathbf{y}}_m|| = 1$ for $m = 1, \ldots, M$:

$$\widehat{\mathbf{y}}_m^\star = \frac{\sum_{i=1}^{N_j} \sum_{j=1}^{N} \kappa_j \alpha_{jim} \mathbf{R}_j^{\star\mathsf{T}} \widehat{\mathbf{x}}_{ji}}{|| \sum_{i=1}^{N_j} \sum_{j=1}^{N} \kappa_j \alpha_{jim} \mathbf{R}_j^{\star\mathsf{T}} \widehat{\mathbf{x}}_{ji}||} \tag{14}$$

Algorithm 1. Joint Rigid Registration of Multiple Generalized Point Sets

---

1 **Inputs:** Multi-dimensional point sets $\mathbf{D}_j = [\mathbf{d}_{j1}...\mathbf{d}_{ji}...\mathbf{d}_{jN_j}] \in \mathbb{R}^{6 \times N_j}$;
2 **Outputs:** $\{\mathbf{R}_j^\star, \mathbf{t}_j^\star\}_{j=1}^N$;
3 **Initialization:** Initialize $\Theta^0 = \{\mathbf{R}_j^0, \mathbf{t}_j^0, \kappa_j^0, \sigma_j^{20}\}_{j=1}^N$, unknown model point set $(\mathbf{Y}, \widehat{\mathbf{Y}})$;
4 **while** *not converged* **do**

    1. *E-step*: Compute posterioriors $\mathbf{P}$ in Eq. (5) given current parameters $\Theta = \{\mathbf{R}_j, \mathbf{t}_j, \kappa_j, \sigma_j^2\}_{j=1}^N$
    2. *M-rigid step*: Update $\{\mathbf{R}_j, \mathbf{t}_j\}_{j=1}^N$ using Eq. (6) and Eq. (10)
    3. *M-var step*: Update$\{\sigma_j^2, \kappa_j\}_{j=1}^N$ using Eq. (11) and Eq. (12)
    4. *M-model step*: Update $\{\mathbf{y}_m, \widehat{\mathbf{y}}_m\}_{m=1}^M$ using Eq. (13) and Eq. (14).

5 **end while**
6 **return** $\{\mathbf{R}_j^\star, \mathbf{t}_j^\star\}_{j=1}^N$;

2.2 Implementation and Initialization Details

As the algorithm iterates, the variance σ_j^2 will become smaller and smaller while the concentration parameter κ_j will become larger and larger. When the posterior probability $P(\mathbf{z}_{ji} = m|\mathbf{d}_{ji})$ is calculated using Eq. (5), κ_j can not be too large in order to make e^{κ_j} computable. Empirically, we set the upper bound for all κ_j as 70. The criteria for the EM steps to terminate includes the follows:

(a) the number of iterations q reaches 100; (b) the largest change of σ_j^2 among $\{\sigma_j^2\}_{j=1}^M$ is less than 10^{-8}; (c) the largest σ_j^2 among $\{\sigma_j^2\}_{j=1}^M$ is less than 10^{-5}. All methods were implemented in MATLAB (R2017b, MathWorks).

We now describe the proper initializations of the model parameters $\Theta^0 = (\{\mathbf{y}_m^0, \widehat{\mathbf{y}}_m^0\}_{m=1}^M, \{\kappa_j^0, {\sigma_j^2}^0, \mathbf{R}_j^0, \mathbf{t}_j^0\}_{j=1}^N)$. All the rotation matrices are initialized to be the identity matrice, i.e. $\mathbf{R}_j^0 = \mathbf{I}_3, \forall j \in [1...N]$. The translation vectors are initialized to be the difference of the observed point set's centroid and the model point set's one [7], i.e. $\mathbf{t}_j^0 = \overline{\mathbf{x}}_j - \overline{\mathbf{y}}$, where $\overline{\mathbf{y}}$ is the GMM centroid and $\overline{\mathbf{x}}_j$ the positional centroid of the j-th generalized point set. The variance σ_j^2 is initialized to be large while the concentration parameter κ_j is initialized to be rather small. In this paper, σ_j^2 is empirically set to be 1000 while κ_j is set to be 10, $\forall j \in [1...N]$. The rational behind this is that at the beginning of EM steps, the error values associated with both the positional and orientational information are quite large. To have a good initialization of $\{\widehat{\mathbf{y}}_m\}_{m=1}^M$, we first generate M vectors whose single element obeys the zero-mean (with 1 deg standard deviation) Gaussian distribution. Then we normalize each vector to produce the *unit* orientation vectors. The number of HMM components M is set to be 450 (referring to the parameter setting in [7]).

3   Results

To verify the proposed algorithm, we use the femur bone's surface points extracted from CT data. The human femur model $\mathbf{D}_2$ consists of $N_2 = 1568$ *generalized points*. The first point set $\mathbf{D}_1$ is generated by random sampling $N_1 = 100$ generalized points in $\mathbf{D}_2$. Positional and orientational errors are added into $\mathbf{D}_1$ to generate the *disturbed* $\mathbf{D}_1$. The error vectors are randomly generated according to Von-Mises-Fisher and Gaussian distributions with $\sigma_j^2 = \frac{1}{3}$, $\kappa_j = 3200$ for $j = 1, \ldots, N$. Moreover, to test the robustness of the proposed algorithm, outliers are further added in the *disturbed* $\mathbf{D}_1$. We denote one test case with specific noise and outliers injected in point sets. The registration accuracy using the proposed algorithm is compared to those using ICP [2], JRMPC [7] and ECMPR [8] methods. For one single registration trial, the 'true' rigid transformation matrix $[\mathbf{R}_{true}, \mathbf{t}_{true}]$ was generated by randomly and uniformly selecting from $[10, 20]°$ and $[10, 20]$ mm. Then $[\mathbf{R}_{true}, \mathbf{t}_{true}]$ is then applied to $\mathbf{D}_2$ to generate the *misaligned* $\mathbf{D}_2$. For each test case, $N_{trial} = 30$ trials are conducted. In one registration trial, the *misaligned* $\mathbf{D}_2$ are registered to the *disturbed* $\mathbf{D}_1$ to recover the rigid transformation $[\mathbf{R}_{cal}, \mathbf{t}_{cal}]$ using all test algorithms. More specifically, in a pair-wise registration, $\mathbf{R}_{cal} = \mathbf{R}_{1,cal}^\top \mathbf{R}_{2,cal}$. The rotational errors in one single trial are calculated as follows:$\mathbf{R}_{err} = ||\mathbf{R}_{cal} - \mathbf{R}_{true}||_F$, where $|| \bullet ||_F$ stands for the Frobenius norm of a matrix. The mean and standard deviation of rotational error computed are recorded since the translational error is not challenging [7] (Fig. 1).

Error Exists in One Point Set. In this case, the *misaligned* $\mathbf{D}_2$ is the model point set without noise injected. Table 1 shows the rotational error statistics.

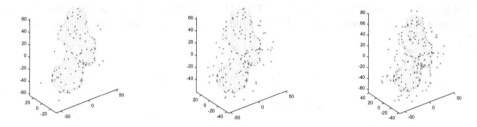

Fig. 1. Femur-bone point sets with 10%, 50% and 90% outliers. All are in mm units. The positions of points in the *model* set, points in the sampled *measured* set, outliers in the *measured* set are represented by *green, blue* and *red* dots, respectively. (Color figure online)

Several observations can be made from Table 1: (a) ICP and JRMPC performs worse with more outliers; (b) ECMPR and the proposed algorithm's performances are quite stable with respect to different percentages of outliers; (c) the proposed algorithm achieves the smallest among the four test algorithms in all test cases. For example, we achieved $\mathbf{R}_{err} = 0.0278 \pm 0.0242$ while JRMPC achieved $\mathbf{R}_{err} = 0.0917 \pm 0.0828$ in the last test case.

Error Exists in Two Point Sets. In this section, error vectors are further injected into the *misaligned* $\mathbf{D}_2$. Thus, both *misaligned* $\mathbf{D}_2$ and *disturbed* $\mathbf{D}_1$ can be considered as observed point set. Table 2 summarizes the registration accuracy. Similar observations can be made like those in Table 1. Comparing the results in Table 1 with those in Table 2, we can conclude that all algorithms achieves larger rotational error when noise exists in both point sets.

Table 1. Rotational errors using ICP, JRMPC, ECMPR and the proposed algorithm. Different ratios of outliers are added into $\mathbf{D}_1$. Isotropic noise are injected into $\mathbf{D}_1$.

Algorithms	10%	30%	50%	70%	90%
ICP	0.0632 ± 0.0496	0.1284 ± 0.1024	0.1942 ± 0.1046	0.1772 ± 0.0982	0.2013 ± 0.1051
JRMPC	0.0322 ± 0.0195	0.0330 ± 0.0264	0.0451 ± 0.0364	0.0813 ± 0.0710	0.0917 ± 0.0828
ECMPR	0.0439 ± 0.0208	0.0416 ± 0.0203	0.0389 ± 0.0170	0.0393 ± 0.0176	0.0369 ± 0.0176
Proposed	$\mathbf{0.0265 \pm 0.0147}$	$\mathbf{0.0255 \pm 0.0208}$	$\mathbf{0.0225 \pm 0.0118}$	$\mathbf{0.0250 \pm 0.0125}$	$\mathbf{0.0278 \pm 0.0242}$

Figure 2 plots the rotational errors with respect to iterations in one random registration trial from the case when 10% outliers exist in $\mathbf{D}_1$, respectively. In all $100 * 0.1 + 100 = 110$ points exist in the *disturbed* outliers. As shown in both plots, the proposed algorithm (a) converges much faster (around 10 iterations) than the other three algorithms do; (b) achieves the smallest rotational error among the four algorithms. With the orientational information incorporated, JRMPC converges even slower than the ICP does.

Table 2. Rotational Errors using ICP, JRMPC, ECMPR and the Proposed Algorithm, Different Ratios of Outliers are added. Isotropic noise are injected into both point sets D_1 and D_2.

Methods	10%	30%	50%	70%	90%
ICP	0.0839 ± 0.0586	0.1281 ± 0.0782	0.2011 ± 0.0984	0.1899 ± 0.0937	0.1985 ± 0.0946
JRMPC	0.0416 ± 0.0208	0.0589 ± 0.0548	0.0478 ± 0.0388	0.0823 ± 0.0633	0.1060 ± 0.0882
ECMPR	0.0463 ± 0.0230	$\mathbf{0.0443 \pm 0.0234}$	0.0417 ± 0.0212	0.0413 ± 0.0202	0.0398 ± 0.0211
Proposed	$\mathbf{0.0397 \pm 0.0222}$	0.0444 ± 0.0273	$\mathbf{0.0396 \pm 0.0237}$	$\mathbf{0.0395 \pm 0.0211}$	$\mathbf{0.0386 \pm 0.0193}$

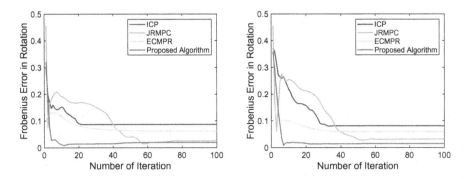

Fig. 2. The convergence rate of rotational error using the four algorithms in one random trial when 10% outliers are added in the into D_1. (Left) Error exists in one point set D_1; (Right) Error exists in both point sets D_1 and D_2.

4   Conclusion and Future Work

In this study, we present a novel joint registration method of multiple generalized point sets under the expectation maximization framework. The orientation information is incorporated into registration and all the point sets to be registered are considered to be observed ones. The experimental results show its promising clinical applications in computer-assisted surgery for its high accuracy and robustness and fast convergence speed.

Acknowledgments. This project is partially supported by the Hong Kong RGC GRF grants #14210117, and Shenzhen Science and Technology Innovation projects JCYJ20170413161616163 awarded to Max Q.-H. Meng.

References

1. Baka, N., Metz, C., Schultz, C.J., van Geuns, R.J., Niessen, W.J., van Walsum, T.: Oriented Gaussian mixture models for nonrigid 2D/3D coronary artery registration. IEEE Trans. Med. Imag. **33**(5), 1023–1034 (2014)
2. Besl, P.J., McKay, N.D., et al.: A method for registration of 3-D shapes. IEEE Trans. Pattern Anal. Mach. Intell. **14**(2), 239–256 (1992)

3. Billings, S., Taylor, R.: Iterative most likely oriented point registration. In: Golland, P., Hata, N., Barillot, C., Hornegger, J., Howe, R. (eds.) MICCAI 2014. LNCS, vol. 8673, pp. 178–185. Springer, Cham (2014). https://doi.org/10.1007/978-3-319-10404-1_23
4. Billings, S., Taylor, R.: Generalized iterative most likely oriented-point (G-IMLOP) registration. Int. J. Comput. Assist. Radiol. Surg. **10**(8), 1213–1226 (2015)
5. Billings, S.D., et al.: Anatomically constrained video-CT registration via the V-IMLOP algorithm. In: Ourselin, S., Joskowicz, L., Sabuncu, M.R., Unal, G., Wells, W. (eds.) MICCAI 2016. LNCS, vol. 9902, pp. 133–141. Springer, Cham (2016). https://doi.org/10.1007/978-3-319-46726-9_16
6. Bishop, C.M.: Pattern Recognition and Machine Learning. Springer, New York (2006)
7. Evangelidis, G.D., Horaud, R.: Joint alignment of multiple point sets with batch and incremental expectation-maximization. IEEE Trans. Pattern Anal. Mach. Intell. **40**(6), 1397–1410 (2017)
8. Horaud, R., Forbes, F., Yguel, M., Dewaele, G., Zhang, J.: Rigid and articulated point registration with expectation conditional maximization. IEEE Trans. Pattern Anal. Mach. Intell. **33**(3), 587–602 (2011)
9. Min, Z., Meng, M.Q.H.: General first-order TRE model when using a coordinate reference frame for rigid point-based registration. In: 2017 IEEE 14th International Symposium on Biomedical Imaging, ISBI 2017, pp. 169–173. IEEE (2017)
10. Min, Z., Ren, H., Meng, M.Q.H.: Estimation of surgical tool-tip tracking error distribution in coordinate reference frame involving pivot calibration uncertainty. Healthc. Technol. Lett. **4**(5), 193–198 (2017)
11. Min, Z., Ren, H., Meng, M.Q.H.: TTRE: a new type of error to evaluate the accuracy of a paired-point rigid registration. In: 2017 IEEE/RSJ International Conference on Intelligent Robots and Systems, IROS 2017, pp. 953–960. IEEE (2017)
12. Min, Z., Wang, J., Meng, M.Q.H.: Robust generalized point cloud registration using hybrid mixture model. In: 2018 IEEE International Conference on Robotics and Automation, ICRA, pp. 4812–4818. IEEE (2018)
13. Ravikumar, N., Gooya, A., Frangi, A.F., Taylor, Z.A.: Generalised coherent point drift for group-wise registration of multi-dimensional point sets. In: Descoteaux, M., Maier-Hein, L., Franz, A., Jannin, P., Collins, D.L., Duchesne, S. (eds.) MICCAI 2017. LNCS, vol. 10433, pp. 309–316. Springer, Cham (2017). https://doi.org/10.1007/978-3-319-66182-7_36
14. Yaniv, Z.: Registration for orthopaedic interventions. In: Zheng, G., Li, S. (eds.) Computational Radiology for Orthopaedic Interventions. LNCVB, vol. 23, pp. 41–70. Springer, Cham (2016). https://doi.org/10.1007/978-3-319-23482-3_3

OCT Segmentation: Integrating Open Parametric Contour Model of the Retinal Layers and Shape Constraint to the Mumford-Shah Functional

Jinming Duan[1]([✉]), Weicheng Xie[2], Ryan Wen Liu[3], Christopher Tench[4], Irene Gottlob[5], Frank Proudlock[5], and Li Bai[1]

[1] School of Computer Science, University of Nottingham, Nottingham, UK
`Jiming.Duan@nottingham.ac.uk`
[2] School of Computer Science and Software Engineering, Shenzhen University, Shenzhen, China
[3] School of Navigation, Wuhan University of Technology, Wuhan, China
[4] School of Medicine, University of Nottingham, Nottingham, UK
[5] Ophthalmology Department, University of Leicester, Leicester, UK

Abstract. In this paper, we propose a novel retinal layer boundary model for segmentation of optical coherence tomography (OCT) images. The retinal layer boundary model consists of 9 open parametric contours representing the 9 retinal layers in OCT images. An intensity-based Mumford-Shah (MS) variational functional is first defined to evolve the retinal layer boundary model to segment the 9 layers simultaneously. By making use of the normals of open parametric contours, we construct equal sized adjacent narrowbands that are divided by each contour. Regional information in each narrowband can thus be integrated into the MS energy functional such that its optimisation is robust against different initialisations. A statistical prior is also imposed on the shape of the segmented parametric contours for the functional. As such, by minimising the MS energy functional the parametric contours can be driven towards the true boundaries of retinal layers, while the similarity of the contours with respect to training OCT shapes is preserved. Experimental results on real OCT images demonstrate that the method is accurate and robust to low quality OCT images with low contrast and high-level speckle noise, and it outperforms the recent geodesic distance based method for segmenting 9 layers of the retina in OCT images.

1 Introduction

Optical coherence tomography (OCT) image segmentation to detect retinal layer boundaries is a fundamental procedure for diagnosing and monitoring the progression of retinal and optical nerve diseases. There exist rich literature on approaches for automatic and semi-automatic OCT image segmentation. Common methods include deformable models [1,2], graph-based and geodesic distance methods [3,4], statistical shape and appearance models [5,6], etc. Very

© Springer Nature Switzerland AG 2018
M. Reuter et al. (Eds.): ShapeMI 2018, LNCS 11167, pp. 178–188, 2018.
https://doi.org/10.1007/978-3-030-04747-4_17

recently, deep neural networks are becoming increasingly popular for OCT segmentation, demonstrating excellent performance [7,8]. However, these deep learning methods usually require the networks to be sufficiently deep to learn all appearance and shape variations of the retinal layers from annotated training sets. Therefore the training set has to be very large and rich to prevent the over-fitting. Large annotated training sets are however difficult to obtain. Existing OCT segmentation algorithms also tend to segment individual retinal layers separately. This form of analysis often fails when there is uncertainty in the image, especially some retinal layers are often difficult to see or missing in OCT images.

We believe that OCT segmentation is more effective by incorporating anatomical shape of the retinal layers and their spatial relations. As such, in this paper we propose a shape-based variational Mumford-Shah (MS) functional for segmentation of up to 9 retinal layer boundaries in OCT images, using only a small training set. We make three distinct contributions to OCT segmentation:

- We introduce a new piecewise constant variational MS functional to evolve a pre-defined retinal layer boundary model for OCT image segmentation. It has a region-based data fidelity term and a hybridised first and second regularisation term. The pre-defined retinal layer boundary model consists of 9 retinal layer boundaries, each is an open explicit parametric contour represented by a set of control points. We then construct two narrowbands around each open contour, within which region-based information is derived to aid contour evolution. We show that by incorporating a retinal layer boundary model our method can segment 9 retinal layers simultaneously, and by utilising regional information, the proposed method has a large convergence range and is robust to initialisation.
- We introduce to the MS functional a shape constraint learnt from a set of training OCT shapes. We then apply the principal component analysis (PCA) to derive the statistical distribution from the training shapes as well as the resulting irregular contours evolved directly from the MS functional. In this way, the irregular contours are restricted to a manifold of familiar shapes and thereby can be pulled back to appropriate positions to allow a faster convergence.
- We apply the proposed method to real OCT dataset acquired from healthy subjects, and demonstrate that the proposed method outperforms the state-of-the-art methods.

2   Methodology

2.1   Intensity-Based Variational MS Functional

We start with a new intensity-based MS segmentation functional, and then apply a learnt shape constraint to the functional. We define a retinal layer boundary model as having 9 retinal layers, each of which is an explicit parametric contour

C. Based on [9], we propose a new piecewise constant MS functional for each of the 9 retinal layers

$$E\left(\{u_i\}, C\right) = \sum_i \int_{\Omega_i} (f - u_i)^2 dx + \frac{\alpha}{2} \int_0^1 |C_s(s)|^2 ds + \frac{\beta}{2} \int_0^1 |C_{ss}(s)|^2 ds, \quad (1)$$

where f is the input image and u_i are the mean grey value of region Ω_i. The first regional energy term follows the Chan-Vese model [2,10]. In the second term, C_s is the first order derivative of the curve C with respect to the arc length s normalized into the region $[0,1]$, and C_{ss} is the second order derivative. α and β are two regularisation coefficients. To segment a retinal layer in OCT, i has two values, namely, $1, 2$. The contour regularisation (last two terms) combines the first and second order derivatives, preventing the contour from bending by introducing elasticity and stiffness to the contour. Each control point of the contour thus can be more equidistant or centred between its neighbourhood points. This makes the functional stable for numerical calculation. C is defined as a parametric contour of a set of control points

$$C(s) = (\boldsymbol{x}, \boldsymbol{y})^T. \quad (2)$$

Here $\boldsymbol{x} = (x_1, \cdots, x_M)$, $\boldsymbol{y} = (y_1, \cdots, y_M)$ are the coordinates of the M control points to represent one retinal layer boundary. The start and end points are $C(0) = (x_1, y_1)^T$ and $C(1) = (x_M, y_M)^T$, respectively.

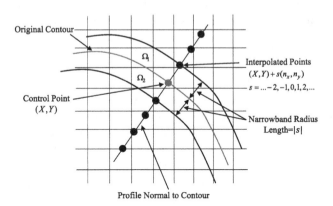

Fig. 1. A strategy to construct a narrowband around an open contour. In the narrowband region information can be utilised.

Variational methods taking into account regional information are generally more robust against noisy and initialisation. In OCT segmentation, we however require the parametric contour C to be an open curve [5]. In this case, $C(0)$ is no longer equal to $C(1)$. This brings difficulties in estimating parameter (u_1, u_2) in (1) due to the vanished image regions Ω_1 and Ω_2. To circumvent this limitation, we propose to construct a narrowband around the open contour C using the method illustrated in Fig. 1:

- For each control point on C, such as the red dot in Fig. 1, we compute its normal using the neighbourhood control points;
- We define a narrowband radius $|s|$, and interpolate new points, as represented by the black dots in Fig. 1, along the two normal directions of the original control points;
- We determine those pixels that have fallen in the narrowband between the two contours in Fig. 1 and afterwards compute (u_1, u_2) as in (3).

2.2   Minimisation of MS by Gradient Descent

We minimise the proposed functional (1) with respect to both the parameter (u_1, u_2) and the contour C, where (u_1, u_2) denote the mean grey values on both sides of contour curve C and have a simple closed-form

$$u_i = \frac{1}{|\Omega_i|} \int_{\Omega_i} f dx, \quad i = 1, 2, \tag{3}$$

where $\Omega_i, i = 1, 2$ are the two regions partitioned by the curve C and they change as the curve evolves. Since we are able to construct regions Ω_i from an open contour C, it is easy to calculate u_i in (3). After u_i are estimated, we fix u_i and use the gradient descent method to minimise the functional (1) with respect to the open contour C. This results in the following contour evolution equation

$$\frac{\partial C(s,t)}{\partial t} = -\frac{\partial E(C)}{\partial C} = \alpha C_{ss}(s,t) - \beta C_{ssss}(s,t) - Q(s,t) \, \boldsymbol{n}(s,t). \tag{4}$$

where $Q(s,t) = (f - u_1)^2 - (f - u_2)^2$, and $\boldsymbol{n}(s,t) = (\boldsymbol{n}_x(s,t), \boldsymbol{n}_y(s,t))$ denotes the outer normal vector of the contour C. The first two terms on the right-hand side of (4) minimise the contour length and thereby enforce an equidistant spacing between the control points. The third term maximises the homogeneity in the adjoining regions in the narrowband, which is measured by the energy density (3). This forces C move towards a retinal layer boundary in the OCT image.

We now need to discretise (4) for numerical implementation. Specifically, for each control point of the contour C, we have the following two semi-implicit iterative schemes

$$\frac{x_i^{k+1} - x_i^k}{\Delta t} = \alpha \partial_{xx} x_i^{k+1} - \beta \partial_{xxxx} x_i^{k+1} - Q(x_i^k, y_i^k) \boldsymbol{n}_x(x_i^k, y_i^k), \tag{5}$$

$$\frac{y_i^{k+1} - y_i^k}{\Delta t} = \alpha \partial_{yy} y_i^{k+1} - \beta \partial_{yyyy} y_i^{k+1} - Q(x_i^k, y_i^k) \boldsymbol{n}_y(x_i^k, y_i^k), \tag{6}$$

where Δt is an artificial time parameter. The superscript k denotes the kth iteration, and the subscript i the ith control point. As compared to explicit iterative methods, semi-implicit relaxation methods allow the use of a relative larger time step Δt, speeding up the convergence rate of contour evolution. We apply the finite difference method with Neumann boundary condition [11] to discretise the 2nd- and 4th-order derivatives $\partial_{xx} x_i$, $\partial_{yy} y_i$, $\partial_{xxxx} x_i$ and $\partial_{yyyy} y_i$.

To iterate (5) and (6), the open contour normals $(\boldsymbol{n}_x, \boldsymbol{n}_y)$ are calculated in Fig. 2. Apart from the two endpoints, for each control point on the contour we first compute its tangent using its neighbours via the centre finite difference scheme. For the start and end points, their tangents are respectively computed with the forward and backward finite differences. The contour normals thereby can be easily derived from the computed tangents because they are perpendicular to each other.

Note that given M control points we have to calculate a set of $2M$ equations as in (5) and (6). Since the 2nd- and 4th-order derivatives are linear differential operators, we can rewrite (5) and (6) to its matrix form as

$$\boldsymbol{x}^{k+1} = (I - \Delta t \mathbf{A})^{-1} \left(\boldsymbol{x}^k - \Delta t Q \left(\boldsymbol{x}^k, \boldsymbol{y}^k \right) \cdot \boldsymbol{n}_x \left(\boldsymbol{x}^k, \boldsymbol{y}^k \right) \right), \qquad (7)$$

$$\boldsymbol{y}^{k+1} = (I - \Delta t \mathbf{A})^{-1} \left(\boldsymbol{y}^k - \Delta t Q \left(\boldsymbol{x}^k, \boldsymbol{y}^k \right) \cdot \boldsymbol{n}_y \left(\boldsymbol{x}^k, \boldsymbol{y}^k \right) \right), \qquad (8)$$

where I is the identity matrix, $\cdot$ denotes pointwise multiplication and $\mathbf{A}$ is an $M \times M$ matrix of the form

$$\begin{pmatrix}
-\alpha - 2\beta & \alpha + 3\beta & -\beta & 0 & 0 & 0 & \cdots & 0 & 0 \\
\alpha + 3\beta & -2\alpha - 6\beta & \alpha + 4\beta & -\beta & 0 & 0 & \cdots & 0 & 0 \\
-\beta & \alpha + 4\beta & -2\alpha - 6\beta & \alpha + 4\beta & -\beta & 0 & \cdots & 0 & 0 \\
0 & -\beta & \alpha + 4\beta & -2\alpha - 6\beta & \alpha + 4\beta & -\beta & \cdots & 0 & 0 \\
0 & 0 & -\beta & \alpha + 4\beta & -2\alpha - 6\beta & \alpha + 4\beta & \cdots & 0 & 0 \\
\vdots & \vdots & \vdots & \vdots & \vdots & \vdots & \ddots & \vdots & \vdots \\
0 & 0 & 0 & 0 & 0 & 0 & \cdots & -2\alpha - 6\beta & \alpha + 3\beta \\
0 & 0 & 0 & 0 & 0 & 0 & \cdots & \alpha + 3\beta & -\alpha - 2\beta
\end{pmatrix}.$$

Matrix $\mathbf{A}$ satisfies the condition that $C(0) \neq C(1)$. It is a sparse matrix and only 5 diagonals have non-zero values so can be inverted efficiently. The Eqs. (7) and (8) are now discretised with a set of control points. The solutions gives the coordinates of all the control points $(\boldsymbol{x}, \boldsymbol{y})$ at $(k + 1)$th iteration.

2.3   Integrating Shape Constraint to Intensity-Based MS

The contour evolution driven by (7) and (8) can become irregular as the MS functional uses only local pixel intensities. To further improve the MS functional we propose to impose some constraint for the functional to control contour evolution. With some manually segmented retinal layer boundaries as training shapes we can derive the statistical distribution of the retinal layer boundaries as a shape constraint on the MS functional. The main idea of this is to project the irregular shapes into a latent space spanned by a few eigenvectors of training shapes with largest eigenvalues. In this way, the resulting irregular shapes are restricted to a manifold of familiar shapes and thereby can be corrected. Note that other dimensionality reduction methods can be also used to derive shape constraint. In this work we found PCA performs reasonably well. Next we detail the use of shape constraint to (1) using PCA. Note that an OCT shape model represents the locations of 9 boundaries.

If one OCT shape model consists of N control points, it can be modelled as a $2N$-dimensional vector $\boldsymbol{z} = (x_1, \cdots, x_N, y_1, \cdots, y_N)^T$, where $N = 9M$ (M

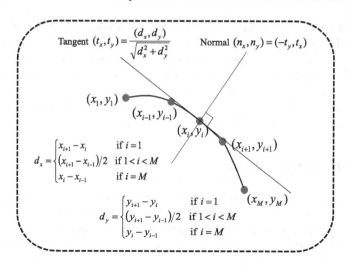

Fig. 2. Computing normals of a discrete point on an open parametric curve.

appears in (2)). Assuming that we have L training shapes manually annotated from L OCT images. We first align all shapes at the centre of coordinate origin by applying the Procrustes transformations. The mean OCT shape is then computed by $\tilde{z} = \frac{1}{L}\sum_{j=1}^{L} z_j$. For each shape z_j in the training set, its deviation from the mean shape $\tilde{z}$ is $dz_j = z_j - \tilde{z}$. Then the $2N \times 2N$ covariance matrix **Cov** can be calculated by $\mathbf{Cov} = \frac{1}{L-1}\sum_{j=1}^{L} dz_j dz_j^T$.

We calculate the eigenvectors v_k and corresponding eigenvalues λ_k of **Cov** (sorted so that $\lambda_k \leq \lambda_{k+1}$). Let $\mathbf{P} = (p_1, \ldots, p_m)$ be the matrix of the first m eigenvectors of v_k. Then we can approximate an OCT shape in the training set by

$$z \approx \tilde{z} + \mathbf{P}b, \qquad (9)$$

where $b = (b_1. b_2, \ldots, b_m)$ defines the parameters for m different deformation patterns. Since $\mathbf{P}$ is an orthogonal matrix, b is given by

$$b = \mathbf{P}^T(z - \tilde{z}). \qquad (10)$$

By varying the parameters b_i, we can generate new examples of the shape. We can also limit each b_i to constrain the deformation patterns of the shape. Typical limits [6] are

$$-3\sqrt{\lambda_i} \leq b_i \leq 3\sqrt{\lambda_i}, \qquad (11)$$

where $i = 1, \ldots, m$.

The use of shape constraint to (1) for segmenting 9 retinal layer boundaries is summarised as follow: $\mathbf{P}$, $\tilde{z}$ and λ_i are first computed from a set of training OCT shapes. After the original OCT shape model (locations of 9 boundaries) is updated with (7) and (8) (each boundary in the shape model is updated separately), it is transformed to approximate the mean shape $\tilde{z}$ with the Procrustes transformation, which forms z. This is followed by updating b using (10) and then projecting it using (11), i.e. the coefficients b obtained with (10) are constrained with equation (11). Next, we correct the original OCT shape using (9) with the projected b and warping the corrected version back to the original location. In this way, the original irregular OCT shape is pulled back to a regular one used for the next iteration of (7) and (8). The whole process is repeated until convergence. The overall numerical optimisation of the proposed method is fast as it only computes a few hundred control points.

3   Experimental Results

Data: 9 retinal layers boundaries were segmented for each image from in vivo OCT B-scans. 30 Spectralis SDOCT (ENVISU C class 2300, Bioptigen, axial resolution = $3.3\,\mu$m, scan depth = 3.4 mm, 32,000 A-scans per second) B-scans from 15 healthy adults were used for the work. The B-scan was imaged from the left and right eye of the healthy adults using a spectral domain OCT device with a chin rest to stabilise the head. The B-scan located at the foveal centre was identified from the lowest point in the foveal pit where the cone outer segments were elongated (indicating cone specialisation). The ground truth boundaries were manually generated by an experienced ophthalmologist. The dataset was randomly split into 20 training and 10 (5 are corrupted with high-level speckle noise using Matlab *imnoise* function with 0.8 variance) validation datasets. For image pre-processing, all images were cropped to extract only region of interest and were flattened using ground truth labels before training. The 9 retinal layer boundaries which can be segmented by the proposed method are shown in Fig. 3.

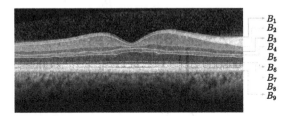

Fig. 3. An example B-Scan OCT image centred at the macula, showing 9 target intra-retinal layer boundaries. The names of these boundaries labelled as notations $B_1, B_2...B_9$ are summarised in Table 1.

Parameters: These parameters in our method are the first and second order regularisation parameters α and β, the artificial time step Δt, the narrowband radius $|s|$, the number of eigenvectors/eigenvalues t, the number of control points for 9 boundaries, and the iteration number (1000).

  These parameters are selected as follows: (1) Large α and β leads to increasingly shorter and finally vanishing segmentation boundaries. Small values may

Table 1. Notations for nine retinal boundaries, their corresponding names and abbreviations

Notation	Name of retinal boundary/surface	Abbreviation
B_1	Internal limiting membrane	ILM
B_2	Outer boundary of the retinal nerve fibre layer	$RNFL_o$
B_3	Inner plexiform layer-inner nuclear layer	IPL-INL
B_4	Inner nuclear layer-outer plexiform layer	INL-OPL
B_5	Outer plexiform layer-outer nuclear layer	OPL-ONL
B_6	Outer nuclear layer-inner segments of photoreceptors	ONL-IS
B_7	Inner segments of photoreceptors-outer segments of photoreceptors	IS-OS
B_8	Outer segments of of photoreceptors-retinal pigment epithelium	OS-RPE
B_9	Retinal pigment epithelium-choroid	RPE-CH

cause control points intersect with each other, thus leading to numerical instabilities. In this work, we fixed $\alpha = \beta = 0.5$; (2) Δt is bounded by the CFL stability condition. Numerical stabilities can be attained by using $\Delta t = 0.01$; (3) $|s|$ was selected according to the initial OCT boundaries. If initialisation is close to the true retinal layer boundaries, $|s|$ is small (10 pixels for Fig. 4 1st row). Otherwise, a large $|s|$ should be used (50 pixels for Fig. 4 last row). Note that we set $|s|$ the same value for each of 9 OCT boundaries; (4) t was confirmed by choosing the first t largest eigenvalues such that $\sum_{i=1}^{t} \lambda_i \geq 0.98 V_T$, where V_T is the total variance of all the eigenvalues. We used the number of training samples as the value of t. Eigenvectors corresponding to small eigenvalues do not contribute much to shape variation; (5) 360 control points in total are used for a whole OCT shape (each retinal layer boundary thus has 40). Overall, we only adjusted $|s|$ for different initialisations (see Fig. 4).

Comparsion: The performance of the proposed segmentation method was evaluated by computing the Hausdorff distance (HD) metric between the automated and ground truth segmentations for different retinal layer boundaries. We compared our method with the geodesic distance method proposed in [4]. In Fig. 5, visual comparison suggests that the proposed method provides significant improvements over intensity-based geodesic distance in OCT segmentation, especially when OCT images are of low contrast and contain high-level speckle noise. In Table 2, we report the HD metric of each boundary as well as the total 9 boundaries over the validation dataset and show that our method outperforms the geodesic distance in terms of the HD metric for all the retinal layer boundaries. The improvements are more evident at IML, $RNFL_\sigma$, IPL-INL, INL-OPL and OPL-ONL boundary locations. Note that in order to compare our results with ground truth labels we fitted a spline curve to each segmentation contour such that the resulting contours run across the entire width of the OCT image.

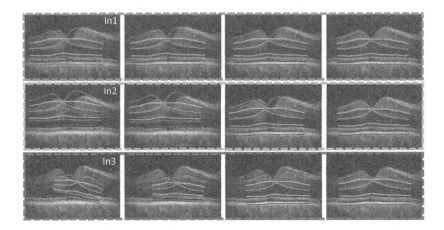

Fig. 4. Experiments of contour evolution with different initialisation conditions for the proposed method. 1st column: three initialisations (i.e. In1, In2 and In3); 2nd-3rd columns: intermediate contour evolution; 4th column: final segmentation results; 5th column: notation abbreviations for 9 retinal layer boundaries (refer to Fig. 3 for their full name). The experiments show that by incorporating region-based information our method has much larger convergence range so it is robust against different initialisations.

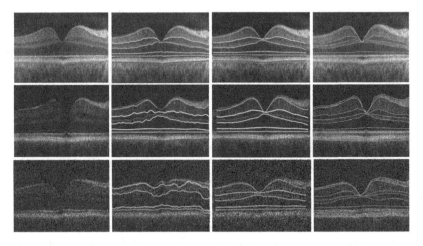

Fig. 5. Visual comparison of segmentation of 9 retinal layer boundaries using the geodesic distance [4] and proposed shape-based MS method. 1st column: input B-scans; 2nd column: geodesic distance results; 3rd column: our results; 4th column: ground truth.

Table 2. Quantitative comparison of segmentation results from the geodesic distance method (GDM) and proposed method for different retinal layer boundary, in terms of Hausdorff distance metric (mean±standard deviation).

	IML	NFL$_\sigma$	IPL-INL	INL-OPL	OPL-ONL
GDM [4]	9.80 ± 2.51	10.2 ± 3.32	25.26 ± 10.5	22.55 ± 8.96	20.46 ± 7.24
Proposed	1.72 ± 0.52	1.68 ± 0.66	1.058 ± 0.12	0.925 ± 0.10	0.863 ± 0.23
	ONL-IS	IS-OS	OS-RPE	RPE-CH	Overall
GDM [4]	2.53 ± 1.05	1.91 ± 1.34	1.21 ± 1.05	1.031 ± 0.98	10.55 ± 4.10
Proposed	0.61 ± 0.05	0.84 ± 0.11	1.61 ± 0.96	0.952 ± 0.78	1.140 ± 0.39

4   Conclusion

We presented a new segmentation method for optical coherence tomography (OCT) images, which allows the integration of statistical shape models learned from a small OCT dataset. To this end, we developed the Mumford-Shah functional in a way which facilitates a parametric representation of open contours. We then constructed narrowbands around the open contours such that regional information can be derived to assist segmentation. We have shown that integrating such information allows the proposed method to have a large convergence range and thus robust against different initialisations. We have also validated that the proposed method is very accurate even OCT images are of low contrast and contain high-level speckle noise, and that the method outperforms the state-of-the-art geodesic distance segmentation method. The proposed method can be readily extended to other segmentation problems involving open contours.

References

1. Rossant, F., Bloch, I., Ghorbel, I., Paques, M.: Parallel double snakes. Application to the segmentation of retinal layers in 2D-OCT for pathological subjects. Pattern Recognit. **48**(12), 3857–3870 (2015)
2. Chan, T.F., Vese, L.A.: Active contours without edges. IEEE Trans. Image Process. **10**(2), 266–277 (2001)
3. Chiu, S.J., Li, X.T., Nicholas, P., Toth, C.A., Izatt, J.A., Farsiu, S.: Automatic segmentation of seven retinal layers in SDOCT images congruent with expert manual segmentation. Opt. Express **18**(18), 19413–19428 (2010)
4. Duan, J., Tench, C., Gottlob, I., Proudlock, F., Bai, L.: Automated segmentation of retinal layers from optical coherence tomography images using geodesic distance. Pattern Recognit. **72**, 158–175 (2017)
5. Xie, W., Duan, J., Shen, L., Li, Y., Yang, M., Lin, G.: Open snake model based on global guidance field for embryo vessel location. IET Comput. Vis. **12**(2), 129–137 (2018)
6. Cootes, T., Baldock, E., Graham, J.: An introduction to active shape models. In: Image Processing and Analysis, pp. 223–248. Oxford University Press, Oxford (2000)

7. Roy, A.G., et al.: Relaynet: retinal layer and fluid segmentation of macular optical coherence tomography using fully convolutional networks. Biomed. Opt. Express **8**(8), 3627–3642 (2017)

8. Fang, L., Cunefare, D., Wang, C., Guymer, R.H., Li, S., Farsiu, S.: Automatic segmentation of nine retinal layer boundaries in oct images of non-exudative amd patients using deep learning and graph search. Biomed. Opt. Express **8**(5), 2732–2744 (2017)

9. Cremers, D., Tischhäuser, F., Weickert, J., Schnörr, C.: Diffusion snakes: introducing statistical shape knowledge into the mumford-shah functional. Int. J. Comput. Vis. **50**(3), 295–313 (2002)

10. Duan, J., Pan, Z., Yin, X., Wei, W., Wang, G.: Some fast projection methods based on chan-vese model for image segmentation. EURASIP J. Image Video Process. **2014**(1), 7 (2014)

11. Noye, B.J., Arnold, R.J.: Accurate finite difference approximations for the neumann condition on a curved boundary. Appl. Math. Model. **14**(1), 2–13 (1990)

Segmenting Bones Using Statistical Shape Modeling and Local Template Matching

Elham Taghizadeh[1], Alexandre Terrier[2], Fabio Becce[3], Alain Farron[4], and Philippe Büchler[1(✉)]

[1] Institute for Surgical Technology and Biomechanics, University of Bern, Bern, Switzerland
philippe.buechler@istb.unibe.ch
[2] Laboratory of Biomechanical Orthopedics,
Ecole Polytechnique Fédérale de Lausanne, Lausanne, Switzerland
[3] Department of Diagnostic and Interventional Radiology,
Lausanne University Hospital, Lausanne, Switzerland
[4] Service of Orthopedics and Traumatology, Lausanne University Hospital,
Lausanne, Switzerland

Abstract. Accurate bone segmentation is necessary to develop chairside manufacturing of implants based on additive manufacturing. Various automatic segmentation techniques have been proposed to streamline the process (e.g. graph-cut or deep-learning), but these techniques do not provide anatomical correspondences during the segmentation process, which makes exploitation of segmentation more difficult to predict missing bone parts in case of fracture or its premorbid shape for degenerative diseases. Bone segmentation using active shape model (ASM) would provide anatomical correspondences. However, this technique is error prone for thin structures, such as the scapular blade or orbital walls. Therefore, we developed a new method relying on shape model fitting and local correction relying on image similarities. The method was evaluated on three challenging anatomical locations: (i) healthy and osteoarthritic scapulae, (ii) orbital bones, and (iii) mandible. On average, results were accurate with surface distance of about 0.5 mm and average Dice coefficients above 90%. This approach was able to separate joint bone surfaces, even in challenging pathological situations such as osteoarthritis. Since anatomical correspondences are propagated during segmentation, the method can directly provide anatomical measurements, define personalized cutting guides, or determine the bone regions to be used to contour patient-specific implants.

Keywords: Segmentation · Bone · Scapula · Mandible · Orbit

This work was supported by the Swiss Innovation Promotion Agency (18060.2 PFIW-IW) and by the Lausanne Orthopedic Research Foundation.

© Springer Nature Switzerland AG 2018
M. Reuter et al. (Eds.): ShapeMI 2018, LNCS 11167, pp. 189–194, 2018.
https://doi.org/10.1007/978-3-030-04747-4_18

1   Introduction

Today orthopedic interventions rely on increased personalization of the intervention based on preoperative images, computer assisted planning and cutting guides [3]. Recently, 3D printing is no longer limited to the fabrication of the cutting guides but has also been employed in the production of personalized implants. Several companies propose solutions to produce patient-specific implants in Titanium, CaP ceramic or polymers (e.g. Trumatch from DePuy Synthes and Materialise, or CT-Bone from Xilloc Medical) based on additive manufacturing techniques, leading the way to chair-side manufacturing of implants. However, new technical solutions are required to enable designing implants directly next to the patient in the operating room.

In this study we develop an automated segmentation method based on statistical shape model (SSM). The proposed approach follows a similar concept as active shape modeling (ASM); information on both shape and image intensity is used for the segmentation. However, in the method proposed in this study, the image intensity is used for local correction, instead of global fitting of SSM parameters. We present results of the method obtained on three anatomical cases - scapula, orbit, and mandible - representing challenging anatomical locations due to the complexity of their shape, proximity of neighboring structures, or imaging artifacts.

2   Methods

The segmentation workflow consists in two main steps; fitting an SSM to the patient's bone followed by correction of the segmentation based on local image registration and template matching.

An initial segmentation of the bone was performed using thresholding. A few pairs of landmarks were then selected on the surface of the reconstructed bone and on the corresponding position of the mean model of the SSM. The landmarks were used to align the sample to the SSM and also to build a posterior shape model to constrain the SSM for a better fitting result [1].

The model fitting is usually not able to accurately reproduce the shape of the bone. To correct the fitting results, we use local template matching. First, we select in the training dataset the five bones that are the most similar to the patient's bone (based on shape parameters). The number of templates was chosen corresponding to an optimal balance between the improved accuracy provided by each sample and the calculation time associated with each additional template. These five samples were then used as templates; for each vertex of the model, a small image patch was extracted from the 3D dataset. The optimal position of the patch in the patient's image is determined using Normalized Correlation Coefficient (NCC), using an image patch selected around the equivalent vertex of the patient's image. A weighted voting was used to find the new location of vertices based on the image; the NCC values for each voxel of the patient's patches was added for the five templates. The values were multiplied by 3D Gaussian filter with sigma equal to the patch size, and the voxel with the maximum similarity was selected as the new location of the vertex.

The segmentation method was implemented on Matlab R2016a and the evaluation was performed on a standard desktop PC having an Intel Core i7 3770 processor at 3.5 GHz and 32 GB of RAM, running Windows 7 Professional.

3   Results

The method was tested on 63 computed tomography (CT) from scapula (combination of healthy and pathological cases), 73 cone beam computed tomography (CBCT) of mandibles, and 50 CT of orbital bones. The datasets resulted from regular clinical practice, with various image resolution and image quality. For each anatomical location, the segmentation of the images was performed by a single experienced operator and verified by a radiologist expert.

The quality of the segmentation was not the same for all the regions on the bone surface. For the scapulae, the most error-prone region was on the acromion, at the point connecting the scapula with the clavicula. Interestingly, the segmentation error on the glenohumeral contact surface was relatively small, about 0.8 mm. The largest average error for mandible was measured where the teeth were removed during the segmentation process. This large error was expected, since it is difficult to systematically remove the teeth from the bone, especially when important artifacts affect patient's images. The method also proved its ability to segment thin structures; the scapula blade as well as the orbita walls showed surface distances below 0.8 mm. Overall, the segmentation error was larger for the region that were also difficult to segment manually, typically because of a fuzzy boundary between the bone and the surrounding tissues.

Quantitatively, the average distance between the automatic and manual segmentation was below 0.5 mm (Fig. 1). More than 95% of the bone surface showed a distance to the manual segmentation below 1.3 mm, and only a few nodes had an error larger than a few millimeters. This observation is confirmed by the Hausdorff distance calculated on these datasets, which is about 1.5 mm and a Dice coefficient above 90%.

The calculation time required for the segmentation varies according to the size of the surface mesh used to represent the bone anatomy, with larger meshes requiring more time to process. Nevertheless, the time per vertex was not identical for all anatomical structures and varies between 4×10^{-2} and 10×10^{-2} seconds per vertex. The complexity of the initial threshold segmentation and the size of the search space used for correction explain this differences. On the opposite, the time for different segmentation of the same anatomical region remain relatively stable, with variations lower than 20% (6% for the mandible, 9% for the scapula, and 20% for the orbit).

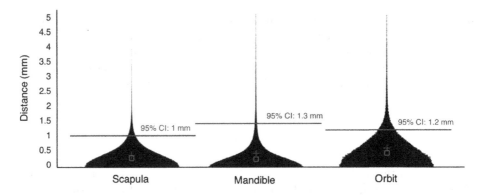

Fig. 1. Violin plots for surface distances on scapular, mandibular and orbital bones. The line on each plot represents the 95% confidence interval, the square is the median and the cross is the average of surface distances.

4   Conclusion

The segmentation approach proposed in this study was successfully tested on a challenging dataset including complex anatomy, difficult structures and very thin anatomy as well as a combination of healthy and pathological datasets.

The proposed technique provides a level of accuracy similar to existing segmentation methods, which typically enable a segmentation of the bones with an average surface distance between 0.2–0.4 mm and a Dice overlap higher than 90% [2,4–6,8–11]. Of course, the quality of the image dataset as well as the anatomical location used to evaluate these algorithms are different, and the test cases are usually limited to normal conditions. Although we believe that the test configurations used in this study represent a challenging environment, the quality of the segmentation is comparable to previous reports, especially considering the limited accuracy of the manual segmentations that represent ground truth.

However, the method presented in this work has a few distinct advantages. On one hand, it provides a precise knowledge on the anatomical position of each vertex of the surface mesh used for segmentation. This contextual information was used in this study to adapt the size of the patches used for the local correction based on the local inter-individual shape variability. This information could also be used to automatically annotate region of interests for the contouring or personalized instrumentation, or to perform automatic anatomical measurements. On the other hand, this technique relies on local correction that enables the segmentation to reach a large range of possible shapes compared to techniques solely based on SSM-based segmentation, since it is not limited to the shape variations provided by the SSM. Global fitting traditionally used tend to provide a reliable overall segmentation accuracy, but might fail to capture local shape change. Therefore, new methods to include additional flexibility to model-based segmentation are required. This feature is important when segmenting pathological structures, where the stability of the shape cannot be guaranteed across the population. As such, the proposed methodology was able to segment both healthy and pathological scapula datasets with a similar level of accuracy.

Alternative methods have been proposed for the deformation of surface models in image segmentation. Similar to the method proposed by Kainmueller [7], the displacement of the vertices are not restricted to moved along a line, but can take any position within the search space. However, the approach chosen here determines the new location of each vertex independently using multiple local registrations rather than based on image intensities and gradients. This registration approach is expected to be more robust for challenging anatomy such as OA, where osteophytes make the delineation of the bone contour difficult.

This automated approach is flexible and the segmentation can be limited to sub-regions of the anatomy of interests (for example, only the orbita was segmented out of the skull). In addition, since it doesn't rely on a label map, the method is able to segment only the outer shell of the bone. This approach represents an additional step towards personalized chair-side implant manufacturing.

References

1. Albrecht, T., Lüthi, M., Gerig, T., Vetter, T.: Posterior shape models. Med. Image Anal. **17**(8), 959–973 (2013). https://doi.org/10.1016/j.media.2013.05.010. http://www.sciencedirect.com/science/article/pii/S1361841513000844
2. Chu, C., Bai, J., Wu, X., Zheng, G.: MASCG: multi-atlas segmentation constrained graph method for accurate segmentation of hip CT images. Med. Image Anal. **26**(1), 173–184 (2015). https://doi.org/10.1016/j.media.2015.08.011. http://www.ncbi.nlm.nih.gov/pubmed/26426453
3. Eraly, K., Stoffelen, D., Vander Sloten, J., Jonkers, I., Debeer, P.: A patient-specific guide for optimizing custom-made glenoid implantation in cases of severe glenoid defects: an in vitro study. J. Shoulder Elbow Surg. **25**(5), 837–45 (2016). https://doi.org/10.1016/j.jse.2015.09.034. http://www.ncbi.nlm.nih.gov/pubmed/26700554
4. Fu, Y., Liu, S., Li, H., Yang, D.: Automatic and hierarchical segmentation of the human skeleton in CT images. Phys. Med. Biol. **62**(7), 2812–2833 (2017). https://doi.org/10.1088/1361-6560/aa6055. http://www.ncbi.nlm.nih.gov/pubmed/28195561
5. Fürnstahl, P., Fuchs, T., Schweizer, A., Nagy, L., Székely, G., Harders, M.: Automatic and robust forearm segmentation using graph cuts. In: 2008 5th IEEE International Symposium on Biomedical Imaging: From Nano to Macro, Proceedings, ISBI, pp. 77–80 (2008). https://doi.org/10.1109/ISBI.2008.4540936
6. Janssens, R., Zeng, G., Zheng, G.: Fully automatic segmentation of lumbar vertebrae from CT Images using cascaded 3D fully convolutional networks. CoRR abs/1712.0 (2017). http://arxiv.org/abs/1712.01509
7. Kainmueller, D., Lamecker, H., Heller, M.O., Weber, B., Hege, H.C., Zachow, S.: Omnidirectional displacements for deformable surfaces. Med. Image Anal. **17**(4), 429–441 (2013). https://doi.org/10.1016/j.media.2012.11.006
8. Lessmann, N., van Ginneken, B., de Jong, P.A., Išgum, I.: Iterative fully convolutional neural networks for automatic vertebra segmentation. In: Proceedings of the SPIE, vol. 10574 (2018). http://arxiv.org/abs/1804.04383

9. Shim, H., Chang, S., Tao, C., Wang, J.H., Kwoh, C.K., Bae, K.T.: Knee cartilage: efficient and reproducible segmentation on high-spatial-resolution MR images with the semiautomated graph-cut algorithm method. Radiology **251**(2), 548–56 (2009). https://doi.org/10.1148/radiol.2512081332. http://www.ncbi.nlm.nih.gov/pubmed/19401579

10. Yang, Z., et al.: Automatic bone segmentation and bone-cartilage interface extraction for the shoulder joint from magnetic resonance images. Phys. Med. Biol. **60**(4), 1441–59 (2015). https://doi.org/10.1088/0031-9155/60/4/1441. http://www.ncbi.nlm.nih.gov/pubmed/25611124

11. Zhang, J., et al.: Joint craniomaxillofacial bone segmentation and landmark digitization by context-guided fully convolutional networks. In: Descoteaux, M., Maier-Hein, L., Franz, A., Jannin, P., Collins, D.L., Duchesne, S. (eds.) MICCAI 2017. LNCS, vol. 10434, pp. 720–728. Springer, Cham (2017). https://doi.org/10.1007/978-3-319-66185-8_81

Shape Analysis of White Matter Tracts via the Laplace-Beltrami Spectrum

Lindsey Kitchell$^{(\boxtimes)}$, Daniel Bullock, Soichi Hayashi,
and Franco Pestilli

Indiana University, Bloomington, IN 47405, USA
{kitchell, franpest}@indiana.edu

Abstract. Diffusion-weighted magnetic resonance imaging (dMRI) allows for non-invasive, detailed examination of the white matter structures of the brain. White matter tract specific measures based on either the diffusion tensor model (e.g. FA, ADC, and MD) or tractography (e.g. volume, streamline count or density) are often compared between groups of subjects to localize differences within the white matter. Less commonly examined is the shape of the individual white matter tracts. In this paper, we propose to use the Laplace-Beltrami (LB) spectrum as a descriptor of the shape of white matter tracts. We provide an open, automated pipeline for the computation of the LB spectrum on segmented white matter tracts and demonstrate its efficacy through machine learning classification experiments. We show that the LB spectrum allows for distinguishing subjects diagnosed with bipolar disorder from age and sex matched healthy controls, with classification accuracy reaching 95%. We further demonstrate that the results cannot be explained by traditional measures, such as tract volume, streamline count, or mean and total length. The results indicate that there is valuable information in the anatomical shape of the human white matter tracts.

Keywords: Shape analysis · White matter · Laplace beltrami spectrum

1 Introduction

The development of diffusion-weighted magnetic resonance imaging (dMRI) has allowed for non-invasive, detailed examination of the white matter structures of the brain. Diffusion tensor imaging (DTI) models the diffusion of water molecules within the tissue of the white matter and provides measures that describe the tissue's microstructure and organization. These measures (such as fractional anisotropy, apparent diffusion coefficient, and mean diffusivity, among others) are often compared between groups of subjects, such as individuals with a neurological disorder and matched healthy controls, to localize differences within the white matter. Tractography can be applied in combination with the dMRI data to map the putative path of neuronal fiber bundles (streamlines) within the white matter. These maps are generally referred to as tractograms and they can be segmented into major white matter tracts. Tract-specific measures (such as volume, streamline density, or streamline count) are also often compared between groups, as well as the diffusion measures along the

© Springer Nature Switzerland AG 2018
M. Reuter et al. (Eds.): ShapeMI 2018, LNCS 11167, pp. 195–206, 2018.
https://doi.org/10.1007/978-3-030-04747-4_19

streamlines. Less commonly examined however, is the anatomical shape of the individual white matter tracts.

Although there are several popular methods for the shape analysis of brain structures (e.g. medial representations, spherical harmonics, deformation-based morphometry, and spectral methods [1–4]), very few have been applied to the segmented tracts of the white matter. This may be because streamlines, rather than a solid structure, are used to represent the white matter tracts, making it difficult to conceptualize the tracts as anatomical objects and to apply the more common brain shape methods. Several techniques specific to the streamline representation of white matter tracts have been developed [e.g. 5–7], however, they may have issues with proper correspondence. These methods typically try to establish correspondence either between the points along the streamlines within a tract or between the streamlines of tracts of different individuals. This can be problematic, as pointed out in Durrleman et al. [8], because it has never been shown that the points on a streamline or the streamlines themselves are homologous anatomical structures. Rather, it is the entire white matter tract that is the homologous structure across populations. Thus, it may be suggested that methods for analyzing the shape of white matter tracts should not rely on point or streamline correspondence, but should instead focus on the boundary and overall shape of the tract.

In this paper, we propose to use the Laplace-Beltrami spectrum as a global shape descriptor of white matter tracts. The Laplace-Beltrami spectrum is isometry invariant and does not require the establishment of correspondence [4, 9]. As such, it can be used to describe the boundary and general shape of the individual tracts (once converted from streamlines to a surface representation) without any registration or alignment. Additionally, the computation of the Laplace-Beltrami spectrum can be automated, making it ideal for large scale analyses, and applied to segmented tracts generated using any tractography algorithm, including probabilistic, deterministic, or ensemble methods. The Laplace-Beltrami spectrum has previously been used for the shape analysis of brain structures [e.g. 4, 10–13], however we believe this is the first study to apply it to segmented white matter tracts. We developed an automated pipeline (Fig. 1) for computing the Laplace-Beltrami spectrum on white matter tracts and make it available as open source code and as cloud-based open services at brainlife.io (see Table 1). We demonstrate the efficacy of the Laplace-Beltrami spectrum as a shape descriptor for white matter tracts using machine learning classification. We show that the Laplace-Beltrami spectrum allows for distinguishing with high accuracy between healthy controls (age and sex matched) and subjects diagnosed with bipolar disorder from the UCLA Consortium for Neuropsychiatric Phenomics LA5c Study [14]. Research on bipolar disorder has consistently demonstrated an association with abnormalities in the white matter [15]. We compare the shape-based results to analyses using volume and other tract-specific measures (e.g. total streamline count, mean length of streamlines, and total length of streamlines). Our results demonstrate that the shape of the human white matter tracts contains important information that allows for the characterization of human individuality and variability between groups of subjects. We show that the Laplace-Beltrami spectrum, when applied to white matter tracts, can be used for discriminating, with high accuracy, between healthy controls and individuals diagnosed with neuropsychiatric disorders.

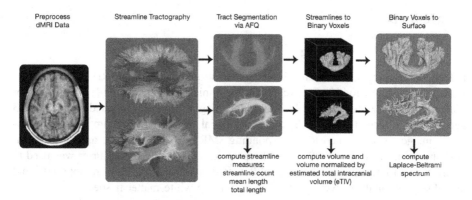

Fig. 1. Automated pipeline for shape analysis of white matter tracts.

Table 1. Links to GitHub repositories and Brainlife.io applications for each step of the pipeline.

Processing step	GitHub repository	Brainlife.io application
Preprocessing of dMRI data	github.com/brain-life/app-datanormalize	https://brainlife.io/app/ 59272453436ee50ffd669a08
	github.com/brain-life/app-splitshells	https://brainlife.io/app/ 592db717b3cd7c00211dc230
	github.com/brain-life/app-dtiinit	https://brainlife.io/app/ 58c56cf7e13a50849b258800
Freesurfer	github.com/brain-life/app-freesurfer	https://brainlife.io/app/ 58c56d92e13a50849b258801
Ensemble tracking	github.com/brain-life/app-ensembletracking	https://brainlife.io/app/ 592dbbccb3cd7c00211dc235
Tract segmentation	github.com/brain-life/app-AFQ_no-life	https://brainlife.io/app/ 59dff93521ff360021b24ebf
Segmentation cleaning	github.com/brain-life/app-AFQclean	https://brainlife.io/app/ 597f8c463a37c7002e39bf77
Binary voxel generation	github.com/kitchell/app-generatetractmasks	https://brainlife.io/app/ 592dc03eb3cd7c00211dc239
Surface generation	github.com/kitchell/app-generatetractsurfaces	https://brainlife.io/app/ 593049d7ff090a00210eff05
LB spectrum	github.com/kitchell/app-LBspectrum_matlab	https://brainlife.io/app/ 5a53b2be56e507002d1a9628
Streamline measures	github.com/kitchell/app-classifiedfibertractstats	https://brainlife.io/app/ 599f2c0a1a12b6002f642c74
Tract volume	github.com/kitchell/app-binvolvolume	https://brainlife.io/app/ 5afe0f2a2e93b90028263655

2   Methods

2.1   Data and Preprocessing

Diffusion-weighted (dMRI) and T1-weighted structural MRI (sMRI) data from the UCLA Consortium for Neuropsychiatric Phenomics LA5c Study [14] were used for this study. We used data from 43 individuals diagnosed with bipolar disorder and 43 age and sex matched controls. The dMRI (spatial resolution of 2 mm^3 and 64 directions) images were aligned to corresponding sMRI, AC-PC aligned, anatomical images, and we utilized the 1,000 s/mm^2 b-value acquisition shell. Freesurfer was used to segment the T1-weighted image into different tissue types and brain regions [16] and all subsequent analyses were performed within the white matter tissue.

2.2   Automated Pipeline for White Matter Tract Shape Analysis

Tractography Generation. For this paper, ensemble tractography methods [17–19] were used to generate a whole brain tractogram of 615,000 streamlines by seeding within the entire white matter segmentation [20]. We combined both probabilistic and deterministic tracking methods, across a range of L_{max} (2–8), a range of curvature (0.25, 0.5, 1, 2, 4), and a fixed step size of 0.2 mm.

Tract Segmentation. Twenty major white matter tracts (9 bi-hemispheric and 2 cross-hemispheric tracts) were segmented using established atlases and segmentation techniques from the Automated Fiber Quantification software (AFQ) [21]. The two cross-hemispheric tracts were the callosum forceps major and callosum forceps minor. The nine bi-hemispheric tracts (18 individual tracts) consisted of the right and left arcuate, cingulum cingulate, cingulum hippocampus, corticospinal, inferior fronto-occipital fasciculus (IFOF), inferior lateral fasciculus (ILF), super lateral fasciculus (SLF), thalamic radiation, and uncinate. An automated cleaning method provided by AFQ was applied to the segmentations to remove stray streamlines that deviate substantially from the core white matter tract path.

Binary Voxel and Surface Generation. To generate surface representations of the segmented white matter tracts, the streamline representations of each tract were first converted into a binary voxel representation. The data was resampled to a higher resolution (2 mm^3 to 0.7 mm^3) in order to create a smoother, more detailed tract. For each streamline comprising the tract, we recorded which voxels of the resampled image contained a streamline node. A smoothing kernel was applied to ensure that the volume was a spatially contiguous, non-porous object. Because this smoothing has the unintended consequence of inflating the object, we removed a proportion of the lowest density voxels (20%). Additionally, a simple masking step was performed with a node count threshold and we removed all voxels with less than 2 nodes. The resulting volume was then passed to the surface generation component of the process.

A discrete marching cubes algorithm was applied to each binary voxel representation to create a triangular surface mesh. The surface was then smoothed for 10 iterations using a windowed sinc function interpolation kernel (a standard signal processing low-pass filter) [22]. This filter essentially relaxed the mesh, making the triangular faces better shaped and the vertices more evenly distributed. After smoothing, any non-connected components of the surface (islands) were removed.

Shape Descriptor Computation. The Laplace-Beltrami (LB) spectrum was used as a shape descriptor of the surface mesh of each white matter tract. The LB spectrum allows for highly discriminative shape comparisons with minimal preprocessing [4, 9]. Importantly, the eigenvalues estimated from the LB spectrum are isometry invariant, therefore requiring no registration or mapping between the surfaces of different tracts or subjects. The eigenvalues of the Laplace-Beltrami operator, Δ, were computed using the first-order finite element method by solving the Laplacian eigenvalue problem on each given surface:

$$\Delta f = -\lambda f. \tag{1}$$

The solution consists of a number (n) of eigenvalue ($\lambda_i \in \mathbb{R}$) and eigenfunction (f_i) pairs, sorted by the eigenvalue magnitude ($0 \leq \lambda_1 \leq \lambda_2 \leq \ldots$). To achieve scale independence and allow a direct shape comparison between tracts irrespective of size, we normalized the eigenvalues by the surface area of the given tract, also known as the Riemannian volume v [9]:

$$\lambda' = vol^{-1/2}\lambda. \tag{2}$$

The normalized LB spectrum was computed on the triangle mesh surfaces of all 20 segmented white matter tracts for all subjects. Similar to spherical harmonics [2], the more eigenvalues included in the spectrum, the more details of the shape are represented (Fig. 2). Because the complexity of the shape of each tract varies widely, we used a range of non-zero eigenvalues of the LB spectrum, dependent on the tract, for the analyses in this paper. All computations of the LB spectrum were done in MatLab (Mathworks, Natick, MA) using the Geometry Processing Toolbox [23].

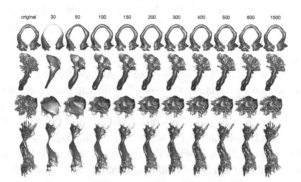

Fig. 2. White matter tracts reconstructed with different amounts of eigenfunctions. The original tract surface is shown in the leftmost column, followed by the tract reconstructed with the number of eigenvalues listed above (30–1500). Top. Callosum forceps minor tract, superior view. Middle. Left corticospinal tract, anterior and superior view. Bottom. Left IFOF tract, left view. Color = z-coordinate of the vertices (yellow - superior, blue - inferior). (Color figure online)

Volume and Streamline Measures Computation. The volume of each white matter tract was computed using the resampled binary voxel representation. To compute the total volume of a tract, the volume of a single voxel was determined based on the resolution of the resampled dMRI data (7 mm^3) and then multiplied by the total number of voxels in the binary voxel representation. The volume was also divided by the estimated total intracranial volume (eTIV) as calculated by Freesurfer [16], to normalize for brain size. Analyses were performed on both the normalized and non-normalized volumes. Additionally, the total number of streamlines, average length of streamlines, and total combined length of the streamlines were computed based on the segmented streamline representation of each tract.

2.3   Statistical Analysis

Permutation tests (20,000 permutations for all tests) were used to compare the volume, streamline measures and eigenvalue spectrums of each segmented white matter tract between the disorder groups and their age/sex matched controls. For the volume and streamline measure values a two-sided, nonparametric, permutation test based on the t-statistic was used. Individual eigenvalues were also compared using independent, two-sided, nonparametric permutation tests, as done in [4, 13], and the false discovery rate method of correction was used to correct for multiple comparisons.

2.4   Machine Learning Experiments

Binary classification (bipolar disorder vs. healthy control) was performed using machine learning algorithms implemented in the Python package scikit-learn [24]. We performed five different machine learning experiments: (1) classification using only the (non-normalized) volume values as features, (2) classification using only the streamline measures as features, (3) classification using the combined LB spectrums of all tracts as features, (4) classification using the LB spectrum of single tracts as features individually, and (5) voting-based ensemble classification based on the results of (4). To prepare the data for classification, we standardized each feature by removing the mean and scaling the values to unit variance. This standardization procedure ensured that each feature had the properties of a standard normal distribution, a requirement for many of the algorithms.

Because this is an initial, exploratory study, we performed an exhaustive grid search using 10-fold cross validation across 7 different machine learning classifier algorithms and classifier hyperparameter sets for each experiment (RandomForestClassifier (RF), AdaBoostClassifier (ABC), SVC (SVM, C-Support Vector Classification), KNeighborsClassifier (KNN), DecisionTreeClassifier (DT), LinearDiscriminantAnalysis (LDA), LogisticRegression (LR) in scikit-learn [24]). In the experiments using the LB spectrum, we also performed the grid search across numbers of eigenvalues (30, 50, 100, 150, 200, 300, 400, 500, 600). The results of the grid search helped us determine which classification algorithms and hyperparameter sets performed best for each feature set, as well as which level of shape detail (number of eigenvalues of the LB spectrum) allowed for the greatest distinction between the two groups. For experiments (1) through (4), the best performing classifier and hyperparameter set was used for a final classification with leave-one-out (LOO) cross validation, repeated 10 times. LOO cross validation was used for the final classification due to the relatively limited number of subjects available in the data set. The average accuracy, sensitivity (true positive rate) and specificity (true negative rate) of the classifications are reported.

For experiment (5), we developed a robust voting-based ensemble classification method that combined the results of the series of weaker classifiers applied to individual white matter tracts in experiment (4) [25]. The results of experiment (4) identified the best performing eigenvalue, classifier, and hyperparameter set for each tract. The classification also provided a predicted classification category (vote) for each subject in the dataset (bipolar disorder or control). The final classification for this experiment is obtained by setting the final category of each subject to the mode of the vote distribution (predicted classification category distribution) across the tracts. In the case of a tie, a null category was reported. This voting-based classification was performed 10 times.

3   Results

3.1   Statistical Analysis

We performed a series of control analyses to show whether the white matter tracts differed between the two groups in a series of properties, such as volume, streamline counts, and length. Results show that only two of the white matter tracts had a statistically significant difference in non-normalized volume between the controls (C) and subjects with bipolar disorder (BD): the right cingulum cingulate ($p = 0.044$, BD > C) and the right uncinate ($p = 0.021$, C > BD). Of the normalized volume (volume/eTIV) comparison, only the right uncinate was statistically significant ($p = 0.007$, C > BD). Four tracts had a statistically significant difference in streamline count between the two groups: the left cingulum hippocampus ($p = 0.015$, BD > C), the left corticospinal tract ($p = 0.020$, C > BD), the right corticospinal tract ($p = 0.013$, C > BD), and the right uncinate ($p = 0.005$, C > BD). One tract had a statistically significant group difference in mean length: the left ILF ($p = 0.005$, BD > C). Three tracts had a statistically significant difference in total length between the two groups: the right cingulum cingulate ($p = 0.048$, BD > C), the left cingulum hippocampus ($p = 0.016$, BD > C), and the right uncinate ($p = 0.016$, C > BD).

We also tested whether single eigenvalues of the individual white matter tracts differed between the two groups. Results of the permutation tests for the eigenvalues are shown in Fig. 3. The right and left cingulum hippocampus, the right and left corticospinal, and the right uncinate all had multiple eigenvalues with p-values that passed the 5% and 15% FDR correction for multiple comparisons, suggesting significant shape differences between the two groups for those tracts. The right arcuate, right SLF, and the right and left ILF had eigenvalues with p-values that passed the 15% FDR correction for multiple comparisons.

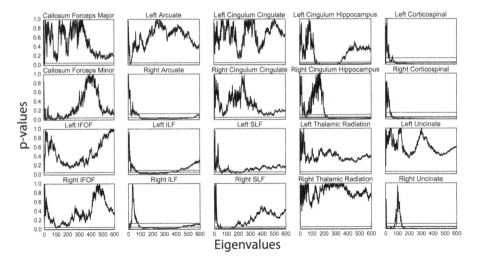

Fig. 3. Results of the permutation tests for the individual eigenvalues of the Laplace-Beltrami spectrum. The p-value of each eigenvalue is plotted for each tract. Red horizontal lines are the 0.05 significance level. If any of the eigenvalues passed FDR correction the FDR significance level is plotted in green (15% FDR) and blue (5% FDR). (Color figure online)

3.2 Machine Learning Classification

(1) **Binary classification using volume only.** For this experiment, we used the non-normalized volume only. The input feature set was 20 volume values for each subject. Using the best classifier and hyperparameter set as determined by the grid search (KNeighborsClassifier), a final classification was performed. The classification accuracy was 54.65%, with a sensitivity of 37.20%, and specificity of 79.09%. The results were the same for all 10 repeats.

(2) **Binary classification streamline measures only.** For this experiment, the input feature set was 20 streamline counts, 20 mean length values, and 20 total length values for each subject. Using the best classifier and hyperparameter set as determined by the grid search (LogisticRegression), a final classification was performed. The classification accuracy was 70.56%, with a sensitivity of 69.76% and specificity of 72.09%. The results were the same for all 10 repeats. Overall classification and specificity was significantly improved using the streamline measures over the volume measures, although specificity was slightly reduced.

(3) **Binary classification using the Laplace-Beltrami spectrum of all tracts.** For these experiments, the input features were the n-number of eigenvalues times 20 tracts across nine different numbers of eigenvalues. The LogisticRegression classifier performed the best in the grid search for all eigenvalue numbers, and therefore was the classifier used for the final classification of all eigenvalue numbers. The results of the final classification using the best performing hyperparameter sets for each eigenvalue number are shown in Table 2. The highest obtained average accuracy was 67.79% (± 1.34) with 200 eigenvalues, a

sensitivity of 67.90% (±0.63), and specificity of 67.67% (±0.87). Overall classification accuracy using the combined LB spectrums of all tracts was better than classification using only the volumes of tracts, but slightly worse than classification using just the streamline measures.

Table 2. Classification results using the combined LB spectrums of all tracts (Experiment 3).

# eigenvalues	30	50	100	150	200	300	400	500	600
Accuracy	62.67 (±2.01)	58.13 (±1.09)	62.79 (±0.00)	64.76 (±1.23)	67.79 (±1.34)	65.58 (±0.98)	65.11 (±0.00)	62.09 (±0.81)	61.97 (±0.95)
Sensitivity	67.67 (±1.19)	65.11 (±0.66)	65.11 (±0.00)	67.90 (±0.42)	67.90 (±0.63)	61.16 (±0.48)	60.46 (±0.00)	59.53 (±0.51)	58.60 (±0.63)
Specificity	57.67 (±0.91)	51.11 (±0.47)	60.46 (±0.00)	61.62 (±0.70)	67.67 (±0.87)	70.00 (±0.73)	69.76 (±0.00)	64.65 (±0.78)	65.34 (±0.56)

(4) **Binary classification using the Laplace-Beltrami spectrum of single tracts**. For these experiments, we performed the final binary classification of each individual tract using the eigenvalue, classifier, and hyperparameter sets that performed best in the grid search. The eigenvalue, average classification accuracy, sensitivity, and specificity of each tract are shown in Figs. 4 and 5. The best overall classification accuracy obtained with a single tract, the left corticospinal tract, was 77.79% (±1.15) (sensitivity = 85.34% (±1.56), specificity = 70.23% (±1.47)), followed by the left arcuate at 76.74% (±0.00) (sensitivity = 79.06% (±0.00), specificity = 74.41% (±0.00)) and the callosum forceps minor at 74.88% (±0.12) (sensitivity = 73.95% (±0.21), specificity = 75.81% (±0.12)). All but one of the white matter tracts achieved an overall accuracy higher than volume based classification (>54%), 6 of the individual tracts achieved an overall accuracy higher than streamline measures based classification (>70%) and 10 achieved an overall accuracy higher than classification based on the combined LB spectrums of all tracts (>67%).

(5) **Voting-based ensemble classification using the Laplace-Beltrami spectrum of each tract.** For this experiment, we used the results of experiment (4) for a voting-based classification. Each tract was used to predict the classification category of each subject. The mode of the classification predictions (votes) across all tracts was computed to assign a final classification category to each subject. The average overall classification accuracy was 95.23% (±0.03), significantly higher than the accuracy of the 4 previous experiments. The average sensitivity was 95.34% (±0.00) and average specificity was 95.11% (±0.06). The average classification accuracy, sensitivity, and specificity are also shown in Figs. 4 and 5.

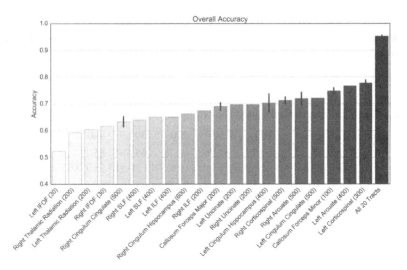

Fig. 4. Average overall accuracy of the classification based on the LB spectrum of individual white matter tracts (Experiment 4) and of the voting-based ensemble classification (Experiment 5), sorted in order of overall accuracy. Black lines represent the standard deviation across the 10 classification repeats; bars with no line had the same result for all repeats. Eigenvalue used for the final classification is listed in parentheses.

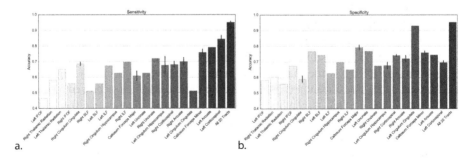

Fig. 5. (a) Average overall sensitivity (true positive rate) and (b) specificity (true negative rate) of the classification based on the LB spectrum of individual white matter tracts (Experiment 4) and of the voting-based ensemble classification (Experiment 5), sorted in the same order as Fig. 4. Black lines represent the standard deviation across the 10 classification repeats; bars with no line had the same result for all repeats.

4   Discussion and Conclusion

In this paper, we proposed the Laplace-Beltrami spectrum be used as a global shape descriptor of white matter tracts. Using the LB spectrum, volume, and streamline measures of segmented white matter tracts, we compared the efficacy of each feature for distinguishing subjects diagnosed with bipolar disorder from age and sex matched controls. Results showed that the shape of the white matter tracts contains important information that allows for a more accurate classification between the two groups. Machine learning classification performed using the LB spectrums of single tracts achieved higher classification accuracy than the volume or streamline measure-based classifications, with 6 of the tracts reaching an overall accuracy above 70%. The individual tract with the highest classification accuracy was the left corticospinal, followed by the left arcuate (comparable to the results of [26]), and the callosum forceps minor. Overall classification accuracy was significantly improved when using a voting-based classification method with the LB spectrums, reaching 95% overall accuracy, 95% sensitivity, and 95% specificity.

Our results illustrate the importance of including shape information in neuroanatomical and neuropsychiatric research for a more complete picture of disorder related differences in the brain. Of the top three performing tracts in the shape classification (all >74% in overall accuracy), only one, the left corticospinal tract, had a significant difference in any of the non-shape measures (streamline count). None of the three had any statistical difference in volume, mean or total streamline length. Analyses based only on volume or streamline measures might mistakenly conclude that there are no disorder related differences in those tracts.

The high classification accuracy we obtained demonstrates that the LB spectrum captures meaningful information about white matter tract morphology. The results suggest that including the shape of white matter tracts in neuropsychiatric research may be useful for narrowing down the etiology of the range of neuropsychiatric and brain disorders known to be accompanied by changes in the white matter [15]. Future research directions include expanding the analyses to incorporate other neuropsychiatric disorders, such as schizophrenia and attention deficit hyperactivity disorder, as well as including comparisons to analyses with diffusion-based microstructure measures.

Acknowledgements. This research was supported by NSF IIS-1636893, NSF BCS-1734853, NIH NIMH ULTTR001108, and a Microsoft Research Award, the Indiana University Areas of Emergent Research initiative "Learning: Brains, Machines, Children", the Pervasive Technology Institute and the Research Technologies Division of University Information Technology Services at Indiana University. The authors thank Yu Wang and Justin Solomon who provided insight and expertise on the Laplace-Beltrami operator.

References

1. Styner, M., et al.: Statistical shape analysis of neuroanatomical structures based on medial models. Med. Image Anal. **7**(3), 207–220 (2003)
2. Styner, M., et al.: Framework for the statistical shape analysis of brain structures using SPHARM-PDM. Insight J. **1071**, 242 (2006)
3. Ashburner, J., Friston, K.J.: Voxel-based morphometry—the methods. Neuroimage **11**(6), 805–821 (2000)
4. Niethammer, M., et al.: Global medical shape analysis using the laplace-beltrami spectrum. In: Ayache, N., Ourselin, S., Maeder, A. (eds.) MICCAI 2007. LNCS, vol. 4791, pp. 850–857. Springer, Heidelberg (2007). https://doi.org/10.1007/978-3-540-75757-3_103

5. Corouge, I., Gouttard, S., Gerig, G.: A statistical shape model of individual fiber tracts extracted from diffusion tensor MRI. In: Barillot, C., Haynor, D.R., Hellier, P. (eds.) MICCAI 2004. LNCS, vol. 3217, pp. 671–679. Springer, Heidelberg (2004). https://doi.org/10.1007/978-3-540-30136-3_82

6. O'Donnell, L.J., et al.: Tract-based morphometry for white matter group analysis. Neuroimage **45**(3), 832–844 (2009)

7. Glozman, T., et al.: Framework for shape analysis of white matter fiber bundles. Neuroimage **167**, 466–477 (2018)

8. Durrleman, S., et al.: Registration, atlas estimation and variability analysis of white matter fiber bundles modeled as currents. Neuroimage **55**(3), 1073–1090 (2011)

9. Reuter, M., et al.: Laplace-Beltrami spectra as 'Shape-DNA' of surfaces and solids. Comput. Aided Des. **38**(4), 342–366 (2006)

10. Shi, Y., Morra, J.H., Thompson, P.M., Toga, A.W.: Inverse-consistent surface mapping with Laplace-Beltrami eigen-features. In: Prince, J.L., Pham, D.L., Myers, K.J. (eds.) IPMI 2009. LNCS, vol. 5636, pp. 467–478. Springer, Heidelberg (2009). https://doi.org/10.1007/978-3-642-02498-6_39

11. Wachinger, C., Golland, P., Kremen, W., Fischl, B., Reuter, M., Initiative, A.D.N.: BrainPrint: a discriminative characterization of brain morphology. NeuroImage **109**, 232–248 (2015)

12. Wachinger, C., et al.: Whole-brain analysis reveals increased neuroanatomical asymmetries in dementia for hippocampus and amygdala. Brain **139**(12), 3253–3266 (2016)

13. Shishegar, R., et al.: Hippocampal shape analysis in epilepsy using Laplace-Beltrami spectrum. In: 2011 19th Iranian Conference on Electrical Engineering (ICEE). IEEE (2011)

14. Poldrack, R.A., et al.: A phenome-wide examination of neural and cognitive function. Sci. Data **3**, 160110 (2016). https://doi.org/10.1038/sdata.2016.110

15. Fields, R.D.: White matter in learning, cognition and psychiatric disorders. Trends Neurosci. **31**(7), 361–370 (2008)

16. Fischl, B.: FreeSurfer. NeuroImage **62**, 774–781 (2012)

17. Takemura, H., Caiafa, C.F., Wandell, B.A., Pestilli, F.: Ensemble tractography. PLoS Comput. Biol. **12**(2), e1004692 (2016)

18. Caiafa, C.F., Pestilli, F.: Multidimensional encoding of brain connectomes. Sci. Rep. **7**(1), 11491 (2017)

19. Pestilli, F., Yeatman, J.D., Rokem, A., Kay, K.N., Wandell, B.A.: Evaluation and statistical inference for human connectomes. Nat. Methods **11**(10), 1058 (2014)

20. Tournier, J.D., Calamante, F., Connelly, A.: MRtrix: diffusion tractography in crossing fiber regions. Int. J. Imaging Syst. Technol. **22**(1), 53–66 (2012)

21. Yeatman, J.D., Dougherty, R.F., Myall, N.J., Wandell, B.A., Feldman, H.M.: Tract profiles of white matter properties: automating fiber-tract quantification. PLoS One **7**(11), e49790 (2012)

22. Taubin, G., Zhang, T., Golub, G.: Optimal surface smoothing as filter design. In: Buxton, B., Cipolla, R. (eds) ECCV 1996. LNCS, vol. 1064, pp. 283–292. Springer, Heidelberg (1996). https://doi.org/10.1007/BFb0015544

23. Jacobson, A., et al.: gptoolbox: geometry processing toolbox (2016). http://github.com/alecjacobson/gptoolbox

24. Pedregosa, F., et al.: Scikit-learn: machine learning in Python. J. Mach. Learn. Res. **12**, 2825–2830 (2011)

25. Dieterich, Thomas G.: Ensemble methods in machine learning. In: Kittler, J., Roli, F. (eds.) MCS 2000. LNCS, vol. 1857, pp. 1–15. Springer, Heidelberg (2000). https://doi.org/10.1007/3-540-45014-9_1

26. Sun, Z.Y., et al.: Shape analysis of the cingulum, uncinate and arcuate fasciculi in patients with bipolar disorder. J. Psychiatry Neurosci.: JPN **42**(1), 27 (2017)

Virtual 2D-3D Fracture Reduction with Bone Length Recovery Using Statistical Shape Models

Ondřej Klíma[1]([⊠])(iD), Roman Madeja[2](iD), Michal Španel[1,3](iD), Martin Čuta[4](iD), Pavel Zemčík[1](iD), Pavel Stoklásek[5], and Aleš Mizera[5](iD)

[1] IT4Innovations Centre of Excellence, Brno University of Technology, Božetěchova 1/2, 612 66 Brno, Czech Republic
{iklima,spanel,zemcik}@fit.vutbr.cz
[2] University Hospital in Ostrava, 17. listopadu 1790, 708 52 Ostrava, Czech Republic
[3] 3Dim Laboratory s.r.o, Kamenice 34, 625 00 Brno, Czech Republic
[4] Laboratory of Morphology and Forensic Anthropology, Department of Anthropology, Masaryk University, Kotlářská 2, 611 37 Brno, Czech Republic
[5] CEBIA-Tech, Faculty of Applied Informatics, Tomas Bata University in Zlín, Nad Stráněmi 4511, 760 05 Zlín, Czech Republic
http://www.3dim-laboratory.cz/

Abstract. Computer-assisted 3D preoperative planning based on 2D stereo radiographs has been brought into focus recently in the field of orthopedic surgery. To enable planning, it is crucial to reconstruct a patient-specific 3D bone model from X-ray images. However, most of the existing studies deal only with uninjured bones, which limits their possible applications for planning. In this paper, we propose a method for the reconstruction of long bones with diaphyseal fractures from 2D radiographs of the individual fracture segments to 3D polygonal models of the intact bones. In comparison with previous studies, the main contribution is the ability to recover an accurate length of the target bone. The reconstruction is based on non-rigid 2D-3D registration of a single statistical shape model onto the radiographs of individual fragments, performed simultaneously with the virtual fracture reduction. The method was tested on a synthetic data set containing 96 virtual fractures and on real radiographs of dry cadaveric bones suffering peri-mortem injuries. The accuracy was evaluated using the Hausdorff distance between the reconstructed and ground-truth bone models. On the synthetic data set, the average surface error reached 1.48 ± 1.16 mm. The method was built into preoperative planning software designated for the selection of the best-fitting fixation material.

Keywords: Preoperative planning · Fracture reduction
Fixation devices · 2D-3D registration · Statistical shape model

© Springer Nature Switzerland AG 2018
M. Reuter et al. (Eds.): ShapeMI 2018, LNCS 11167, pp. 207–219, 2018.
https://doi.org/10.1007/978-3-030-04747-4_20

1   Introduction

Plain radiography plays a key role in bone fracture diagnosis and treatment. In the case of surgical intervention, plain radiographs enable basic preoperative planning, such as bone fracture classification and the determination of an appropriate fixation technique for its stabilization. More advanced, computer-assisted planning of the osteosynthesis provides a virtual simulation of the intervention, which typically includes situating the fracture segments into anatomically correct and mechanically stable poses, measuring the bone morphology, or placing fixation devices [9]. The virtual simulations rely on 3D polygonal models of individual bone fragments, which are conventionally obtained from volumetric images provided by computed tomography (CT). However, during the CT examinations, the patients are exposed to substantially higher doses of radiation in comparison with plain radiography. Therefore, the indication of CT examinations is generally restricted only to cases of severe or complex fractures, while the treatment of rather common cases depends on plain radiographs. Nevertheless, computer-assisted planning can be still beneficial even for rather routine fractures, especially for long bone fractures of the lower limbs. One important contribution is the possibility of preoperative measurement of patient-specific bone morphology with aim of determining the features of the best-fitting fixation devices, such as the length of the intramedullary nail [8], the size of the bone plate, or the number and placement of bone screws. Therefore, a reconstruction of a 3D patient-specific anatomy based only on plain, clinically available radiographs instead of volumetric images is of great importance for the application of virtual planning in a broader spectrum of bone fracture treatment procedures.

In this paper, we propose a semi-automatic 3D virtual fracture reduction method, which is able to reconstruct a polygonal model of an intact bone from stereo radiographic images of the individual fracture segments. The method is focused on displaced diaphyseal fractures of the simple or wedge type.

2   Related Work

In the field of orthopedic surgery, a somewhat similar challenge of computer-assisted 3D preoperative planning based only on plain radiographs was recently addressed by several projects [1,2] focusing on total hip arthroplasty (THA), total knee arthroplasty (TKA), and lower extremity osteotomy. Other studies were focused on observing 3D joint kinematics from fluoroscopy sequences without the requirement of CT image acquisition [5,17,18]. Instead of CT scans, a non-rigid registration of 3D bone atlases onto the stereo radiographs was exploited to reconstruct polygonal models of the bones. As proposed in works such as [15], statistical shape models were involved as the atlases to perform a shape-constrained 2D-3D registration. With respect to the statistical shape models, this reconstruction approach is straightforward when the target bone is not suffering any injuries, which is fulfilled for the total joint arthroplasty or observation of joint kinematics. However, arbitrarily shaped fracture segments make reconstruction based on statistical shape models a challenging task.

The first attempt to reconstruct injured bones using statistical atlases was proposed in a study focused on the reduction of multi-fragment fractures of the distal radius [7]. The goal of the study was to obtain a polygonal model of an intact bone from plain radiographs of the fracture segments. The reconstruction, together with the fracture reduction, were achieved at the same time by a 2D-3D registration of a single statistical appearance model of an intact distal radius into individual fracture segments. Splitting the statistical appearance model into fracture segments was performed automatically by the registration. The method was evaluated *in silico* using simulated fractures, concluding that the atlas-based reconstruction may provide a more accurate distal radius template than the conventionally used mirrored model obtained from the contralateral limb.

A later study, using a similar principle of a multi-fragment 2D-3D registration of a statistical shape model, focused on diaphyseal fractures of the long bones of the lower limbs [16]. In contrast with the previous work, its aim was to determine the rotation alignment between the proximal and distal fragments along the longitudinal axis. In addition to the rotation angles, the study considered the reconstruction of surface models of the individual fracture segments. However, the approach was unable to perform virtual fracture reduction and to provide a model of the intact bone, as the method was unable to determine the correct length of the target bone. Moreover, the shape model had to be divided into fragments in advance, without further refinement during the registration process. The bone length also had to be provided manually in a study focused on automatic fracture reduction using statistical atlases, working with mesh models of fracture segments obtained from CT scans [3].

In this paper, we address the challenge of accurate bone length recovery. Unlike [16], the division of the statistical shape model into segments is performed automatically by the registration, enabling optimization of the shape model length. In consequence, the proposed method is able to perform virtual fracture reduction and provide a 3D model of the intact bone.

3   Method

The method is based on a multi-fragment registration of a statistical shape model into stereo radiographs of individual fracture segments, extended by simultaneous optimization of the shape model length.

3.1   Statistical Shape Models

The statistical shape models involved in this study work as elastic tetrahedral models of bones. As their elasticity is shape-constrained, it is ensured the models always represent anatomically reasonable bones. The shape models involved were created using a procedure detailed in [12]. As the models are based on probabilistic principal component analysis (PPCA), they are represented by the following generative model:

$$S = \phi \mathbf{b} + \overline{S} + \omega \tag{1}$$

Table 1. Characteristics of involved statistical shape models.

Statistical shape model	Size of training set	Modes of variation	Tetrahedral vertices	Tetrahedra
Femur	43 bones	41	20,843	93,480
Tibia	42 bones	40	22,003	106,436

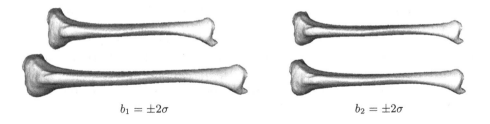

$$b_1 = \pm 2\sigma \qquad\qquad b_2 = \pm 2\sigma$$

Fig. 1. Statistical shape model of the tibia. The instances were generated by setting the first *(left)* and the second *(right)* parameter to $\pm 2\sigma$. The rest of the modes were set to zero.

where S is a vector containing tetrahedral vertices of the model, the shape of which is determined by independent modes of variation $\mathbf{b}$; $\overline{S}$ is a tetrahedral model of the mean bone; ϕ is a matrix of the principal components; and ω describes zero-meaned Gaussian noise.

Two statistical shape models, representing the femur and tibia, were created using CT images of intact bones, provided by the University Hospital in Ostrava. The characteristics of the models are shown in Table 1. Both tetrahedral models include a polygonal surface, formed by $19,996$ faces and by a subset counting $10,000$ tetrahedral vertices.

As previously described in [3], the length of the femoral or tibial shaft is relatively independent of the shape of the joint regions. Considering the statistical shape models of the involved bones, the length of the shaft is controlled mainly by the first mode b_1, while features such as the size or shape of the joint regions are modeled in particular by the rest of the modes $b_2 \ldots b_n$ (Fig. 1). Therefore, it is impossible to determine the length of a bone based only on the shape of its distal and proximal parts.

3.2 Reconstruction

The reconstruction outcome comprises a model of a patient-specific intact bone, described by shape modes $\mathbf{b}$, and poses $p_{\mathrm{prox}}, p_{\mathrm{dist}}$ of both fracture segments, forming a vector $\mathcal{P} = (\mathbf{b}, p_{\mathrm{prox}}, p_{\mathrm{dist}})$. The results are obtained by minimization of the reprojection error, evaluated using a nonoverlapping area measure (NOA), together with a length criterion (LC):

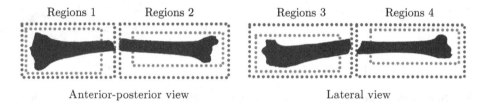

Fig. 2. The input radiographs are divided into different regions of interest. The regions related to nonoverlapping area evaluation *(orange)* border the maximal intact parts of the bones. The boundaries of regions for length estimation *(blue)* are determined with respect to the detachement point of the bone fragments. The regions are estimated as scaled-up bounding boxes of the fragment segmentations, except the sides nearest to the fracture, which are set interactively by the user. (Color figure online)

$$(\mathcal{P}^*) = \arg\min_{\mathcal{P}} \left[\mathrm{NOA}(\mathcal{P}) + \mathrm{LC}(\mathcal{P}) \right] \tag{2}$$

Both terms are evaluated using the input radiographs, though with different regions of interest (Fig. 2).

Nonoverlapping Area. The measure is evaluated between binary segmentations of the input digital radiographs (DR) and digitally reconstructed radiographs (DRR) [12] with a reprojected statistical shape model, using only the intact regions of the bones. The nonoverlapping area is defined as the area that the segmentations do not have in common (Fig. 3). As shown in [13], it can be evaluated as a sum of the squared pixel differences (PD) between the input and virtual segmentations:

$$d(\mathcal{P}, x, y) = \mathrm{DR}(x, y) - \mathrm{DRR}(\mathcal{P}, x, y) \tag{3}$$
$$\mathrm{PD}(\mathcal{P}) = \big(d(x_1 \ldots x_n, y_1 \ldots y_m) \big) \tag{4}$$
$$\mathrm{NOA}(\mathcal{P}) = \|\mathrm{PD}(\mathcal{P})\|^2 \tag{5}$$

Instead of a count of different pixels, it is convenient to express the size of the nonoverlapping area relatively as $\frac{\mathrm{NOA}(\mathcal{P})}{\mathrm{NOA}(\mathcal{P}) + \mathrm{OA}(\mathcal{P})}$, where $\mathrm{OA}(\mathcal{P})$ is the size of the overlapping area. The measure is an intensity-based similarity metric in the sense that the evaluation is performed directly with the input and reprojected pixels, leading to correspondence-free registration [13]. In contrast, the feature-based methods [5,6] usually require establishing correspondences between the shape model vertices and the contours detected in the radiographs, which is a challenging and error-prone task.

Bone Length Recovery. As the method works with simple or wedge fractures, the injured bone is split into two main fragments. Each fragment is captured in two regions of interest forming a stereo pair, as shown in Fig. 2. The key idea of the recovery is to assign each vertex of the shape model to only one of the

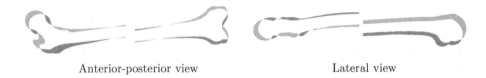

Anterior-posterior view   Lateral view

Fig. 3. Nonoverlapping area between the input *(red)* and virtual *(green)* segmentations. The size of the depicted nonoverlapping area is 28.5%. (Color figure online)

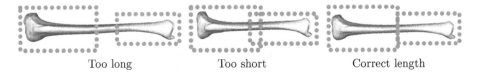

Too long   Too short   Correct length

Fig. 4. Relation between vertex assignment and resulting bone length. No assignment of the vertices in the middle of the shaft to any of the fragments leads to a bone that is too long *(left)*. Assignment of the vertices to both fragments results in a bone that is too short *(middle)*. The correct length is ensured by assigning each vertex to exactly one fragment *(right)*.

main fragments. In consequence, each vertex should be reprojected in precisely two regions, which is achieved by minimizing the length criterion:

$$\text{RV}(\mathcal{P}) = \big(\text{r}(\mathcal{P}, v_1 \ldots v_n) - 2\big) \tag{6}$$

$$\text{LC}(\mathcal{P}) = \|\text{RV}(\mathcal{P})\|^2 \tag{7}$$

where $\text{r}(\mathcal{P}, v)$ is the number of reprojections of the current vertex v. The relation between misassigned vertices and bone length is shown in Fig. 4. The regions of interest for the length recovery must be set with respect to a point of detachement (Fig. 2).

Optimization Scheme. The registration is solved as a non-linear least squares (NLS) problem, using a numerical Levenberg-Marquardt optimizer [10]. Although a computationally demanding approximation of the Jacobian matrix is required, due to its high rate of convergence, the optimizer is able to outperform stochastic gradient-free methods [14]. The Jacobian matrix J_F has the following form:

$$J_F = \begin{pmatrix} \partial\text{PD}_{\text{prox}}(\mathcal{P})/\partial p_{\text{prox}} & 0 & \partial\text{PD}_{\text{prox}}(\mathcal{P})/\partial\mathbf{b} \\ 0 & \partial\text{PD}_{\text{dist}}(\mathcal{P})/\partial p_{\text{dist}} & \partial\text{PD}_{\text{dist}}(\mathcal{P})/\partial\mathbf{b} \\ \partial\text{RV}(\mathcal{P})/\partial p_{\text{prox}} & \partial\text{RV}(\mathcal{P})/\partial p_{\text{dist}} & \partial\text{RV}(\mathcal{P})/\partial\mathbf{b} \end{pmatrix} \tag{8}$$

where the partial derivatives are approximated using central differences as $\partial f(t)/\partial t \approx f(t+\epsilon) - f(t-\epsilon)/2\epsilon$.

The reconstruction is divided into three subsequent optimizations. At first, only poses $p_{\text{prox}}, p_{\text{dist}}$ are considered. Next, the first five shape modes $b_1 \ldots b_5$ are optimized together with the poses. Finally, all modes $\mathbf{b}$ are involved in the last stage. Before the optimization, a rough initial pose of the statistical shape model together with the regions of interest must be set interactively by the user, or estimated from the segmentations, as described in the following sections. The binary segmentations of the input radiographs are performed manually. The modes of variation of the shape model are initialized to zeros.

4   Results

The accuracy and performance of the proposed method were evaluated on synthetic X-ray images of simulated fractures and on real radiographs of dry cadaveric bones suffering perimortem injuries. To evaluate the accuracy, the differences between the polygonal models reconstructed by the proposed method, and ground-truth surfaces obtained from CT data sets were measured using the symmetric Hausdorff distance [4]. The CT data sets of ground-truth bones were never included into the training sets of the statistical shape models. Following the reconstruction convergence criterion stated in [6], the method converged in each evaluated case, as the RMS error was always lower than 3 mm. The ϵ for the Jacobian matrix approximation was set to 1 mm or 1° in the case of pose parameters and to 1 standard deviation σ for shape modes b, as previously proposed in [12].

The evaluations were performed using a 64-bit Windows 7 desktop machine, equipped with an Intel i5 processing unit, NVidia GTX 980Ti 6 GB graphics adapter and 24 GB DDR4 RAM.

4.1   Simulated Injuries

For the *in silico* evaluation of the fracture reduction, we adopted a data set of virtual X-ray images, previously presented in [12]. The virtual radiographs were ray-casted from 8 already segmented CT images of femoral bones obtained from the Virtual Skeleton Database (VSD) [11]. From each CT image, 12 virtual stereo pairs of orthogonal radiographs were created, resulting in 96 cases in total. As the bones were rotated 30° along the longitudinal axis between the individual renderings, the data set contained X-ray images captured even from arbitrary views, in addition to standard anterior-posterior and lateral radiographs. The source-image distance (SID) was set to exactly 1 m; the pixel spacing of the radiographs was set to 0.75 mm. To simulate transversal fractures of the femoral shaft, each radiograph was split into proximal and distal parts. A sample test case chosen from the evaluation data set is shown in Fig. 5.

Initial poses of the statistical shape model were generated randomly, with uniform distribution and maximum difference to the ground-truth poses limited to ±10 mm and ±10°, respectively.

Figure 5 shows the result of the virtual fracture reduction of the sample test case. As the virtual radiographs and the reference polygonal models were obtained from the same CT images, the reconstructed bones were compared directly with ground-truth surfaces. The accuracy evaluation for each bone, together with the size of the nonoverlapping area, the number of misassigned

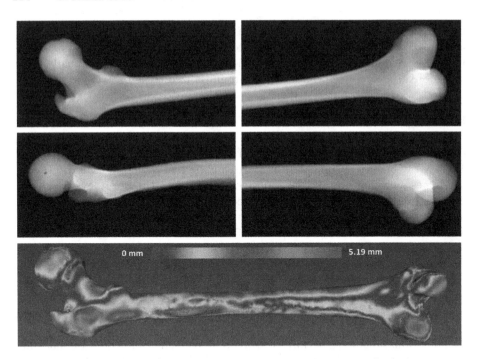

Fig. 5. A sample test case of stereo radiographs with simulative transversal fracture of the femoral shaft, chosen from the virtual data set *(top)*. Accuracy of the sample case reconstruction *(bottom)*. The heatmap shows the differences between reconstructed and ground-truth surfaces, evaluated using the symmetric Hausdorff distance.

tetrahedral vertices, and the length error, as well as the performance evaluation, including the overall reconstruction time, number of iterations in each stage and a total number of rendered images, are shown in Table 2. The results for each bone were averaged from 12 evaluations using different stereo radiographic pairs.

The virtual reduction method extends the *Black & White Pixel Differences* (BW-PD) approach proposed in [12], designated for a single-fragment 2D-3D reconstruction of the uninjured bones. Evaluated on the same synthetic data set, the BW-PD method reached an average accuracy of 1.02 ± 1.35 mm when reconstructing the uninjured bones, while the proposed method reached 1.48 ± 1.16 mm when performing virtual reduction of simulated shaft fractures.

4.2   Dry Cadaveric Bones Study

The cadaveric study involved archeological bones, two femoral and one tibial, suffering peri-mortem diaphyseal fractures. A sample bone from the study is shown in Fig. 6. The radiographs of individual fragments were taken sequentially, using a Kodak Carestream Directview DR 9500 System imaging system. Two CR X-ray cassettes with dimensions of 35×43 cm and 0.168 mm pixel spacing were exploited for the captures. The source-image distance was set to approximately

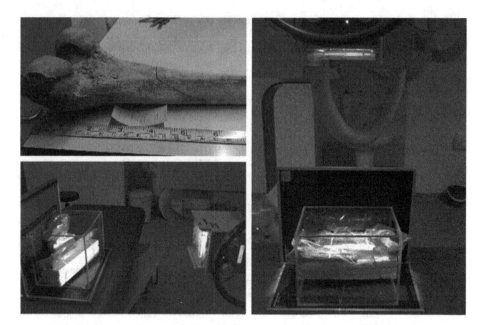

Fig. 6. Physically reduced dry cadaveric femur involved in the study *(top-left)*, capturing an anterior-posterior radiograph of the experimental setup *(right)*, taking a lateral radiograph *(bottom-left)*.

1 m. The radiographs were calibrated using a custom made radiostereometric biplanar calibration box, described in detail in [13]. The complete experimental set up for capturing radiographs is shown in Fig. 6. Individual bone fragments, sealed in a foil sleeve, were placed approximately in the center of the box, on Styrofoam underlays. Contrary to the synthetic data set, the radiographs were taken only from the anterior-posterior and lateral views. After capturing the radiographs, the fractures were actually reduced and fixed by gluing individual fragments together. Then, the reference polygonal models were obtained from CT images of the reduced bones. The poses of the statistical shape model were initialized interactively in a custom viewer.

In contrast with the *in silico* study, rigid registration of the reconstructed bones onto the reference models had to be performed before the Hausdorff distance evaluation. The results of the evaluation are shown in Table 2, revealing a slight decrease in accuracy for the cadaveric bones. The accuracy was affected by the manual segmentation and the real-world calibration of the radiographic images; the higher RMS error in comparison with the simulative data set was caused by certain degradations of the archeological bones involved. The higher number of misassigned tetrahedral vertices was related to a user estimation of the separation spot, which was, by contrast, ideal in the case of the *in silico* study.

Table 2. Results of the reconstruction accuracy and performance evaluation.

Bone	Nonoverlapping area (%)	Misassigned vertices	Length error (mm)	Mean Hausdorff distance (mm)	RMS error
VSD identif.	*Simulated fractures*				
226	2.34	11.0	0.57	1.28	0.99
230	2.38	6.3	1.06	1.23	0.95
238	2.60	10.3	0.49	1.61	1.27
254	2.56	13.3	2.16	1.54	1.20
5900	2.85	6.7	4.07	1.31	1.02
5953	2.60	3.7	2.77	1.41	1.09
6009	2.85	8.1	1.44	1.70	1.35
5939	3.33	15.0	0.94	1.78	1.43
	Perimortem fractured dry cadaveric bones				
Femur 1	3.41	86	3.8	1.89	2.16
Femur 2	2.33	50	3.1	1.38	1.70
Tibia	3.50	131	2.0	1.73	2.16

Bone	Overall time (mm:ss)	Iterations			Renderings
		Stage 1	Stage 2	Stage 3	
VSD identifier	*Simulated fractures*				
226	1:54.4	55.6	16.3	12.9	9,609
230	1:59.0	48.8	21.7	14.8	10,454
238	2:15.2	63.3	21.1	15.0	11,248
254	3:55.2	84.0	79.6	22.5	20,550
5900	3:04.5	80.2	66.3	12.7	15,387
5953	2:11.1	56.5	20.1	15.9	11,149
6009	2:57.6	66.1	58.5	16.3	15,343
5939	2:11.9	67.9	40.3	10.6	11,583
	Perimortem fractured dry cadaveric bones				
Femur 1	3:49.3	11	48	38	19,752
Femur 2	2:16.7	42	24	21	12,684
Tibia	1:13.0	17	34	13	9,160

4.3 Preoperative Planning Software

The method has been built into preoperative planning software, which provides a large database of 3D models capturing bone plates and intramedullary nails. The user is able to select the intended device from the database, place it interactively onto the reconstructed bone model, possibly to perform a virtual bending of the bone plate, and finally refine its pose using an automatic procedure. The application also provides the cutting planes of the obtained polygonal model as a tentative approximation of the fracture detachment sites, or measurements of required screw lengths (Fig. 7). A mutual pose of stereo radiographs is determined using a calibration marker, which is usually attached to a lower limb splint. The shape model is initially aligned with the longitudinal axes of fragments, which are reconstructed in 3D from the binary segmentations.

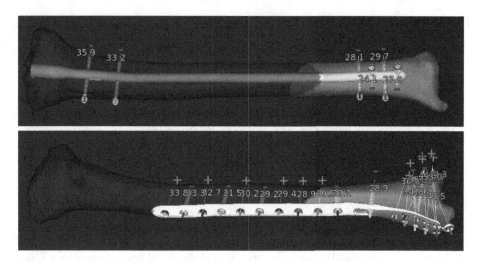

Fig. 7. A virtual simulation of intramedullary nailing of a tibial shaft fracture *(top)*, and a virtual placement of a distal tibial bone plate *(bottom)*. The bone model was reconstructed from radiographs of a real traumatology case.

5   Discussion and Conclusions

In this paper, we proposed a method for a virtual 2D-3D reduction of shaft fractures of the lower limbs. To the best of our knowledge, no other method considering multifragment 2D-3D reconstruction with a focus on accurate length estimation has been proposed so far. The accuracy of the method is comparable even with single-fragment reconstruction approaches, presented in a brief summary in [6]. The results revealed that the accuracy and performance are sufficient for involvement in preoperative planning software designed for the selection of the best-fitting fixation material. To omit the manual segmentation of input radiographs, which is a time-consuming and subjective task, the future work will focus on replacing the nonoverlapping area measure with density-based registration. We assume that the length estimation based on assigning the statistical shape model vertices to individual bone fragments is straightforwardly generalizable, even for application in virtual fracture reduction using 3D models of the fragments obtained from CT images, as proposed e.g. in [3]. The reconstruction method is distributed as open-source library and front-end application at https://github.com/klepo/libmultifragmentregister.

Acknowledgements. This work was supported by the Technology Agency of the Czech Republic Grant No. TE01020415 V3C - Visual Computing Competence Center and by the Ministry of Education, Youth and Sports of the Czech Republic within the National Sustainability Programme project No. LO1303 (MSMT-7778/2014).

References

1. iJoint: 2D/3D reconstruction of patient-specific hip joint from conventional X-ray radiographs. http://www.istb.unibe.ch/research/information_processing_in_medical_interventions/ijoint/index_eng.html. Accessed 08 Aug 2018
2. iLeg: 2D/3D reconstruction of lower extremity from clinically available X-rays. http://www.istb.unibe.ch/research/information_processing_in_medical_interventions/ileg/index_eng.html. Accessed 08 Aug 2018
3. Albrecht, T., Vetter, T.: Automatic fracture reduction. In: Levine, J.A., Paulsen, R.R., Zhang, Y. (eds.) MeshMed 2012. LNCS, vol. 7599, pp. 22–29. Springer, Heidelberg (2012). https://doi.org/10.1007/978-3-642-33463-4_3
4. Aspert, N., Santa-Cruz, D., Ebrahimi, T.: MESH: measuring errors between surfaces using the Hausdorff distance. In: Proceedings of the 2002 IEEE International Conference on Multimedia and Expo. ICME 2002, vol. 1, pp. 705–708 (2002)
5. Baka, N., et al.: Statistical shape model-based femur kinematics from biplane fluoroscopy. IEEE Trans. Med. Imaging **31**(8), 1573–1583 (2012)
6. Baka, N., et al.: 2D–3D shape reconstruction of the distal femur from stereo X-ray imaging using statistical shape models. Med. Image Anal. **15**, 840–850 (2011)
7. Gong, R.H., Stewart, J., Abolmaesumi, P.: Reduction of multi-fragment fractures of the distal radius using atlas-based 2D/3D registration. Proc. SPIE **7261**, 7261–7261-9 (2009)
8. Issac, R.T., Gopalan, H., Abraham, M., John, C., Issac, S.M., Jacob, D.: Preoperative determination of tibial nail length: an anthropometric study. Chin. J. Traumatol. **19**(3), 151–155 (2016)
9. Jiménez-Delgado, J.J., Paulano-Godino, F., PulidoRam-Ramírez, R., Jiménez-Pérez, J.R.: Computer assisted preoperative planning of bone fracture reduction: simulation techniques and new trends. Med. Image Anal. **30**, 30–45 (2016)
10. Kelley, C.T.: Iterative Methods for Optimization. Frontiers in Applied Mathematics. SIAM, Philadelphia (1999)
11. Kistler, M., Bonaretti, S., Pfahrer, M., Niklaus, R., Büchler, P.: The virtual skeleton database: an open access repository for biomedical research and collaboration. J. Med. Internet Res. **15**(11), e245 (2013)
12. Klima, O., Kleparnik, P., Spanel, M., Zemcik, P.: Intensity-based femoral atlas 2D/3D registration using Levenberg-Marquardt optimisation. Proc. SPIE **9788**, 9788–9788-12 (2016)
13. Klima, O., et al.: Intensity-based nonoverlapping area registration supporting "Drop-Outs" in terms of model-based radiostereometric analysis. J. Healthc. Eng. **2018**, 1–10 (2018)
14. Klima, O., Chromy, A., Zemcik, P., Spanel, M., Kleparnik, P.: A study on performace of Levenberg-Marquardt and CMA-ES optimization methods for atlas-based 2D/3D reconstruction. IFAC-PapersOnLine **49**(25), 121–126 (2016). 14th IFAC Conference on Programmable Devices and Embedded Systems PDES 2016
15. Markelj, P., Tomaževič, D., Likar, B., Pernuš, F.: A review of 3D/2D registration methods for image-guided interventions. Med. Image Anal. **16**(3), 642–661 (2012). Computer Assisted Interventions
16. Schumann, S., Bieck, R., Bader, R., Heverhagen, J., Nolte, L.P., Zheng, G.: Radiographic reconstruction of lower-extremity bone fragments: a first trial. Int. J. Comput. Assist. Radiol. Surg. **11**(12), 2241–2251 (2016)

17. Smoger, L.M., Shelburne, K.B., Cyr, A.J., Rullkoetter, P.J., Laz, P.J.: Statistical shape modeling predicts patellar bone geometry to enable stereo-radiographic kinematic tracking. J. Biomech. **58**, 187–194 (2017)
18. Valenti, M., et al.: Fluoroscopy-based tracking of femoral kinematics with statistical shape models. Int. J. Comput. Assist. Radiol. Surg. **11**(5), 757–765 (2016)

Shape Classification and Deep Learning

Deep Shape Analysis on Abdominal Organs for Diabetes Prediction

Benjamín Gutiérrez-Becker[1]([✉]), Sergios Gatidis[2], Daniel Gutmann[2],
Annette Peters[3], Christopher Schlett[4], Fabian Bamberg[2],
and Christian Wachinger[1]

[1] Artificial Intelligence in Medical Imaging (AI-Med), KJP, LMU München,
Munich, Germany
benjamin.gutierrez_becker@med.uni-muenchen.de
[2] Department of Diagnostic and Interventional Radiology, University of Tübingen,
Tübingen, Germany
[3] Institute of Epidemiology, Helmholtz Zentrum München, Munich, Germany
[4] Department of Diagnostic and Interventional Radiology,
University Hospital Heidelberg, Heidelberg, Germany

Abstract. Morphological analysis of organs based on images is a key
task in medical imaging computing. Several approaches have been proposed for the quantitative assessment of morphological changes, and they
have been widely used for the analysis of the effects of aging, disease
and other factors in organ morphology. In this work, we propose a deep
neural network for predicting diabetes on abdominal shapes. The network directly operates on raw point clouds without requiring mesh processing or shape alignment. Instead of relying on hand-crafted shape
descriptors, an optimal representation is learned in the end-to-end training stage of the network. For comparison, we extend the state-of-the-art
shape descriptor BrainPrint to the AbdomenPrint. Our results demonstrate that the network learns shape representations that better separates
healthy and diabetic individuals than traditional representations.

1 Introduction

Shape models have been widely used in medical imaging, not only as a prior
for segmentation algorithms, but also as a powerful tool to assess morphological
differences between subjects [8]. A critical element in shape analysis is the choice
of a numerical representation which can be used for a quantitative analysis of
shape. Multiple shape representations have been previously explored, ranging
from very basic volumetric and thickness measurements [6,19], to more complex
models such as Point Distribution Models [2], spectral signatures [20], spherical
harmonics [4], medial representations [5], and diffeomorphisms [13].

Despite the ample success of deep learning for many medical imaging tasks,
their application for medical shape analysis is still largely unexplored; mainly
because typical shape representations such as point clouds and meshes do not
possess an underlying Euclidean or grid-like structure. Deep networks can learn

© Springer Nature Switzerland AG 2018
M. Reuter et al. (Eds.): ShapeMI 2018, LNCS 11167, pp. 223–231, 2018.
https://doi.org/10.1007/978-3-030-04747-4_21

complex, hierarchical feature representations from data that typically outperforms hand-crafted features, which are not optimal for the given task.

Recently, we have introduced the Multi-Structure PointNet (MSPNet) [7], which is able to learn shape representations directly on point clouds and can predict a label given the shape of multiple brain structures. To the best of our knowledge MSPNet is the first deep end-to-end learning system used to perform prediction based on organ shapes. MSPNet operates directly on point clouds, without the need to create meshes and it does not require computing point correspondences between different shapes.

As most work on shape analysis, we have used MSPNet in the study brain morphology; however, the use of shape models to analyze other anatomical regions remains a relatively unexplored area. In an effort to fill this gap, we propose the deep shape analysis of abdominal anatomy. Our main interest lies on the use of MSPNet to learn shape representations which are able to measure morphological differences in the liver and spleen of healthy subjects when compared to individuals diagnosed with diabetes mellitus. Diabetes mellitus is a worldwide prevalent condition, which is defined by levels of hyperglycaemia giving rise to risk of microvascular damage and its diagnosis is associated with complications, which lead to reduced life expectancy and diminished quality of life [15].

Concretely, we propose the first deep learning approach operating on the shape of abdominal organs for the prediction of diabetes. Further, we extend the state-of-the-art shape representation BrainPrint [20] to the abdomen, yielding the AbdomenPrint. Finally, we compare MSPNet and AbdomenPrint in the challenging task of predicting diabetes directly from the shape of the liver and spleen.

1.1 Related Work

The use of shape models for the analysis of morphological changes associated with disease or other factors has mainly been explored in neuroimaging. Significant relationships between measurements of brain morphology and a variety of factors such as age [1] and neurodegenerative diseases [20] have been thoroughly explored. In this work, we focus on the abdominal organs liver and spleen. Previous approaches have explored the morphological analysis of the liver based on imaging data. Lamecker et al. [11] present for the first time a statistical shape model of the liver. Dura et al. [3] present the construction of a probabilistic liver atlas. In terms of using shape models for the diagnosis of liver related diseases, Kohara et al. [10] use a statistical shape model of the liver to assess differences between healthy subjects and individuals diagnosed with cirrhosis. A similar approach is proposed by Mukherjee et al. [14] for the discrimination of chronic liver disease from CT Data and by Hori et al. [9] where a statistical shape model is used to evaluate differences in liver shape caused by hepatic fibrosis.

Shape analysis of the spleen is a far less explored area of research. Tateyama et al. [18] present the use of a Point Distribution Model (PDM) for the analysis of spleen shape. Yates et al. [24] present a morphological study of the spleen, relating the principal components obtained from a statistical shape model to anthropometric and demographic information.

In this work, we deviate from these previous approaches in the methodology used to assess relationships between abdominal morphology and clinical variables. Instead of modeling shape variation using the commonly used features derived from Point Distribution Models, we evaluate the use of two state-of-the-art approaches: MSPNet [7] and BrainPrint [20]. These two approaches have previously been used for the morphological analysis of brain structures, but they have yet to be applied for the analysis of abdominal structures.

2 Method

The usual pipeline of shape analysis of anatomical structures consists of extracting a binary segmentation of the structure of interest from an image (either manually or automatically) followed by the extraction of a shape descriptor vector $S \in \mathbb{R}^{dim}$ which can be used to quantitatively model the shape of an organ of interest. In the case of a classification task, we can then find a function $f(S) \mapsto y$ mapping shape descriptors S to a label y. Which corresponds to the variable to be predicted. In our case $y \in \{0, 1\}$ is an indicator variable which determines if a particular subject is healthy $(y = 0)$ or has been diagnosed with a diabetic condition $(y = 1)$.

In our experiments, we evaluate the use of two different shape representations S. In both cases, independent shape representations S_l and S_s are calculated independently for the liver and spleen, and are afterwards concatenated to obtain a global shape descriptor S.

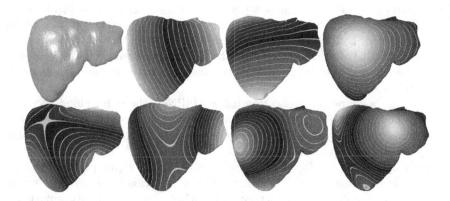

Fig. 1. Liver surface and first seven non-constant eigenfunctions of the Laplace-Beltrami operator (sorted left to right, top to bottom) calculated on the surface. Increasing positive values of the eigenfunctions are shown in the color gradient from red to yellow and decreasing negative values are shown from dark blue to light blue. (Color figure online)

2.1   AbdomenPrint

The AbdomenPrint **S** is the analogy of the BrainPrint [20], which has been successfully used to associate morphological changes in the brain correlated to Alzheimer's disease [21–23], but in our case we apply it to the analysis of abdominal organs. AbdomenPrint uses the shapeDNA [17] as shape descriptor, which is computed from the intrinsic geometry of organs by calculating the Laplace-Beltrami spectrum. Considering the Laplace-Beltrami operator Δ, the spectrum is obtained by solving the Laplacian eigenvalue problem:

$$\Delta f = -\lambda f. \tag{1}$$

The solution of this problem consists of a series of eigenvalues $\lambda_i \in \mathbb{R}$ and eigenfunctions f_i (see Fig. 1). The first l non-zero eigenvalues, computed with the finite element method, form the ShapeDNA: $\lambda = (\lambda_1, \ldots, \lambda_l)$. We further linearly re-weight the eigenvalues, $\hat{\lambda}_i = \lambda_i/i$, to balance the impact of higher eigenvalues that show higher variance [20]. The shape of an organ can then be represented by the vector of normalized eigenvalues $\mathbf{S} = \hat{\lambda}$. For the computation of shapeDNA, triangular meshes are constructed from organ segmentations via marching cubes.

2.2   MSPNet

We have recently introduced Multi-structure PointNet (MSPNet) [7] for shape analysis of brain structures. MSPNet is a network architecture based on Point-Net, a state of the art deep learning approach for point cloud classification [16]. In MSPNet, a shape representation can be learned in an end-to-end fashion directly from a point cloud $\mathbf{P} = [x_0, y_0, z_0, x_1, y_1, z_1, \ldots, x_n, y_n, z_n]$ where x_i, y_i, z_i correspond to the cartesian coordinates of the points representing the surface of the organ of interest. Different to other shape representations based on point clouds such as Point Distribution Models, in MSPNet it is not required for the points in **P** to be ordered, which means that no anatomical correspondences between shapes are needed.

To obtain a shape representation using MSPNet, the point cloud vector **P** is fed to the network (see Fig. 2). The first stage of the network corresponds to a transformation network which corresponds to a function $f(\mathbf{P}) \to \mathbf{T}$ mapping the input point cloud to a transformation matrix $\mathbf{T} \in \mathbb{R}^{3x3}$. This transformation matrix is applied to the input point cloud, so that the input point clouds are aligned before further processing is done. This transformation layer is known as T-Net [16], and is similar in structure to PointNet. After this transformation is applied to the input point cloud, the representation **S** is obtained by applying $l = 1 \ldots L$ layers:

$$\mathbf{S}^{(l)} = \mathbf{max}(\{g(W^{(l)}a_i^{(l-1)} + b^{(l)})\}_{i=1}^N) \tag{2}$$

where $W^{(l)}$ corresponds to the shared weights of the lth layer, g is a non linear activation function and $a_i^{(l-1)}$ correspond to the activation of the ith point of the previous layer. By processing the point cloud $\mathbf{P}$ through these shared weight layers, MSPNet obtains a global feature vector $\mathbf{S}$ at the last shared weight layer corresponds to a feature representation of each organ. This feature vector is then connected to a fully connected multilayer perceptron corresponding to a function $f(\mathbf{S}) \mapsto y$. It is important to notice that since this network is trained in an end-to-end fashion, the feature vector $\mathbf{S}$ is optimized for the diabetes classification task.

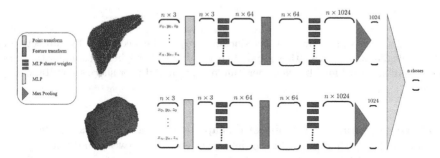

Fig. 2. MSPNet architecture for abdominal structures. The network consists of one branch per structure, one for the liver and one for the spleen, which are fused before the final multilayer perceptron (MLP). Each structure is represented by a point cloud with n points that pass through transformer networks and multilayer perceptrons at each individual branch. Numbers over each layer correspond to their sizes.

3   Experiments

Experiments are performed on a set of whole-body Magnetic Resonance Images (MRI) obtained from the Cooperative Health Research in the Region Augsburg project (KORA). Manual segmentations of the liver and the spleen were obtained from 359 images, 228 corresponding to healthy controls and 131 corresponding to subjects diagnosed with either pre-diabetes or diabetes according to definitions by the world health organization [15]. From these segmentations, point clouds are obtained by uniformly sampling the surface area of each organ.

3.1   Diabetes Classification

For a first experiment we evaluate the ability of each shape representation for the problem of discriminating between shapes of organs obtained from healthy individuals compared to subjects diagnosed with pre-diabetes or diabetes. Our set of 359 images is split divided in training and testing sets (50/50) and classification performance is evaluated in terms of Area Under the Curve (AUC) (Table 1) of the Receiver Operating Characteristic (ROC) curves shown in Fig. 3. For comparison we compute AbdomenPrint features, and a gradient boosting classifier

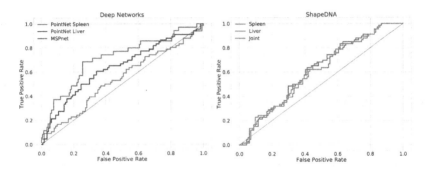

Fig. 3. ROC curves showing the classification results between healthy subjects and individuals diagnosed with either pre-diabetes or diabetes. Higher area under the curve values were obtained for MSPNet operating on spleen and liver shapes simultaneously.

is trained to operate on the obtained shape descriptors. Our results show that although both methods are able to detect differences between diabetic and control patients, MSPNet presents a higher classification performance. It is also worth mentioning that using joint shape descriptors of both the spleen and the liver did not improve classification for AbdomenPrint, whereas MSPNet was able to leverage on joint information obtained from both organs simultaneously.

Table 1. Area under the curve values for the diabetes classification experiment.

	Liver	Spleen	Abdomen
AbdomenPrint	0.61	0.60	0.62
MSPNet	0.69	0.61	**0.74**

3.2   Visualization of the Shape Feature Spaces

One of the main advantages of using representations that are trained in an end-to-end fashion for classification is that the obtained shape representation is specifically optimized for a particular task. In the case of MSPNet, we expect the shape descriptors **S** to lie on a space where shapes of organs of healthy patients are clustered close to each other and separated to the shapes of organs of patients diagnosed with diabetes. To have a better understanding of the properties of these learned representations, we visualize 2D projections of the shape descriptors **S** by embedding them into a two dimensional space using t-Distributed Stochastic Neighbor Embedding (t-SNE) [12]. These embeddings can be observed in Fig. 4, where we present embeddings on the 2D space for the liver using both AbdomenPrint and MSPNet. In this figure we can observe that the feature space obtained using MSPNet leads to clusters which group together either healthy subjects or individuals diagnosed with pre-diabetes or diabetes. This can be explained by the fact that the shape descriptors **S** of MSPNet are specifically optimized for the separation between these two classes as opposed to AbdomenPrint, which uses standard descriptors that are not targeted to a specific task.

4 Conclusions

We have proposed the use of a deep learning based representation for the morphological analysis of abdominal organs, and we have applied this representation for the task of diabetes classifications. Our results show that the use of learning representations based on deep networks have the potential to uncover shape deformations correlated to disease, and potentially to other factors. Compared to other methods, which rely on engineered features, the shape descriptors learned by MSPNet are optimized for the task of diabetes classification and are based on a simple point cloud representation without the need of calculating meshes or finding points correspondences between subjects.

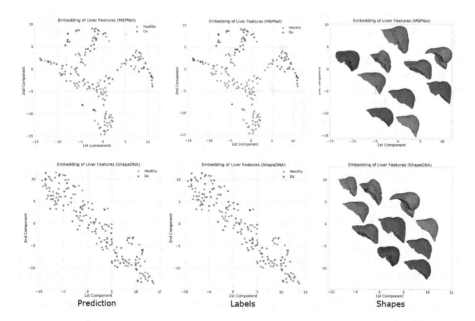

Fig. 4. Embedding of the shape descriptors **S** into a 2D space using t-SNE. Each point corresponds to a different subject. The color coding on the left corresponds to the real diagnosis for each subject and the coding in the middle to the label assigned by the classifier. Liver shapes on the right column are shown according to their location in the t-SNE space (the color of the surfaces of the livers is just used for visualization purposes and is not related to the labels).

Acknowledgments. This work was supported in part by DFG, SAP SE and the Bavarian State Ministry of Education, Science and the Arts in the framework of the Centre Digitalisation.Bavaria (ZD.B).

References

1. Cole, J.H., Franke, K.: Predicting age using neuroimaging: innovative brain ageing biomarkers. Trends Neurosci. **40**(12), 681–690 (2017)
2. Cootes, T., Taylor, C., Cooper, D., Graham, J.: Active shape models-their training and application. Comput. Vis. Image Underst. **61**(1), 38–59 (1995)
3. Dura, E., Domingo, J., Ayala, G., Marti-Bonmati, L., Goceri, E.: Probabilistic liver atlas construction. Biomed. Eng. Online **16**(1), 15 (2017)
4. Gerardin, E., et al.: Multidimensional classification of hippocampal shape features discriminates Alzheimer's disease and mild cognitive impairment from normal aging. Neuroimage **47**(4), 1476–1486 (2009)
5. Gorczowski, K., et al.: Statistical shape analysis of multi-object complexes. In: Computer Vision Pattern Recognition, pp. 1–8 (2007)
6. Gutierrez-Becker, B., Klein, T., Wachinger, C., Initiative, A.D.N., et al.: Gaussian process uncertainty in age estimation as a measure of brain abnormality. NeuroImage **175**, 246–258 (2018)
7. Gutierrez-Becker, B., Wachinger, C.: Deep multi-structural shape analysis: application to neuroanatomy. In: International Conference on Medical Image Computing and Computer Assisted Interventions (2018). https://arxiv.org/abs/1806.01069
8. Heimann, T., Meinzer, H.P.: Statistical shape models for 3D medical image segmentation: a review. Med. Image Anal. **13**(4), 543–563 (2009)
9. Hori, M., et al.: Quantitative imaging: quantification of liver shape on CT using the statistical shape model to evaluate hepatic fibrosis. Acad. Radiol. **22**(3), 303–309 (2015). https://doi.org/10.1016/j.acra.2014.10.001
10. Kohara, S., et al.: Application of statistical shape model to diagnosis of liver disease. In: 2010 2nd International Conference Software Engineering and Data Mining (SEDM), vol. 1, pp. 680–683 (2010)
11. Lamecker, H., Lange, T., Seebass, M.: Segmentation of the liver using a 3D statistical shape model (2004)
12. van der Maaten, L., Hinton, G.: Visualizing data using t-SNE. J. Mach. Learn. Res. **9**(Nov), 2579–2605 (2008)
13. Miller, M.I., Younes, L., Trouvé, A.: Diffeomorphometry and geodesic positioning systems for human anatomy. Technology **2**(01), 36–43 (2014)
14. Mukherjee, D.P., et al.: Utilizing disease-specific organ shape components for disease discrimination: application to discrimination of chronic liver disease from CT Data. In: Mori, K., Sakuma, I., Sato, Y., Barillot, C., Navab, N. (eds.) MICCAI 2013. LNCS, vol. 8149, pp. 235–242. Springer, Heidelberg (2013). https://doi.org/10.1007/978-3-642-40811-3_30
15. World Health Organization, et al.: Definition, diagnosis and classification of diabetes mellitus and its complications: report of a who consultation. Part 1, diagnosis and classification of diabetes mellitus (1999)
16. Qi, C.R., Su, H., Mo, K., Guibas, L.J.: Pointnet: deep learning on point sets for 3D classification and segmentation. In: Proceedings Computer Vision and Pattern Recognition (CVPR), vol. 1, no. 2, p. 4. IEEE (2017)
17. Reuter, M., Wolter, F.E., Peinecke, N.: Laplace-Beltrami spectra as shape-DNA of surfaces and solids. Comput. Aided Des. **38**(4), 342–366 (2006)

18. Tateyama, T., Foruzan, A., Chen, Y.W.: PCA based statistical shape model of the spleen. In: 5th International Conference Natural Compututation ICNC 2009, 6 January 2009
19. Valizadeh, S., Hänggi, J., Mérillat, S., Jäncke, L.: Age prediction on the basis of brain anatomical measures. Hum. Brain Mapp. **38**(2), 997–1008 (2017)
20. Wachinger, C., Golland, P., Kremen, W., Fischl, B., Reuter, M.: Brainprint: a discriminative characterization of brain morphology. NeuroImage **109**, 232–248 (2015)
21. Wachinger, C., Nho, K., Saykin, A.J., Reuter, M., Rieckmann, A.: A longitudinal imaging genetics study of neuroanatomical asymmetry in Alzheimers disease. Biol. Psychiatry **84**(7), 522–530 (2018)
22. Wachinger, C., Reuter, M.: Domain adaptation for Alzheimer's disease diagnostics. Neuroimage **139**, 470–479 (2016)
23. Wachinger, C., Salat, D.H., Weiner, M., Reuter, M.: Whole-brain analysis reveals increased neuroanatomical asymmetries in dementia for hippocampus and amygdala. Brain **139**(12), 3253–3266 (2016)
24. Yates, K.M., Lu, Y.C., Untaroiu, C.D.: Statistical shape analysis of the human spleen geometry for probabilistic occupant models. J. Biomech. **49**(9), 1540–1546 (2016). https://doi.org/10.1016/j.jbiomech.2016.03.027

Nonparametric Aggregation of Geodesic Trends for Longitudinal Data Analysis

Kristen M. Campbell$^{(\boxtimes)}$ and P. Thomas Fletcher

Scientific Computing and Imaging Institute, University of Utah,
Salt Lake City, UT, USA
kris@sci.utah.edu

Abstract. We propose a technique for analyzing longitudinal imaging data that models individual changes with diffeomorphic geodesic regression and aggregates these geodesics into a nonparametric group average trend. Our model is specifically tailored to the unbalanced and sparse characteristics of longitudinal imaging studies. That is, each individual has few data points measured over a short period of time, while the study population as a whole spans a wide age range. We use geodesic regression to estimate individual trends, which is an appropriate model for capturing shape changes over a short time window, as is typically found within an individual. Geodesics are also adept at handling the low sample sizes found within individuals, and can model the change between as few as two timepoints. However, geodesics are limited for modeling longer-term trends, where constant velocity may not be appropriate. Therefore, we develop a novel nonparametric regression to aggregate individual trends into an average group trend. We demonstrate the power of our method to capture non-geodesic group trends on hippocampal volume (real-valued data) and diffeomorphic registration of full 3D MRI from the longitudinal OASIS data.

1 Introduction

Quantifying anatomical shape changes due to disease progression is an important step towards improving early disease detection, tracking treatment efficacy, and generally understanding disease processes. While cross-sectional studies have yielded some insights into disease progression, such as understanding atrophy in Alzheimer's, these methods cannot explain the changes that individuals undergo. Longitudinal studies, on the other hand, measure changes within individuals by repeating measurements for each participant over time. This allows estimation of individual trajectories, as well as the average trajectory for a group.

Semiparametric mixed effect models have been used to analyze longitudinal data such as height changes over time [3]. These mixed effect models have been used to analyze longitudinal neuroimaging data by looking at summary measures like volume of the brain or its various substructures. However these summaries cannot give a detailed picture of where or how the shape changes over time. Other methods have extended this analysis to look at longitudinal change of

© Springer Nature Switzerland AG 2018
M. Reuter et al. (Eds.): ShapeMI 2018, LNCS 11167, pp. 232–243, 2018.
https://doi.org/10.1007/978-3-030-04747-4_22

substructure surfaces [12,17]. This requires segmenting the structures of interest beforehand and finding correspondences between points on the surface. Work has also been done to analyze longitudinal change of measures like fractional anisotropy along DTI fiber tracts [18]. Allowing the measures to vary along the tracts is valuable, but it requires measurements along the length of the tract and alignment of tracts across subjects. In fact, many of the existing methods are designed to work with this kind of balanced data where all subjects have measurements across the entire duration of the period of interest.

Some analysis has been done on longitudinal univariate manifold data, in particular trying to find alignment of time of disease onset [14]. We want to go beyond the univariate measures and characterize shape changes over time. Methods for looking at shape change over time [4,5,8,10] look for geodesic group trends and geodesic subject trends. However, as pointed out in [7], a geodesic model is not sufficient to explain shape change during periods of significant growth or atrophy. This is because a geodesic must be constant velocity, whereas anatomical shape changes typically exhibit acceleration or deceleration.

We develop a longitudinal data analysis that has the flexibility to model complex, non-constant speed trends at the group level. At the same time, we can handle individual data that is sparsely sampled in time, and unbalanced, that is, individuals are not sampled at the same timepoints, and may even have different numbers of measurements. To do this, we model the individual trends with a geodesic, which is adept at sparsely sampled, short-term shape trends. Next, we develop a novel method called Aggregation of Longitudinal Geodesics (ALG) for averaging the geodesic trends into a nonparametric group trend that can capture accelerating or decelerating shape changes. We perform experiments with 3D brain MRI and associated univariate measurements to show that the group trends are not constant speed and that our approach captures these complexities.

2   Methods

We consider longitudinal data lying on a Riemannian manifold M. In the present paper, we will analyze univariate measurements ($M = \mathbb{R}$), as well as 3D MR images under the LDDMM metric. However, our method is generally applicable to other manifolds. Let $y_{ij} \in M$ denote the jth measurement from the ith subjects, taken at time t_{ij}, and let N be the number of subjects, each with P_i measurements. The full data set spans an age range, $[t_{\min}, t_{\max}]$, while each individual subject spans a much smaller age range, i.e., $t_{i,P_i} - t_{i,1} \ll t_{\max} - t_{\min}$.

Individual Geodesic Trends. We start by modeling the subject-specific trajectories as geodesic curves, $\gamma_i : [t_{i1}, t_{iP_i}] \to M$. These geodesic trends are fit to the subject data, (t_{ij}, y_{ij}) using geodesic regression. A geodesic can be parameterized by its initial position $p = \gamma_i(t_{i1}) \in M$ and velocity $v = \gamma_i'(t_{i1}) \in T_p M$ (tangent space to p). Geodesic regression [6] solves the least-squares problem:

$$(\hat{p}_i, \hat{v}_i) = \arg \min_{(p,v) \in TM} d(y_{ij}, \mathrm{Exp}_p (t_{ij} v))^2,$$

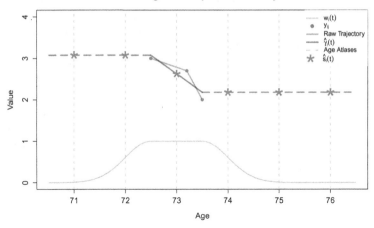

Fig. 1. Illustration showing the contributions from one subject's longitudinal measurements, weighted by the kernel function $w_i(t)$.

where Exp is the Riemannian exponential map, which converts an inital position and velocity into a geodesic curve, i.e., $\gamma(t) = \text{Exp}_p(tv)$, and $d(\cdot, \cdot)$ is the Riemannian distance on M. The end result, for each subject i, is an estimated geodesic trend $\hat{\gamma}_i$, parameterized by its initial position $\hat{p}_i$ and velocity $\hat{v}_i$.

For univariate data, a geodesic is a straight line, and geodesic regression is simply ordinary least-squares regression. Whereas, for images, we use diffeomorphic geodesic regression [11]. For this work, we used the vector momenta formulation [15] of LDDMM to perform the geodesic regression. In order to define kernel-weighted averaging of trends, we need a definition of an individual's trend over time extending for the full support of the kernel, which will generally extend beyond the time interval of a subject. To do this, we define a constant extension of the data at the endpoints for a subject. Thus, the ith subject's trend is given by

$$\hat{s}_i(t) = \begin{cases} \hat{\gamma}_i(t_{i1}) & \text{if } t < t_{i1}, \\ \hat{\gamma}_i(t) & \text{if } t_{i1} \leq t \leq t_{iP_i}, \\ \hat{\gamma}_i(t_{iP_i}) & \text{otherwise.} \end{cases} \tag{1}$$

Nonparametric Group Trend. We build a group trend of age-specific atlases as a nonparametric kernel regression of the subject-specific models' predictions. We then compute a weighted average of the data (univariate or images) at that age where the weight for a subject's interpolated image is 1 when the age falls between the time of the first and last measurement for that subject. Outside of that window, the weight for an age, t, decreases according to a Gaussian kernel of the form

$$K_l(t, i) = e^{\frac{-(t - t_{i,1})^2}{2\sigma^2}}, K_r(t, i) = e^{\frac{-(t - t_{i,P_i})^2}{2\sigma^2}} \tag{2}$$

where $K_l(t, i)$ is used when age $t < t_{i,1}$ and $K_r(t, i)$ is used when the age $t > t_{i,P_i}$. These kernels are used to compute the weight function, w_i for each subject:

$$w_i(t) = \begin{cases} K_l(t, i) & \text{if } t < t_{i,1}, \\ 1 & \text{if } t_{i,1} \leq t \leq t_{i,P_i}, \\ K_r(t, i) & \text{otherwise.} \end{cases} \tag{3}$$

To construct an age atlas, a_t, at age t, we compute the weighted Fréchet mean:

$$a_t = \arg\min_{a \in M} \sum_{i=1}^{N} w_i(t) d(\hat{s}_i(t), a)^2. \tag{4}$$

For univariate data ($M = \mathbb{R}$), the solution to this minimization problem is the weighted average. For images under the LDDMM metric, we follow the approach in [2], by constructing the weighted diffeomorphic atlas a_t by gradient descent optimization. In Fig. 1, we illustrate how one subject would contribute to the age atlases constructed every year between 71 and 76.

3   Experiments

3.1   Simulated Univariate Data

Before applying ALG to real data, we wanted to understand how well it can reconstruct a known nonlinear group trend in longitudinal data. We start by simulating univariate data with a ground truth group trend of $y = 4x^2 - 8x + 4$ in the range $[0, 1]$ with slope $y' = 8x - 8$. We simulate longitudinal data for $N = 100$ subjects by generating $P_i = 3$ time points for each subject that follow a noisy y-shifted version of the group trend. We draw the middle age for a subject, $t_{i,2} \sim \text{Unif}(0, 1)$, and compute the group slope and intercept at this point. We then choose a random first and last age not too far away in time, $t_{i,1} = t_{i,2} - \delta_{i,1}, t_{i,3} = t_{i,2} + \delta_{i,2}$ where $\delta_{i,j} \sim N(0, 0.05)$. From these time points we generate the associated measurements $m_{i,j} = y'(t_{i,2}) * t_{i,j} + y(t_{i,2}) - y'(t_{i,2}) * t_{i,2} + \eta_i + \epsilon_{i,j}$ where $\eta_i \sim N(0, 1)$ and $\epsilon_{i,j} \sim N(0, 0.1)$.

We apply ALG with $\sigma = 0.1$ for 10 equally spaced age atlases, a_t. Figure 2 shows all 100 subjects and the age atlases showing the estimated group trend. Notice that the estimated group trend closely follows the nonlinear ground truth trend.

3.2   Simulated Images

We tested ALG with simulated images by creating a longitudinal version of the cross-sectional bulls-eye experiment from [2]. We generate 256×256 2D bulls-eye images at 4 different time points for each of 173 individuals where the 3 radii that define each bulls-eye evolve in time according to known processes. The innermost radius, $R1$, follows a logistic decay process from 18 pixels at age

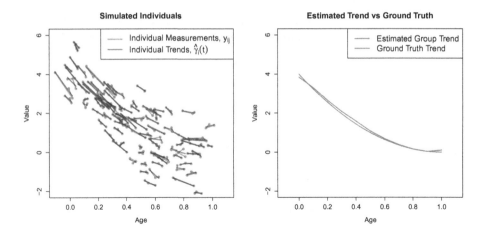

Fig. 2. Left: longitudinal data simulated to follow a nonlinear group trend. Right: atlas values computed by ALG recover the ground truth trend.

65 to 12 at age 95. The middle radius, $R2$, grows logistically from 25 to 45 pixels over the same time, and the outer radius, $R3$, grows linearly from 70 to 90 pixels.

The starting age for the i-th subject is drawn from $t_{i,0} \sim \mathrm{Unif}(0,1)$. The ages for each of the subsequent 3 time points for that subject are $t_{i,j+1} = t_{i,j} + \delta_{i,j}$ where $\delta_{i,j} \sim N(1,0.5)$. The radii for the i-th subject at the j-th time point are calculated as

$$R_{1,i,j}(t_{i,j}) = f_1(t_{i,j}) + \eta_{1,i} + \epsilon_{1,i,j} \tag{5}$$

$$R_{2,i,j}(t_{i,j}) = f_2(t_{i,j}) + \eta_{2,i} + \epsilon_{2,i,j} \tag{6}$$

$$R_{3,i,j}(t_{i,j}) = f_3(t_{i,j}) + \eta_{3,i} + \epsilon_{3,i,j}, \tag{7}$$

where the k-th radius has a subject-specific noisy shift, $\eta_{k,i} \sim N(0,2)$, and also timepoint-specific noise, $\epsilon_{k,i,j} \sim N(0,1)$. Once the images are created, zero-mean Gaussian noise with standard deviation $= 0.03$ is added to the image intensities.

Figure 3 shows the results of univariate ALG with $\sigma = 3$ performed separately on each of the radii measurements to create an age atlas for each year between 65 and 95. We then apply ALG with the same sigma value to the 173 sets of 4 longitudinal 2D images (see Fig. 4 for a representative selection of these images). As shown in Fig. 5, we compared the estimated atlases and associated momenta with the ground truth atlases and found that the original atlases are recovered and that the momenta between atlases change nonlinearly over time.

To quantify the dynamics of the shape change, we looked at two properties of the estimated paths: the norm of the momenta at each time point and also the deviation of the velocity from a geodesic (see Fig. 6). A geodesic satisfies the equation, $\frac{dv}{dt} + \mathrm{ad}_v^\dagger v = 0$. So, if we compute the left-hand side, we can measure how "non-geodesic" the path is, and we call this value the curvature of the path. This is the covariant derivative of the velocity along the path, i.e., $\nabla_{v(t)} v(t)$. If

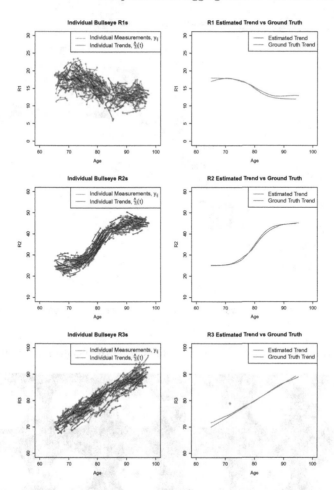

Fig. 3. Univariate ALG analysis of bulls-eye radii.

the norm is nearly constant and the curvature is nearly 0 everywhere then the longitudinal trend is linear. Notice that our results have a large increase in both the norm and curvature around age 80, consistent with the logistic processes for R1 and R2 that change the fastest at their halfway point. ALG successfully models this nonlinear group trend in the image data and provides atlases for each age that match the ground truth image for that age.

3.3   Real Data

We used T1 MRIs for 142 adults with and without Alzheimer's disease from the longitudinal OASIS database [9] with 72 Nondemented (Clinical Dementia Rating, CDR = 0) subjects between the ages of 60 and 93, 56 Demented (CDR ≥ 0.5) subjects between the ages of 61 and 96 and 14 Converted subjects (CDR

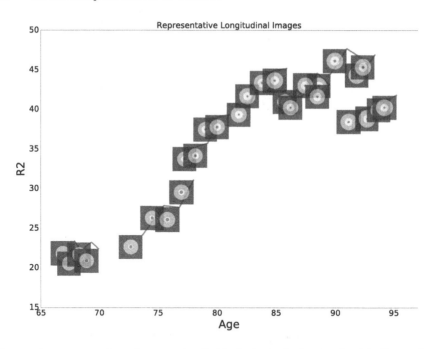

Fig. 4. A representative selection of individuals from the longitudinal bulls-eye data.

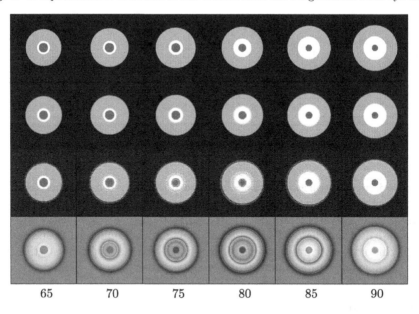

Fig. 5. Columns 1–6: 2D bullseye atlases at a selection of ages. First row: ground truth images. Second row: Estimated atlases. Third row: estimated atlases with initial momenta overlaid as red arrows. Last row: estimated atlases with the log jacobian determinant of the deformations from one atlas to the next overlaid. Blue is contraction (negative values), white is 0 and red is expansion (postive values). (Color figure online)

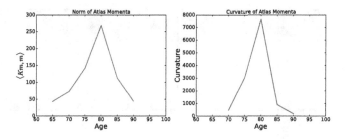

Fig. 6. Momenta norm and curvature of estimated bulls-eye atlases.

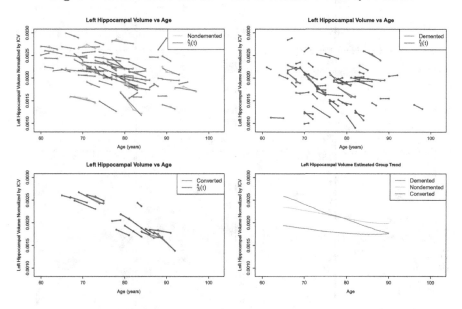

Fig. 7. Left hippocampal volumes normalized by inter-cranial volume (ICV).

changed from 0 to 0.5 over course of the study) between the ages of 65 and 87. The subjects had between 1 and 5 MRI scans taken with a time between first and last scans of between 1 and 7 years.

All images were processed using longitudinal Freesurfer to do skull stripping and intensity normalization and to measure left and right hippocampal volumes [13]. Geodesic regression was then performed on the processed images for each subject individually as described in [16]. We use the vector momenta implementation of geodesic shooting to shoot the initial momenta from the individual geodesic regressions in order to find an image for a subject at a particular age. We chose to use the "Goldie Locks" sigma of 6 years for the kernel which was also used by [2].

First, we look at the left and right hippocampal volumes computed by longitudinal Freesurfer. Figure 7 shows the results of ALG applied to left hippocampal

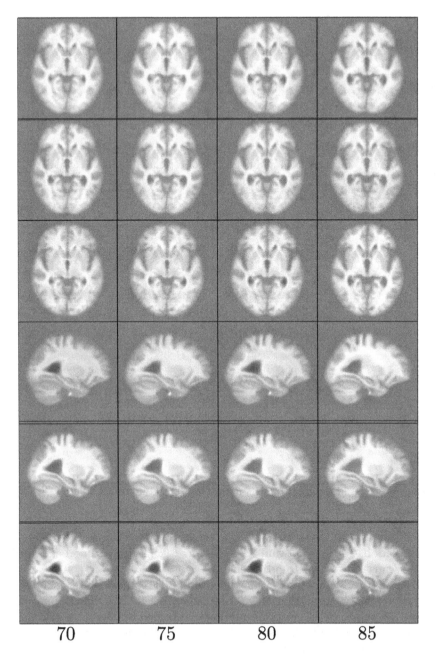

70   75   80   85

Fig. 8. Columns 1–4: atlases of 3D OASIS data at a selection of ages. Rows 1–3: 2D axial view of nondemented, demented and converted atlases respectively. Rows 4–6: 2D sagittal view of nondemented, demented and converted atlases respectively. The log jacobian determinant of the deformations from one atlas to the next are overlaid with a colormap, where blue is contraction, white is 0 and red is expansion. (Color figure online)

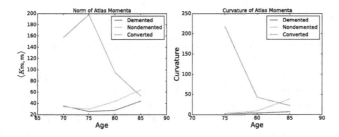

Fig. 9. Momenta norm and curvature of OASIS atlases.

volumes normalized by inter-cranial volume (ICV). Similar results were found for the right hippocampus. Note in particular that our method captures the nonlinear nature of the volume change over time.

Now let's look how the diffeomorphisms change over time. In Fig. 8, we show the age atlases overlaid with the initial momenta at each age. Notice that the location and magnitude of the shape change changes over time, especially around the ventricles and hippocampi. This is consistent with the literature [1,12,17]. We quantified this nonlinearity by computing the norm and curvature of the momenta between estimated atlases as shown in Fig. 9. Since the norm is non-constant and the curvature is nonzero, the shape change of these images is nonlinear. The age-specific atlases generated by ALG capture this acceleration and deceleration in shape change over time.

4   Discussion

We presented ALG, a method that can aggregate longitudinal measurements across subjects, where the measurements for an individual span a small time window compared to the aggregated time window. ALG works for any manifold data that can be modelled by a geodesic regression.

We applied ALG to simulated univariate and image data and were able to recover the underlying group trend in both cases. We then applied ALG to the longitudinal OASIS data and saw that the group trends for atrophy are nonlinear, with different structures atrophying at different rates and different times in the disease progression, which is consistent with the literature [1]. This demonstrates that ALG is indeed able to capture accelerating and decelerating anatomical shape changes.

Acknowledgements. This work was supported by NIH grant R01EB022876. The OASIS data was provided by the following grants: P50 AG05681, P01 AG03991, R01 AG021910, P20 MH071616, U24 RR021382. Thanks to Nikhil Singh for providing the preprocessed Freesurfer data and subject-specific geodesic regressions.

References

1. Braak, H., Braak, E.: Evolution of the neuropathology of Alzheimer's disease. Acta Neurol. Scand. **94**(S165), 3–12 (1996)
2. Davis, B., Fletcher, P., Bullitt, E., Joshi, S.: Population shape regression from random design data. Int. J. Comput. Vis. **90**(2), 255–266 (2010)
3. Durbán, M., Harezlak, J., Wand, M., Carroll, R.: Simple fitting of subject-specific curves for longitudinal data. Stat. Med. **24**(8), 1153–1167 (2005)
4. Durrleman, S., Pennec, X., Trouvé, A., Braga, J., Gerig, G., Ayache, N.: Toward a comprehensive framework for the spatiotemporal statistical analysis of longitudinal shape data. Int. J. Comput. Vis. **103**(1), 22–59 (2013)
5. Fishbaugh, J., Prastawa, M., Durrleman, S., Piven, J., Gerig, G.: Analysis of longitudinal shape variability via subject specific growth modeling. In: Ayache, N., Delingette, H., Golland, P., Mori, K. (eds.) MICCAI 2012. LNCS, vol. 7510, pp. 731–738. Springer, Heidelberg (2012). https://doi.org/10.1007/978-3-642-33415-3_90
6. Fletcher, T.: Geodesic regression on Riemannian manifolds. In: MFCA, pp. 75–86 (2011)
7. Gerig, G., Fishbaugh, J., Sadeghi, N.: Longitudinal modeling of appearance and shape and its potential for clinical use. Med. Image Anal. **33**, 114–121 (2016)
8. Hadj-Hamou, M., Lorenzi, M., Ayache, N., Pennec, X.: Longitudinal analysis of image time series with diffeomorphic deformations: a computational framework based on stationary velocity fields. Frontiers Neurosci. **10**, 236 (2016)
9. Marcus, D., Fotenos, A., Csernansky, J., Morris, J., Buckner, R.: Open access series of imaging studies: longitudinal MRI data in nondemented and demented older adults. J. Cogn. Neurosci. **22**(12), 2677–2684 (2010)
10. Muralidharan, P., Fletcher, P.: Sasaki metrics for analysis of longitudinal data on manifolds. In: CVPR, pp. 1027–1034. IEEE (2012)
11. Niethammer, M., Huang, Y., Vialard, F.-X.: Geodesic regression for image time-series. In: Fichtinger, G., Martel, A., Peters, T. (eds.) MICCAI 2011. LNCS, vol. 6892, pp. 655–662. Springer, Heidelberg (2011). https://doi.org/10.1007/978-3-642-23629-7_80
12. Qiu, A., Younes, L., Miller, M., Csernansky, J.: Parallel transport in diffeomorphisms distinguishes the time-dependent pattern of hippocampal surface deformation due to healthy aging and the dementia of the alzheimer's type. NeuroImage **40**(1), 68–76 (2008)
13. Reuter, M., Schmansky, N., Rosas, H., Fischl, B.: Within-subject template estimation for unbiased longitudinal image analysis. Neuroimage **61**(4), 1402–1418 (2012)
14. Schiratti, J., Allassonniere, S., Colliot, O., Durrleman, S.: Learning spatiotemporal trajectories from manifold-valued longitudinal data. In: NIPS, pp. 2404–2412 (2015)
15. Singh, N., Hinkle, J., Joshi, S., Fletcher, P.: A vector momenta formulation of diffeomorphisms for improved geodesic regression and atlas construction. In: ISBI, pp. 1219–1222. IEEE (2013)
16. Singh, N., Hinkle, J., Joshi, S., Fletcher, P.: Hierarchical geodesic models in diffeomorphisms. Int. J. Comput. Vis. **117**(1), 70–92 (2016)

17. Tang, X., Holland, D., Dale, A., Younes, L., Miller, M.: The diffeomorphometry of regional shape change rates and its relevance to cognitive deterioration in mild cognitive impairment and Alzheimer's disease. Hum. Brain Mapp. **36**(6), 2093–2117 (2015)
18. Zhu, H., et al.: Fadtts: functional analysis of diffusion tensor tract statistics. NeuroImage **56**(3), 1412–1425 (2011)

DeepSSM: A Deep Learning Framework for Statistical Shape Modeling from Raw Images

Riddhish Bhalodia[1,2]([✉]), Shireen Y. Elhabian[1,2,3], Ladislav Kavan[2], and Ross T. Whitaker[1,2,3]

[1] Scientific Computing and Imaging Institute, University of Utah, Salt Lake City, USA
riddhishb@gmail.com
[2] School of Computing, University of Utah, Salt Lake City, USA
[3] Comprehensive Arrhythmia Research and Management Center, University of Utah, Salt Lake City, USA

Abstract. Statistical shape modeling is an important tool to characterize variation in anatomical morphology. Typical shapes of interest are measured using 3D imaging and a subsequent pipeline of registration, segmentation, and some extraction of shape features or projections onto some lower-dimensional shape space, which facilitates subsequent statistical analysis. Many methods for constructing compact shape representations have been proposed, but are often impractical due to the sequence of image preprocessing operations, which involve significant parameter tuning, manual delineation, and/or quality control by the users. We propose DeepSSM: a deep learning approach to extract a low-dimensional shape representation directly from 3D images, requiring virtually no parameter tuning or user assistance. DeepSSM uses a convolutional neural network (CNN) that simultaneously localizes the biological structure of interest, establishes correspondences, and projects these points onto a low-dimensional shape representation in the form of PCA loadings within a point distribution model. To overcome the challenge of the limited availability of training images with dense correspondences, we present a novel data augmentation procedure that uses existing correspondences on a relatively small set of processed images with shape statistics to create plausible training samples with known shape parameters. In this way, we leverage the limited CT/MRI scans (40–50) into thousands of images needed to train a deep neural net. After the training, the CNN automatically produces accurate low-dimensional shape representations for unseen images. We validate DeepSSM for three different applications pertaining to modeling pediatric cranial CT for characterization of metopic craniosynostosis, femur CT scans identifying morphologic deformities of the hip due to femoroacetabular impingement, and left atrium MRI scans for atrial fibrillation recurrence prediction.

© Springer Nature Switzerland AG 2018
M. Reuter et al. (Eds.): ShapeMI 2018, LNCS 11167, pp. 244–257, 2018.
https://doi.org/10.1007/978-3-030-04747-4_23

1 Introduction

Since the pioneering work of D'Arcy Thompson [30], statistical shape models (SSM), also called morphological analysis, have evolved into an important tool in medical and biological sciences. A classical approach to comprehend a large collection of 2D or 3D shapes is via landmark points, often corresponding to distinct anatomical features. More recently, shape analysis for medical images is conducted with dense sets of correspondences that are placed automatically to capture the statistics of a population of shapes [8,9,28] or by quantifying the differences in coordinate transformations that align populations of 3D images [4]. The applications of these statistical shape methods are diverse, finding uses in orthopedics [16], neuroscience [13], and cardiology [12].

The goals of these kinds of analyses vary. In some cases, the analysis may be toward a clinical diagnosis, a task that might lend itself to a detection or classification strategy, which may bypass the need for any explicit quantification of shape. However, in many cases the goals include more open-ended questions, such as the formulation or testing of hypotheses or understanding/communicating pathological morphologies. Furthermore, training a state-of-the-art classifier for a specific disease would typically require (on the order of) thousands of samples/images for training, which becomes a significant burden for many clinical or biological applications, especially those involving human subjects.

Therefore, in this paper we address the problem of generating a rich set of shape descriptors in the form of PCA loadings on a shape space and an associated set of dense (i.e., thousands) correspondence points. The goal is to design a system that bypasses the typical pipeline of segmenting and/or registering images/shapes and the associated optimization (and associated parameter tuning)—and instead produces shape information directly from images via a deep (convolutional) neural network. This shape information can then be used to study pathologies, perform diagnoses, and/or visualize or study properties of populations or individuals.

Another contribution of this paper is the overall system architecture (and the demonstration of its efficacy on cranial, left atria and femur morphologies), which provides a blueprint for building other systems that could be built/trained to perform image-to-shape analyses with relative ease. Another contribution is the particular strategy we have used for training, which relies on a conventional shape analysis on relatively small set of images to produce a very large training/validation data set, sufficient to train a convolutional neural network (CNN).

2 Related Work

The proposed system learns the projection of images onto a shape space, which is built using correspondences between surfaces. Explicit correspondences between surfaces have been done using geometric parameterizations [10,27] as well as functional maps [23]. In this work, we rely on a discrete, dense set of samples, whose positions are optimized across a population to reduce the statistical complexity of the resulting model. The resulting point sets can be then turned into a low-dimensional shape representation by principal component analysis (PCA), as in the method of point distribution models (PDMs) [15]. For this optimization of correspondences, we use the open-source *ShapeWorks* software [7,8], which requires extensive pre-processing of input 3D images including: registration, segmentation, anti-aliasing (including a topology-preserving smoothing) and conversion to a signed distance transform. These image processing steps require well-tuned parameters, which, in practice, precludes a fully automatic analysis of unseen scans.

Also related is the work on atlas building and computational anatomy using methods of deformable registration (e.g., diffeomorphisms derived from flows) [4]. Here, we pursue the correspondence-based approach because many applications benefit from explicit correspondences, exact matching of surfaces, and modes of variation and shape differences that can be easily computed and visualized for the surfaces under study (e.g., [32]). While DeepSSM may be relevant for such registration-based methods, such an approach would likely build on the many proposed neural-net solutions to image registration [26].

DeepSSM builds on various works that have applied convolution neural networks (CNNs) to 3D images [19]. More recently, deep learning is being generalized to mesh-based representations, with applications e.g., in shape retrieval [31]. While much has been done in detection [33], classification [20], and segmentation (e.g., pixel classification) [3,24], more directly relevant is the work on regression from 3D images. For instance, in [18] they regress the orientation and position of the heart from 2D ultrasound. Another recent work [22] demonstrates the efficacy of PCA loadings in regressing for landmark position, being used for ultrasound segmentation task. DeepSSM extends this idea to 3D volumes and an extensive evaluation using it is performed on different datasets. DeepSSM proposes a novel data-augmentation scheme to counter limited-data availability in medical imaging applications. Furthermore, we employ the use of existing shape modeling tools to generate point distribution model and leverage the shape statistics for direct prediction of general shape parameters using CNN.

3   Methods

DeepSSM, unlike standard statistical shape modeling methods, is not a generative framework. It focuses on minimal pre-processing and direct computation of shape descriptors from raw images of anatomy that can be further used for shape analysis applications; some of which are described in the results section. Figure 1 illustrates the training and usage of DeepSSM. In this section, we outline the data augmentation procedure, the CNN architecture and the learning protocols.

3.1   Training Data Augmentation

We start with a dataset with about 40–50 data samples, which are either CT or MRI images. These images are rigidly registered and downsampled to make

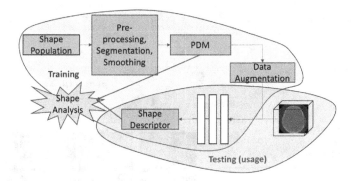

Fig. 1. Illustration of how DeepSSM is trained and used for getting shape descriptors for shape analysis directly from images.

the CNN training times manageable on current hardware, while still allowing for morphology characterization. Because a set of 40–50 data samples is not large enough for CNN training, we propose a new data augmentation method. First, we construct a statistical shape model from surfaces extracted from the original data. We place a dense set of 3D correspondence points on each of the shapes using *ShapeWorks* software [7,8], even though any method of producing a PDM is applicable. We reduce this high dimensional PDM to M dimensions using PCA, producing M−dimensional "loading vectors", where M between 10–15 is usually sufficient to capture 99% of the data variability. This corresponds to a multivariate (M−dimensional) Gaussian distribution, $\mathcal{N}(\mu, \Sigma)$. To generate a new synthetic image, we first draw a random sample $s \in \mathbb{R}^M$ from the $\mathcal{N}(\mu, \Sigma)$ distribution. This random sample s corresponds to a statistically plausible shape. To obtain a realistic 3D image associated with s, we find the closest example (denoted n) from input images. For this shape n, we already have a set of correspondences, C_n and an associated image, I_n. We use the correspondences $C_n \leftrightarrow C_s$ to construct a thin-plate spline (TPS) warp [6] of I_n to obtain a synthetic image I_s, which has the intensity profile of I_n but the cranial shape s. The amount of TPS deformation is typically small, and using this method, we can generate thousands of new images that are consistent with the PCA space and intensity characteristics of the original dataset (see Fig. 3). We also employ an add-reject strategy to prevent extreme outliers from being created. In particular, we find the nearest neighbour of each generated sample from the original shapes and we reject the sample if the Euclidean distance between the two shapes exceeds a specified threshold.

3.2   Network Architecture

We use a CNN architecture with five convolution layers followed by two fully connected layers to produce the output regression coefficients, see Fig. 3. The input to our network is a 3D image and the output is a set of ordered PCA loadings with respect to the shape space constructed in Sect. 3.1. We found that in

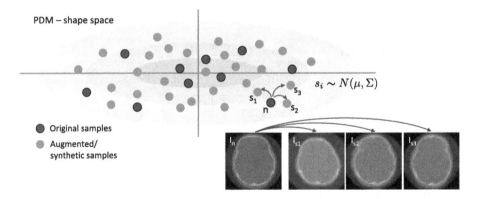

Fig. 2. Top: Shapes given by the original input CT scans (red dots) are augmented by sampling in the PDM shape space, from a normal distribution. Bottom-right: The resulting correspondences are used to transform original images of nearby samples (with a TPS warp) to create new images with known shape parameters. (Color figure online)

our setting, parametric ReLU [17] outperforms the traditional ReLU as a nonlinear activation function. We also perform batch normalization for all convolution layers. The weights of the network are initialized by Xavier initialization [14].

3.3   Learning Protocol

We use 4000–5000 training data points and 1000–2000 validation images generated as described in Sect. 3.1. We use TensorFlow [1] for constructing and training DeepSSM with a training batch size 10, which results in optimal saturation of the GPU (NVIDIA-Tesla K40c). The loss function is defined by taking $\mathbb{L}_2$ norm between the actual PCA loadings and the network output, and Adagrad [11] is used for optimization. We use average root mean square error per epoch to evaluate convergence. We observed empirically that, in all datasets, this error becomes level after 50 epochs staying in range between $1.9 - 2.5$. Based on these observations we train our network for 60 epochs.

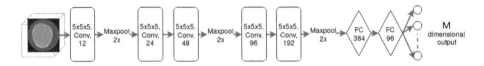

Fig. 3. The architecture of the CNN network.

4   Results and Discussion

We apply DeepSSM on three different datasets pertaining to three different applications: (i) Pediatric cranial CT scans (ages : 5–15 months) for metopic craniosynostosis characterization, (ii) Left Atrium MRI data for prediction for the atrial fibrillation recurrence, and, (iii) Femur CT Data for the characterization of morphologic deformities of the hip due to femoroacetabular impingement. For each application, we divide the data into two categories, one which is used to generate the original PDM to be used for data augmentation, and the other data is completely quarantined and will be used to check the generalizablity of DeepSSM, we will refer to this data as "unseen" data. We would like to stress that the unseen data is not part of the original data used for data augmentation or the PDM formation making it completely isolated. Further, we divide the data used for getting the PDM and it's accompanying augmented data into standard training, validation, and testing datasets. Another aspect to note is we perform a rigid ICP pre-alignment of all the images before computing it's PDM. It is important to note that DeepSSM is not an approach to discriminate between normal and pathological morphology, but an approach for reconstruction of shape representation from images that enables shape population statistics.

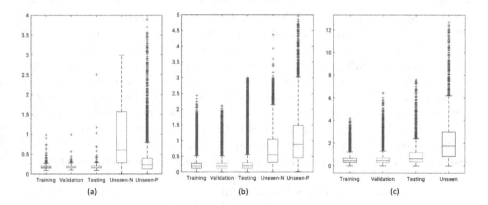

Fig. 4. Shape reconstruction errors in mm. Each boxplot shows the error per-point per-shape in each category, for training, testing, and validation datasets. As ground truth correspondences are available, the error is simple Euclidean distance (in mm). For the unseen normal (unseen-N) and unseen pathological (unseen-P), the error is the minimum projection distance of the predicted point to original surface mesh (again in mm). (a) Metopic Craniosynostosis data, (b) Femur data, and (c) Left Atrium data.

4.1   Metopic Craniosynostosis

Metopic craniosynostosis is a morphological disorder of cranium in infants caused by premature fusion of the metopic suture, see Fig. 5(metopic head). The characterization of the severity of the condition is hypothesized to be dependent on the deviation of skull shape from a normal phenotypical pediatric skull morphology. We aim to use DeepSSM to characterize this deviation. We use a dataset of 74 cranial CT scans of children with age between 5 to 15 months with 58 representing normal phenotypical skull morphology and 16 with metopic craniosynostosis, i.e., pathological skull deformities. 50 normative CT scans from the dataset were used in constructing our point distribution model, where each shape is represented by 1024 3D points; the vector of all these points is projected onto a 15-dimensional PCA subspace. We use this PDM to augment the data and train DeepSSM. We use the PCA loading predictions from a trained DeepSSM to reconstruct the 1024 correspondences and compare it with the original correspondences for obtaining the training, testing, and validation losses. To evaluate the accuracy of DeepSSM in predicting correspondences for unseen data, we use the remaining 8 CT scans of normal pediatric head shapes and 16 CT scans of children diagnosed with metopic craniosynostosis. We extract the outer skull surface from the unseen CT scans from a user-aided segmentation and render it as a triangle mesh using marching cubes. To account for an unknown coordinate system used in the unseen CT scan, we rigidly register this mesh to the 1024 3D correspondence points produced by DeepSSM from the raw CT scan. We then project these registered points to the surface of the mesh, these projection distances forms the error for evaluation on unseen data. The box plot representing the per-point per-shape Euclidean distance error, correspondence difference error for training, validation and testing data and the point to mesh projection error for the unseen cases, is shown in Fig. 4(a). We observe that even though there is significant variability in skull shapes, the average error (across both data inclusive and exclusive to the data augmentation method) does not exceed 1 mm. Our original CT scans were 1 mm isotropic and they were downsampled by a factor of 4 making the voxel size to be 4 mm, which means that DeepSSM predicts the correspondences with subvoxel accuracy. It is encouraging that even though our initial shape space was constructed for only normal head shapes, DeepSSM generalizes well also to skulls with abnormal morphology resulting from metopic craniosynostosis. Next, we use this to explore an example application of automatic characterization of metopic craniosynostosis. We take 16 CT scans of pediatric patients diagnosed with metopic craniosynostosis and processed through DeepSSM, which produces their PCA loadings in the normative skull-shape space. We hypothesize that the skull shapes affected by metopic craniosynostosis will be statistically different from normal skull shapes. We compute the Mahalanobis distance between each of our head shapes (both normal and metopic ones) and our normative statistical shape model $\mathcal{N}(\mu, \Sigma)$. The histograms of these Mahalanobis distances for our datasets are shown in Fig. 5. We can see that the histograms of training, validation, and testing images are closely overlapping, which is not surprising because these data sets correspond to normal phenotypical shape variations. However, the histogram of the metopic skull shapes indicates much larger Mahalanobis distance on average (yellow bars; the bars are wider and longer because no data augmentation was performed on the metopic craniosynostosis CT scans, and we have just 16 scans). The histograms of metopic-craniosynostosis and normal-skulls do overlap to some extent; this is indicative of mild cases of metopic craniosynostosis, which do not differ significantly from normal population and often do not require surgical intervention (unlike severe cases where surgery is often recommended [21]).

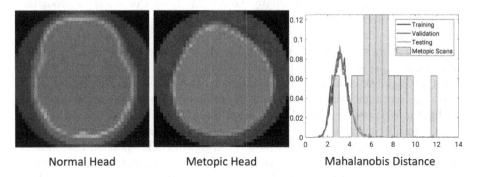

Normal Head   Metopic Head   Mahalanobis Distance

Fig. 5. (Left) CT scan of a normal head. (Middle) CT scan of a head shape affected by metopic craniosynostosis. (Right) The histograms of Mahalanobis distance for training, validation and testing datasets and the metopic-heads dataset (yellow bars, no data augmentation was performed). (Color figure online)

4.2   Cam-Type Femoroacetabular Impingement (cam-FAI)

cam-FAI is a primary cause of hip osteoarthritis and is characterized by an abnormal bone growth of the femoral head (see Fig. 6). Statistical shape modeling could quantify anatomical variation in normal/FAI hips, thus providing an objective method to characterize cam-lesion and an anatomical map to guide surgical correction [2]. We follow a very similar approach to that described in the Sect. 4.1. Our dataset comprises of 67 CT scans with 57 femurs of normal patients and 10 pathological femurs. We start with 50 CT scans of femurs of normal patients which forms our control group. We reflect all the femurs to a consistent frame and then rigidly register them to a reference, the reflection is necessary as our data consists of both left and right femur bones. We use this set of 50 CT scans to form the PDM of 1024 3D correspondences, followed by its subsequent data augmentation. We again use 15 PCA loadings which captures $\sim 99\%$ of shape variability, and we train the DeepSSM to regress for these PCA loadings for 45 epochs. We use PCA loading predictions from the trained network to reconstruct the 1024 correspondences and compare it with the original correspondences. The box plot representing the Euclidean distance error (in mm) per-point per-shape is shown in Fig. 4(b). For the unseen data (data which have no initial PDM on them), the error is again computed using the projection distance of the predicted correspondence from the original mesh. The femurs are also downsampled from 1 mm isotropic voxel spacing by a factor of 4, making the voxel spacing 4 mm. Our unseen data consists of the remaining 7 normal CT scans of femurs and 10 pathological femurs, We generate the correspondences from the PCA loading predicted by the DeepSSM and again evaluate the accuracy of the predictions using the maximal projected distance to the original mesh. The surface-to-surface distances for the unseen as well as seen scans are shown in Fig. 7. We want to evaluate the sensitivity of DeepSSM in predicting the subtle dysmorphology in the femoral head. As such, we compute the mean and standard deviation of the errors (i.e., surface to surface distances) for unseen normal and unseen pathological femurs and show them as a heatmap on a mean femur mesh. This is shown on the right in Fig. 7. A critical observation to note is that in Fig. 7[B], which is the mean error of the unseen pathological scans, the orange rectangle highlights the region of interest in characterization of the cam lesion. We observe that in this region, DeepSSM—trained only on normal femurs—results in a reconstruction error with sub-voxel accuracy, which is not as accurate as some other (irrelevant to surgical treatment) regions of morphology. Aspect being stressed here is that pathological variation is not being captured by the training data, and hence the loss in reconstruction accuracy on pathologic cases. In particular, the network is learning a prior based on how a standard femur shape should look like and, it being trained on data augmented using a normative shape space, the pathological mode is not represented. Due to constraints in the data, we refrained from jointly modeling the initial PDM, which is essential if the pathological mode is to be captured using DeepSSM.

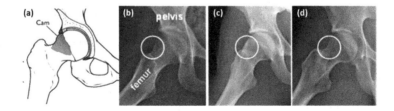

Fig. 6. (a) Schematics of cam-FAI. Normal femur (b) compared to a cam femur (c); circles show location of deformity. (d) – cam FAI patient post-surgery. Surgical treatment aims to remove bony deformities. (Color figure online)

4.3   Atrial Fibrillation

Left atrium (LA) shape has been shown to be an independent predictor of recurrence after atrial fibrillation (AF) ablation [29]. Our dataset contains 100 MRIs of left atrium of paitents with AF. We start from 75 MRI scans from teh original dataset, and use them to form the initial PDM with 1024 points. We use 10 PCA components to capture 90% of shape variability and use our data augmentation and train DeepSSM for 50 epochs. We use PCA loading predictions from the trained network to reconstruct the 1024 correspondences and compare

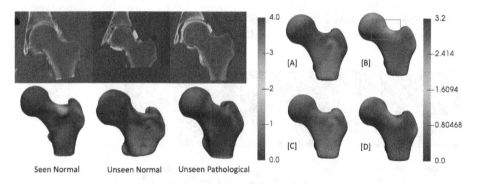

Fig. 7. The left two rows represent the images (seen normal femur, unseen normal femur and unseen pathological femur) and the corresponding shape reconstruction error (Hausdorff distance in mm) interpolated as a heatmap on the original meshes. On the right: [A] mean error of unseen normal femurs overlayed on mean shape, [B] mean error of unseen pathological femurs overlayed on mean shape, [C] standard deviation of error of unseen normal femurs overlayed on mean shape, [D] standard deciation of error of unseen pathological femurs overlayed on mean shape

it with the original correspondences. The box plot representing the Euclidean distance error (in mm) per-point per-shape is shown in Fig. 4(c). The remaining 25 forms the unseen data (data which have no initial PDM on them), the error is again computed using the projection distance of the predicted correspondence from the original mesh. The MRI are downsampled from 1 mm isotropic voxel spacing with a factor of 2 which leads to 2 mm voxel spacing. We can see that DeepSSM performs poorly as compared to the other two applications on the unseen data. The reason for this is the huge variability in the intensity profile of the left atrium MRI, this is shown in Fig. 8. We linearly scale the intensity range between 0–255 for training DeepSSM, but other then this there is no intensity equalization/correction is performed. It's encouraging that DeepSSM can still achieve an on average sub-voxel accuracy, and with smart subset selection, we believe the accuracy will increase substantially. Also in this analysis, we only use 10 PCA modes because, empirical observation of the other modes shows that they correspond to variations in the pulmonary veins, which is not important in AF recurrence prediction [5], this also translates in the most error being concentrated in the pulmonary veins region Fig. 8(leftmost). Furthermore, we want to see that how does DeepSSM work in predicting AF recurrence. We use the PCA loadings from the original PDM on the data and use them to perform multi-layer perceptron (MLP) regression against the AF recurrence data. We use this trained MLP and perform the same prediction, but now using the input data as the PCA loadings predicted using DeepSSM. We observe that the predicted recurrence probability using the PCA loadings from PDM and from DeepSSM are statistically same by T-Test with a confidence of 79.6%. The recurrence probability difference from both inputs can be seen in Fig. 8. We also perform a two one-sided test (TOST) [25] for equivalence, we find that the recurrence prediction by DeepSSM and PDM PCA loadings are equivalent with a confidence of 88% with the mean difference bounds of ±0.1.

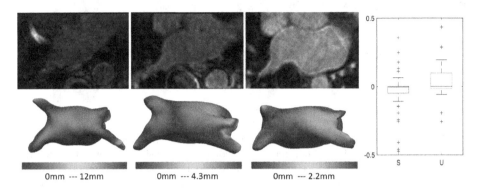

Fig. 8. Bottom row represent representative sample of different image types in our database, going from worst to best (left to right). Top row represent shape derived from corresponding image using the proposed method, with a distance map overlay from particle modeling shape reconstruction. (Right) S: "Seen" Data U: "Unseen" Data: Boxplot for AF recurrence probability difference using PCA loadings using the PDM directly and those estimated by DeepSSM

5   Conclusion

DeepSSM provides a complete framework to extract low-dimensional shape representation directly from a shape population represented by 3D images. It provides a novel method to augment data from a small subset of images, and it's subsequent training. In contrast to previous methods which achieve similar functionality via a sequence of image processing operations and involve significant parameter tuning and/or user assistance, DeepSSM directly consumes raw images and produces a sub-voxel accurate shape model, with virtually no user intervention required for pre-processing the images unlike other shape modeling methods. We believe this functionality may enable new clinical applications in the future. We evaluate DeepSSM on both MRI as well as CT modalities, being applied to three different applications indicating that the framework is applicable to any collection of shapes. Our preliminary analysis showing the efficacy of DeepSSM in pathology characterization for femoral heads and metopic craniosynostosis, even if it's trained on normal morphology, and opens up pathways to more detailed clinical analysis with DeepSSM on joint shape models. We hope that automatic shape assessment methods will contribute to new computerized clinical tools and objective metrics, ultimately translating to improved standards of medical care accessible to everyone.

Acknowledgment. This work was supported by the National Institutes of Health [grant numbers R01-HL135568-01, P41-GM103545-19 and R01-EB016701]. This material is also based upon work supported by the National Science Foundation under Grant Numbers IIS-1617172 and IIS-1622360. Any opinions, findings, and conclusions or recommendations expressed in this material are those of the author(s) and do not necessarily reflect the views of the National Science Foundation. The authors would like to thank the Comprehensive Arrhythmia Research and Management (CARMA) Center (Nassir Marrouche, MD), Pittsburgh Children's Hospital (Jesse Goldstein, MD) and the Orthopaedic Research Laboratory (Andrew Anderson, PhD) at the University of Utah for providing the left atrium MRI scans, pediatric CT scans, and femur CT scans, and their corresponding segmentations.

References

1. Abadi, M., et al.: Tensorflow: a system for large-scale machine learning. In: OSDI. vol. 16, pp. 265–283 (2016)
2. Atkins, P.R., et al.: Quantitative comparison of cortical bone thickness using correspondence-based shape modeling in patients with cam femoroacetabular impingement. J. Orthop. Res. **35**(8), 1743–1753 (2017)
3. Badrinarayanan, V., Handa, A., Cipolla, R.: Segnet: a deep convolutional encoder-decoder architecture for robust semantic pixel-wise labelling. arXiv preprint arXiv:1505.07293 (2015)
4. Beg, M.F., Miller, M.I., Trouvé, A., Younes, L.: Computing large deformation metric mappings via geodesic flows of diffeomorphisms. Int. J. Comput. Vision **61**(2), 139–157 (2005)
5. Bieging, E.T., Morris, A., Wilson, B.D., McGann, C.J., Marrouche, N.F., Cates, J.: Left atrial shape predicts recurrence after atrial fibrillation catheter ablation. J. Cardiovasc. Electrophysiol. (2018)
6. Bookstein, F.L.: Principal warps: thin-plate splines and the decomposition of deformations. IEEE Trans. Pattern Anal. Mach. Intell. **11**(6), 567–585 (1989)
7. Cates, J., Elhabian, S., Whitaker, R.: Shapeworks: particle-based shape correspondence and visualization software. In: Statistical Shape and Deformation Analysis, pp. 257–298. Elsevier (2017)
8. Cates, J., Fletcher, P.T., Styner, M., Shenton, M., Whitaker, R.: Shape modeling and analysis with entropy-based particle systems. In: Karssemeijer, N., Lelieveldt, B. (eds.) IPMI 2007. LNCS, vol. 4584, pp. 333–345. Springer, Heidelberg (2007). https://doi.org/10.1007/978-3-540-73273-0_28
9. Davies, R.H., Twining, C.J., Cootes, T.F., Waterton, J.C., Taylor, C.J.: A minimum description length approach to statistical shape modeling. IEEE Trans. Med. Imag. **21**(5), 525–537 (2002)
10. Davies, R.H., Twining, C.J., Cootes, T.F., Waterton, J.C., Taylor, C.J.: 3D statistical shape models using direct optimisation of description length. In: Heyden, A., Sparr, G., Nielsen, M., Johansen, P. (eds.) ECCV 2002. LNCS, vol. 2352, pp. 3–20. Springer, Heidelberg (2002). https://doi.org/10.1007/3-540-47977-5_1
11. Duchi, J., Hazan, E., Singer, Y.: Adaptive subgradient methods for online learning and stochastic optimization. J. Mach. Learn. Res. **12**, 2121–2159 (2011)
12. Gardner, G., Morris, A., Higuchi, K., MacLeod, R., Cates, J.: A point-correspondence approach to describing the distribution of image features on anatomical surfaces, with application to atrial fibrillation. In: 2013 IEEE 10th International Symposium on Biomedical Imaging, pp. 226–229, April 2013

13. Gerig, G., Styner, M., Jones, D., Weinberger, D., Lieberman, J.: Shape analysis of brain ventricles using spharm. In: Proceedings IEEE Workshop on Mathematical Methods in Biomedical Image Analysis (MMBIA 2001), pp. 171–178 (2001)
14. Glorot, X., Bengio, Y.: Understanding the difficulty of training deep feedforward neural networks. In: Proceedings of the Thirteenth International Conference on Artificial Intelligence and Statistics. Proceedings of Machine Learning Research, PMLR. vol. 9, pp. 249–256, May 2010
15. Grenander, U., Chow, Y., Keenan, D.M.: Hands: A Pattern Theoretic Study of Biological Shapes. Springer, New York (1991). https://doi.org/10.1007/978-1-4612-3046-5
16. Harris, M.D., Datar, M., Whitaker, R.T., Jurrus, E.R., Peters, C.L., Anderson, A.E.: Statistical shape modeling of cam femoroacetabular impingement. J. Orthopaedic Research **31**(10), 1620–1626 (2013). https://doi.org/10.1002/jor.22389
17. He, K., Zhang, X., Ren, S., Sun, J.: Delving deep into rectifiers: surpassing human-level performance on imagenet classification. CoRR abs/1502.01852 (2015). http://arxiv.org/abs/1502.01852
18. Huang, W., Bridge, C.P., Noble, J.A., Zisserman, A.: Temporal heartnet: towards human-level automatic analysis of fetal cardiac screening video. In: Descoteaux, M., Maier-Hein, L., Franz, A., Jannin, P., Collins, D.L., Duchesne, S. (eds.) MICCAI 2017. LNCS, vol. 10434, pp. 341–349. Springer, Cham (2017). https://doi.org/10.1007/978-3-319-66185-8_39
19. Lecun, Y., Bottou, L., Bengio, Y., Haffner, P.: Gradient-based learning applied to document recognition. Proc. IEEE **86**(11), 2278–2324 (1998)
20. Li, Q., Cai, W., Wang, X., Zhou, Y., Feng, D.D., Chen, M.: Medical image classification with convolutional neural network. In: 2014 13th International Conference on Control Automation Robotics Vision (ICARCV), pp. 844–848, December 2014
21. McCarthy, J.G., et al.: Parameters of care for craniosynostosis. Cleft Palate Craniofac. J. **49**(1–suppl), 1–24 (2012)
22. Milletari, F., Rothberg, A., Jia, J., Sofka, M.: Integrating statistical prior knowledge into convolutional neural networks. In: Descoteaux, M., Maier-Hein, L., Franz, A., Jannin, P., Collins, D.L., Duchesne, S. (eds.) MICCAI 2017. LNCS, vol. 10433, pp. 161–168. Springer, Cham (2017). https://doi.org/10.1007/978-3-319-66182-7_19
23. Ovsjanikov, M., Ben-Chen, M., Solomon, J., Butscher, A., Guibas, L.: Functional maps: a flexible representation of maps between shapes. ACM Trans. Graph. (TOG) **31**(4), 30 (2012)
24. Ronneberger, O., Fischer, P., Brox, T.: U-net: convolutional networks for biomedical image segmentation. CoRR abs/1505.04597 (2015). http://arxiv.org/abs/1505.04597
25. Schuirmann, D.J.: A comparison of the two one-sided tests procedure and the power approach for assessing the equivalence of average bioavailability. J. Pharmacokinet. Biopharm. **15**(6), 657–680 (1987)
26. Sokooti, H., de Vos, B., Berendsen, F., Lelieveldt, B.P.F., Išgum, I., Staring, M.: Nonrigid image registration using multi-scale 3D convolutional neural networks. In: Descoteaux, M., Maier-Hein, L., Franz, A., Jannin, P., Collins, D.L., Duchesne, S. (eds.) MICCAI 2017. LNCS, vol. 10433, pp. 232–239. Springer, Cham (2017). https://doi.org/10.1007/978-3-319-66182-7_27
27. Styner, M., Brechbuhler, C., Szekely, G., Gerig, G.: Parametric estimate of intensity inhomogeneities applied to MRI. IEEE Trans. Med. Imaging **19**(3), 153–165 (2000)

28. Styner, M., et al.: Statistical shape analysis of brain structures using SPHARM-PDM. The insight J. **1071**, 242–250 (2006)

29. Bieging, E.T., Morris, A., Wilson, B.D., McGann, C.J., Marrouche, N.F., Cates, J.: Left atrial shape predicts recurrence after atrial fibrillation catheter ablation. J.Cardiovasc. Electrophysiol. **29**(7), 966–972. https://doi.org/10.1111/jce.13641

30. Thompson, D.W., et al.: On Growth and Form. Cambridge University Press, Cambridge (1942)

31. Xie, J., Dai, G., Zhu, F., Wong, E.K., Fang, Y.: Deepshape: deep-learned shape descriptor for 3D shape retrieval. IEEE Trans. Pattern Anal. Mach. Intell. **39**(7), 1335–1345 (2017)

32. Zachow, S.: Computational planning in facial surgery. Facial Plast. Surg. **31**(05), 446–462 (2015)

33. Zheng, Y., Liu, D., Georgescu, B., Nguyen, H., Comaniciu, D.: 3D deep learning for efficient and robust landmark detection in volumetric data. In: Navab, N., Hornegger, J., Wells, W.M., Frangi, A.F. (eds.) MICCAI 2015. LNCS, vol. 9349, pp. 565–572. Springer, Cham (2015). https://doi.org/10.1007/978-3-319-24553-9_69

Combining Deep Learning and Shape Priors for Bi-Ventricular Segmentation of Volumetric Cardiac Magnetic Resonance Images

Jinming Duan[1,2(✉)], Jo Schlemper[1], Wenjia Bai[1], Timothy J. W. Dawes[2,3], Ghalib Bello[2], Carlo Biffi[1,2], Georgia Doumou[2], Antonio De Marvao[2], Declan P. O'Regan[2], and Daniel Rueckert[1]

[1] Biomedical Image Analysis Group, Imperial College London, London, UK
j.duan@imperial.ac.uk
[2] MRC London Institute of Medical Sciences, Imperial College London, London, UK
[3] National Heart and Lung Institute, Imperial College London, London, UK

Abstract. In this paper, we combine a network-based method with image registration to develop a shape-based bi-ventricular segmentation tool for short-axis cardiac magnetic resonance (CMR) volumetric images. The method first employs a fully convolutional network (FCN) to learn the segmentation task from manually labelled ground truth CMR volumes. However, due to the presence of image artefacts in the training dataset, the resulting FCN segmentation results are often imperfect. As such, we propose a second step to refine the FCN segmentation. This step involves performing a non-rigid registration with multiple high-resolution bi-ventricular atlases, allowing the explicit shape priors to be inferred. We validate the proposed approach on 1831 healthy subjects and 200 subjects with pulmonary hypertension. Numerical experiments on the two datasets demonstrate that our approach is capable of producing accurate, high-resolution and anatomically smooth bi-ventricular models, despite the artefacts in the input CMR volumes.

1 Introduction

Cardiac magnetic resonance (CMR) imaging is a non-invasive and non-ionising imaging technique that produces good image quality and excellent soft tissue contrast. Among existing imaging techniques, it has established itself as the gold standard for assessing cardiac chamber volume and mass for a wide range of cardiovascular diseases [1]. CMR imaging techniques, together with semi-automated or automated CMR segmentation algorithms [2–11], have shown a great impact on studying, understanding and diagnosing cardiovascular diseases. However, there are still limitations in current CMR segmentation methods.

Anatomically, a human heart is composed of the left ventricle (LV) and the right ventricle (RV). Each ventricle can be subdivided into the cavity region (left ventricular cavity [LVC] and right ventricular cavity [RVC]) and the wall

© Springer Nature Switzerland AG 2018
M. Reuter et al. (Eds.): ShapeMI 2018, LNCS 11167, pp. 258–267, 2018.
https://doi.org/10.1007/978-3-030-04747-4_24

region (left ventricular wall [LVW] and right ventricular wall [RVW]). Most of the segmentation techniques have only focused on the LVC and LVW [3,4] (or at most the LVC, LVW and RVC [2,5–10]). Few studies have attempted a full bi-ventricular segmentation (i.e. LVC + LVW + RVC + RVW) due to the narrow structure of RVW (sometimes less than one millimetre in thickness). This prohibits accurate cardiac assessments involving coupled bi-ventricular cardiac motion. In addition, due to the limitations of standard clinical acquisition protocols, the raw volumetric CMR images acquired often contain several artefacts [12], including intensity inhomogeneity, inter-slice shift (i.e. respiratory motion), large slice thickness, lack of slice coverage, etc. Most existing segmentation methods [3–11] deal with CMR volumes directly without taking the artefacts into account. As such, the resulting segmentation inevitably inherit these artefacts. Building an accurate, motion-free, automatically meaningful bi-ventricular segmentation model therefore remains an open problem.

To overcome the aforementioned limitations of current approaches, in this paper we propose a novel approach that addresses the problem of bi-ventricular segmentation of short-axis CMR volumetric images. We make the following three distinct contributions. First, the proposed approach segments an input cardiac volume into LVC, LVW, RVC and RVW. The technique introduced herein is the first one capable of producing a full high-resolution bi-ventricular segmentation in 3D. Second, we introduce anatomical shape prior knowledge (via image registration) to a deep learning approach by using a cohort of high-resolution atlas shapes. As such, the proposed approach is capable to produce an accurate, motion-free and clinically meaningful bi-ventricular segmentation model, despite the existing artefacts in the input volume. Third, we thoroughly assess the effectiveness and robustness of proposed method using two datasets, including high- and low-resolution cardiac volumes from 1831 healthy subjects and 200 pathological subjects, respectively. To our knowledge, this is one of the first CMR segmentation studies utilising datasets of this scale. To quantitatively evaluate our proposed segmentation algorithm, we also develop a method that is able to simulate the artefacts in CMR volumes.

2   Methodology

Fully Convolutional Network: We treat the problem of predicting segmentation maps as the multi-class classification problem. First, let us formulate the learning problem as follows: we denote the input training dataset by $S = \{(U_i, R_i), i = 1, \ldots, N_t\}$, where N_t is the number of training data, $U_i = \{u_j^i, j = 1, \ldots, |U_i|\}$ is the raw input CMR volume, $R_i = \{r_j^i, j = 1, \ldots, |R_i|\}$, $r_j^i \in \{1, \ldots, N_r\}$ is the ground truth region labels for volume U_i ($N_r = 5$ representing the LVC, LVW, RVC, RVW and background regions). Note that $|U_i| = |R_i|$ stands for the total number of voxels in a CMR volume. We then define all network layer parameters as $\mathbf{W}$. In a supervised setting, we propose to solve the following minimisation problem via standard (back-propagation) stochastic gradient descent (SGD)

$$\mathbf{W}^* = \operatorname{argmin}(L_S(\mathbf{W}) + \alpha L_D(\mathbf{W}) + \beta\|\mathbf{W}\|_F^2), \tag{1}$$

where α and β are weight coefficients balancing the three terms. $L_S(\mathbf{W})$ and $L_D(\mathbf{W})$ are the region associated losses that enable the network to predict segmentation maps. $\|\mathbf{W}\|_F^2$, known as the weight decay term, represents the Frobenius norm on the weights $\mathbf{W}$. This term is used to prevent over-fitting in the network. The training problem is to estimate the parameters $\mathbf{W}$ associated with all the convolutional layers and by minimising (1) the network is able to predict segmentation maps. The definitions of $L_S(\mathbf{W})$ and $L_D(\mathbf{W})$ are given separately as follows:

$$L_S(\mathbf{W}) = -\sum_i \sum_k \sum_{j \in X_k^i} \log P(r_j^i = k | U_i, \mathbf{W}), \tag{2}$$

where i, k and j respectively denote the training sample index, the region label index and the voxel index. X_k^i represents the voxels in training sample i that fall in the region for which the label value is k. $P(r_j^i = k | U_i, \mathbf{W})$ corresponds to the softmax probability estimated by the network for a specific voxel j (subject to the restriction $r_j^i = k$), given the training volume U_i and network weights $\mathbf{W}$. Note that (2) is known as the categorical cross-entropy loss or multi-class logistic loss, in which the summations are carried out over all voxels, labels and training samples.

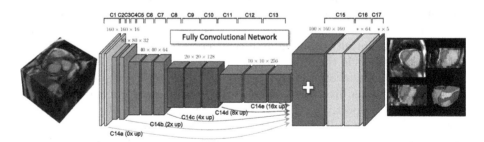

Fig. 1. The architecture of a fully convolutional network with 17 convolutional layers. The network takes the CMR volume as input, applies a branch of convolutions, learns image features from fine to coarse levels, concatenates multi-scale features and finally segments the image into 5 disjoint regions. (Color figure online)

Along with (2) for predicting segmentation maps, we use the Dice loss that evaluates spatial overlap with ground truth region labels. More specifically, we use a differentiable approximation of Dice loss, defined as follows:

$$L_D(\mathbf{W}) = -\sum_i \frac{2\sum_k \sum_j 1_{\{r_j^i=k\}} \cdot P(r_j^i = k | U_i, \mathbf{W})}{\sum_k \sum_j \left(1_{\{r_j^i=k\}}^2 + P^2(r_j^i = k | U_i, \mathbf{W})\right)}, \tag{3}$$

where $1_{\{\cdot\}}$ is the indicator function and other notations in (3) have the same meanings as those in (2).

In Fig. 1, we show the proposed network architecture for automatic CMR segmentation, which is a fully convolutional network (FCN). It is adapted from [10] and similar to the U-net architecture [13]. Batch-normalisation (BN) is used after each convolutional layer, and before a rectified linear unit (ReLU) activation. The last layer is followed by the channel-wise softmax function. In the FCN, input images have pixel dimensions of 192×192. Every layer whose label is prefixed with 'C' performs the operation: convolution $\rightarrow$ BN $\rightarrow$ ReLU, except C17. The (filter size/stride) is $(3 \times 3/1)$ for layers from C1 to C16, excluding layers C3, C5, C8 and C11 which are $(3 \times 3/2)$. The arrows represent $(3 \times 3/1)$ convolutional layers (C14a–e) followed by a transpose convolutional (up) layer with a factor necessary to achieve feature map volumes with size $160 \times 160 \times 32$, all of which are concatenated into the red feature map volume. Finally, C17 applies a $(1 \times 1/1)$ convolution with a softmax activation, producing the blue feature map volume with a depth 5, corresponding to 5 segmented regions of an input volume.

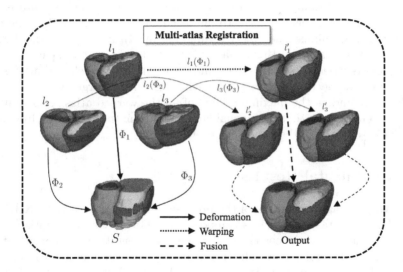

Fig. 2. Incorporation of shape constraints by multi-atlas registration. l_1, l_2 and l_3 are high-resolution bi-ventricular atlas shape models. They are warped to l'_1, l'_2 and l'_3 using the transform between the FCN result S and each atlas. The warped results are finally fused together to generate a smooth high-resolution output.

Multi-atlas Registration: As Fig. 1 shows, the segmentation produced by FCN is influenced by respiratory motion artefact. Moreover, as the CMR volume are low resolution in the long-axis, the 3D segmentation model is not smooth. Further, due to the narrow structure of the RVW, the segmentation model is incomplete. By incorporating shape prior knowledge with the following image registration, as also shown in Fig. 2, these artefacts can be resolved.

Since the correspondences of structures across both target and atlas volumes are explicitly encoded in their segmentations, we only use segmentations for the following non-rigid registration. Let S and l_n ($n = 1, \ldots, L$) be the network segmentation and the nth atlas segmentation (i.e. shape, respectively. Note that here we use a cohort of high-resolution atlases, each of which has an image resolution of $1.25 \times 1.25 \times 2.0$ mm. Let $P_{S,l_n}(i,j)$ be the joint probability of labels i and j in S and l_n, respectively. It is estimated as the number of voxels with label i in S and label j in l_n divided by the total number of voxels in the overlap region of both segmentations. We then maximise the overlap of structures denoted by the same label in both S and l_n by minimising the following objective function

$$\Phi_n^* = \arg\min \mathcal{C}\left(S, l_n(\Phi_n)\right) \tag{4}$$

where Φ_n is the transformation between S and l_n, which is modelled by a free-form deformation (FFD) based on B-splines [14]. $\mathcal{C}(S, l_n) = \sum_{i=1}^{N_r} P_{S,l_n}(i,i)$, representing the label consistency [15]. $\mathcal{C}$ in (4) is a similarity measure of how many labels of all the labels in the atlas segmentation are correctly mapped into the target segmentation. The measure is zero when none of the atlas labels has been correctly mapped into the target segmentation. The measure is one when all reference labels are correctly matched. A multi-scale gradient descent is then used to minimise the objective function in (4). After the optimal Φ_n^* is found, the segmentation in the nth atlas is warped to the target space (i.e. l_n'). The process is repeated several times until after all the pre-selected atlases are warped. Lastly, the resulting label at each voxel in the target volume can be calculated by finding the maximum label of all the warped atlas segmentations at that voxel. We note that six manual landmarks from the target and from each atlas shape to initialise the non-rigid registration.

3   Experimental Results

For the training and evaluation of the proposed method, we use the UK Digital Heart Project Dataset[1], which is composed of 1831 cine high-resolution CMR volumetric images and the corresponding dense segmentation annotations at the end-diastolic (ED) and end-systolic (ES) frames. These volumes are derived from healthy subjects, scanned at Hammersmith Hospital, Imperial College London using a 3D cine balanced steady-state free precession (b-SSFP) sequence [16] and has a resolution of $1.25 \times 1.25 \times 2$ mm. The high-resolution imaging technique enables us to characterise the cardiac shape in great detail. Moreover, it requires only one single breath-hold of a subject during each scan and thereby does not produce the artefacts (i.e. inter-slice shift, large slice thickness, lack of slice coverage, etc.) [16], which are commonly seen when low-resolution imaging techniques [12] are used. Figure 3a shows a long-axis view of a high-resolution volume at the ED frame, and the corresponding ground truth 2D and 3D segmentation labels are given in c and d, respectively.

To quantitatively study our proposed segmentation algorithm, we develop a method to simulate the artefacts in low-resolution cardiac volumes. Specifically,

---

[1]   https://digital-heart.org/.

the original high-resolution volume and its segmentation are first downsampled from $1.25 \times 1.25 \times 2$ mm to $1.25 \times 1.25 \times 10$ mm, as shown in the second row of Fig. 3. As evident, after this step the segmentation shape takes on the staircase artefacts as now the downsampled versions have a relatively low long-axis resolution. Moreover, the segmentation around the apical region becomes incomplete due to the lack of slice coverage of the whole heart. We further simulate inter-slice shift artefact by randomly translating each 2D short-axis slice independently. After this step the cardiac volume and its segmentation become misaligned, as shown in the last row of Fig. 3. Next, for training the network the low-resolution volume g and its segmentation h are used as inputs. Note that our method is capable of producing a high-resolution smooth segmentation model even through the input volume is like g. Since we have the smooth ground truth c for g, we can quantitatively compare the output of our method with the ground truth c.

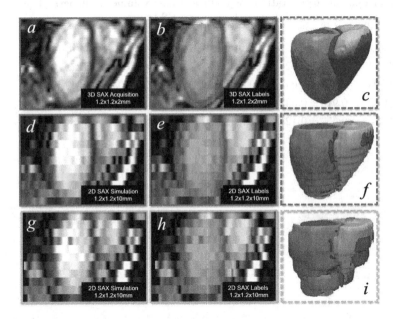

Fig. 3. Simulating cardiac artefacts in real scenarios. 1st row: artefact-free high-resolution cardiac volume and ground truth labels. 2nd row: downsampled versions of volumes in the 1st row. 3rd row: inter-slice shift is added to the downsampled volumes in the 2nd row.

We then randomly split the 1831 dataset into three sets of 1000/600/231. The first two sets are then corrupted with the simulated artefacts introduced above, which are respectively used for training the neural network in Fig. 1 and evaluating the proposed segmentation algorithm. The last set remains unchanged and is used as a cohort of high-resolution atlas shapes for refining the network segmentation. Note that we intend to segment a cardiac volume into the left ventricular cavity (LVC), right ventricular cavity (RVC), left ventricular wall (LVW) and right ventricular wall (RVW).

Table 1 reports the Dice metric and Hausdorf distance between automated and manual segmentations, evaluated on the test set of 600 subjects at ED and ES. The mean Dice values of LVC, LVW and RVC demonstrate an excellent agreement between automated and manual segmentations for these structures. However, for RVW its mean Dice values at ED and ES are only 0.557 and 0.608. This is due to its thin structure (only two or three voxels in thickness) and the Dice index is more sensitive to errors in this structure. However, in terms of the Hausdorff distance for RVW, the mean value is relatively small. Hence, our method achieves a better performance for all the four structures.

Table 1. The Dice metric and Hausdorf distance (HD) between automated segmentation and manual segmentation for 600 short-axis volumetric images. The mean ± standard deviation are reported at the ED and ES frames.

Region	Dice (ED)	HD in mm (ED)	Dice (ES)	HD in mm (ES)
LVC	0.940 ± 0.024	4.045 ± 0.675	0.910 ± 0.028	4.127 ± 0.632
LVW	0.863 ± 0.049	4.394 ± 0.841	0.892 ± 0.033	4.231 ± 0.797
RVC	0.914 ± 0.033	5.039 ± 1.218	0.901 ± 0.038	5.333 ± 1.253
RVW	0.557 ± 0.121	7.119 ± 2.956	0.608 ± 0.123	6.778 ± 2.717

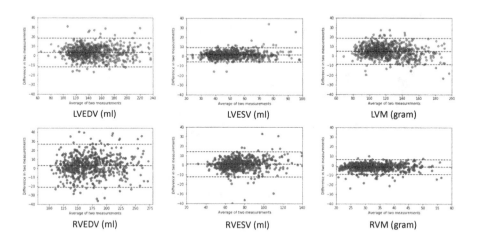

Fig. 4. Bland-Altman plots of clinical measures between automated measurement and manual measurement. The LV end-diastolic volume (LVEDV), end-systolic volume (LVESV), LV myocardial mass (LVM), RV end-diastolic volume (RVEDV), end-systolic volume (RVESV), and RV myocardial mass (RVM) are derived from our segmentation method and the manual segmentation.

To further quantitatively evaluate the proposed method, Fig. 4 shows the Bland-Altman plots of the clinical measures. The Bland-Altman plot is commonly used for analysing agreement and bias between two measurements. This figure compares automated measurements to manual measurements on the evaluation set, which shows that the mean difference is centred close to zero, indicating that the automated measurement is almost unbiased relative to the observer. Also, there is no evidence of bias over hearts of difference sizes or volumes. In particular, RVM shows a very good consistency between the two measurements, validating an accurate segmentation of RVW despite relatively lower Dice values.

Finally, the proposed method was evaluated on a dataset of 200 patients with pulmonary hypertension. Greyscale volumetric images were acquired at low resolution ($1.38 \times 1.38 \times 10$ mm) and segmented into high-resolution smooth 3D models. Results were visually assessed by one clinician with over five years' experience of CMR imaging and judged satisfactory in all cases. In Fig. 5, we present an exemplary segmentation of a cardiac volume in a pulmonary hypertension patient. We visually compare the proposed method with the vanilla deep learning method without shape prior knowledge [10]. As the figure shows, the proposed method gives a better 3D phenotype result which is smooth, accurate and artefact-free. This is due to the application of shape prior information. Our method thus outperforms the vanilla FCN in this regard.

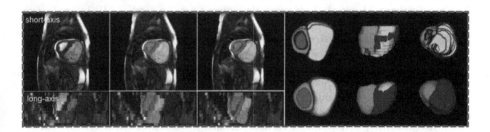

Fig. 5. Visual comparison of segmentation results from the vanilla FCN and the proposed method on a pathological case. 1st column: original short- and long-axis CMR slices. 2nd column: vanilla FCN results. 3rd column: results by the proposed method. Last column: FCN results (top) and our results (bottom). The 5 segmented regions are respectively RVC (yellow), LVC (red), RVW (blue), LVW (green) and background. (Color figure online)

4   Conclusion

In this paper, we developed a shape-based CNN-based method for bi-ventricular segmentation of cardiac MR volumetric images. The method first employs a fully convolutional network (FCN) to segment the volume at a low-resolution level. Based on the FCN results, the method then performs the non-rigid registration by using multiple high-resolution atlas shapes, thereby imposing shape constraints explicitly and effectively. Extensive experiments have showed that the method has capability of producing smooth bi-ventricular segmentation results that follow the global anatomical properties of the underlying anatomy, even through the input volumetric images contain several unpleasant artefacts. In addition, we have also showed that the method has a very good generalisation ability for segmentation of pathological cases. Future work will focus on statistical shape analysis using the smooth results produced by the method.

Acknowledgements. The research was supported by the British Heart Foundation (NH/17/1/32725, RE/13/4/30184); National Institute for Health Research (NIHR) Biomedical Research Centre based at Imperial College Healthcare NHS Trust and Imperial College London; and the Medical Research Council, UK. We would like to thank Dr Simon Gibbs, Dr Luke Howard and Prof Martin Wilkins for providing the CMR image data. The TITAN Xp GPU used for this research was kindly donated by the NVIDIA Corporation.

References

1. Ripley, D., Musa, T., Dobson, L., Plein, S., Greenwood, J.: Cardiovascular magnetic resonance imaging: what the general cardiologist should know. Heart (2016). Heartjnl-2015
2. Bai, W., Shi, W., Ledig, C., Rueckert, D.: Multi-atlas segmentation with augmented features for cardiac MR images. Med. Image Anal. **19**(1), 98–109 (2015)
3. Nasr-Esfahani, M., et al.: Left ventricle segmentation in cardiac MR images using fully convolutional network. arXiv:1802.07778 (2018)
4. Ngo, T., Lu, Z., Carneiro, G.: Combining deep learning and level set for the automated segmentation of the left ventricle of the heart from cardiac cine magnetic resonance. Med. Image Anal. **35**, 159–171 (2017)
5. Patravali, J., Jain, S., Chilamkurthy, S.: 2D–3D fully convolutional neural networks for cardiac MR segmentation. arXiv:1707.09813 (2017)
6. Baumgartner, C., Koch, L., Pollefeys, M., Konukoglu, E.: An exploration of 2D and 3D deep learning techniques for cardiac MR image segmentation. arXiv:1709.04496 (2017)
7. Isensee, F., Jaeger, P., Full, P., Wolf, I., Engelhardt, S., Maier-Hein, K.: Automatic cardiac disease assessment on cine-MRI via time-series segmentation and domain specific features. arXiv:1707.00587 (2017)
8. Zheng, Q., Delingette, H., Duchateau, N., Ayache, N.: 3D consistent & robust segmentation of cardiac images by deep learning with spatial propagation. IEEE Trans. Med. Imaging (2018)
9. Tran, P.: A fully convolutional neural network for cardiac segmentation in short-axis MRI. arXiv:1604.00494 (2016)
10. Bai, W., et al.: Human-level CMR image analysis with deep fully convolutional networks. arXiv:1710.09289 (2017)
11. Duan, J., et al.: Deep nested level sets: fully automated segmentation of cardiac MR images in patients with pulmonary hypertension. In: Frangi, A.F., Schnabel, J.A., Davatzikos, C., Alberola-López, C., Fichtinger, G. (eds.) MICCAI 2018. LNCS, vol. 11073, pp. 595–603. Springer, Cham (2018). https://doi.org/10.1007/978-3-030-00937-3_68
12. Petersen, S., et al.: UK biobank's cardiovascular magnetic resonance protocol. J. Cardiovasc. Magn. Reson **18**(1), 8 (2015)

13. Ronneberger, O., Fischer, P., Brox, T.: U-net: convolutional networks for biomedical image segmentation. In: Navab, N., Hornegger, J., Wells, W.M., Frangi, A.F. (eds.) MICCAI 2015. LNCS, vol. 9351, pp. 234–241. Springer, Cham (2015). https://doi.org/10.1007/978-3-319-24574-4_28

14. Rueckert, D., Sonoda, L., Hayes, C., Hill, D., Leach, M., Hawkes, D.: Nonrigid registration using free-form deformations: application to breast MR images. IEEE Trans. Med. Imaging **18**(8), 712–721 (1999)

15. Frangi, A., Rueckert, D., Schnabel, J., Niessen, W.: Automatic construction of multiple-object three-dimensional statistical shape models: application to cardiac modeling. IEEE Trans. Med. Imaging **21**(9), 1151–1166 (2002)

16. De Marvao, A., et al.: Population-based studies of myocardial hypertrophy: high resolution cardiovascular magnetic resonance atlases improve statistical power. J. Cardiovasc. Magn. Reson **16**(1), 16 (2014)

Deep Learning for Quality Control of Subcortical Brain 3D Shape Models

Dmitry Petrov[1,2]($\boxtimes$), Boris A. Gutman[1,2,9]($\boxtimes$), Egor Kuznetsov[8],
Christopher R. K. Ching[1], Kathryn Alpert[3], Artemis Zavaliangos-Petropulu[1],
Dmitry Isaev[1], Jessica A. Turner[4], Theo G. M. van Erp[5], Lei Wang[3],
Lianne Schmaal[6,7], Dick Veltman[7], and Paul M. Thompson[1]

[1] Imaging Genetics Center, Stevens Institute for Neuroimaging and Informatics,
University of Southern California, Los Angeles, USA
to.dmitry.petrov@gmail.com
[2] The Institute for Information Transmission Problems, Moscow, Russia
[3] Department of Psychiatry, Northwestern University, Chicago, USA
[4] The Mind Research Network, Albuquerque, USA
[5] Clinical Translational Neuroscience Laboratory, Department of Psychiatry,
University of California, Irvine, Irvine, USA
[6] Orygen, The National Centre of Excellence in Youth Mental Health,
Melbourne, Australia
[7] Department of Psychiatry, VU University Medical Center,
Amsterdam, The Netherlands
[8] Skolkovo Institute of Science and Technology, Moscow, Russia
[9] Department of Biomedical Engineering, Illinois Institute of Technology,
Chicago, USA

Abstract. We present several deep learning models for assessing the morphometric fidelity of deep grey matter region models extracted from brain MRI. We test three different convolutional neural net architectures (VGGNet, ResNet and Inception) over 2D maps of geometric features. Further, we present a novel geometry feature augmentation technique based on parametric spherical mapping. Finally, we present an approach for model decision visualization, allowing human raters to see the areas of subcortical shapes most likely to be deemed of failing quality by the machine. Our training data is comprised of 5200 subjects from the ENIGMA Schizophrenia MRI cohorts, and our test dataset contains 1500 subjects from the ENIGMA Major Depressive Disorder cohorts. Our final models reduce human rater time by 46–70%. ResNet outperforms VGGNet and Inception for all of our predictive tasks.

Keywords: Deep learning · Subcortical shape analysis
Quality checking

D. Petrov and B. A. Gutman—These authors contributed equally.

© Springer Nature Switzerland AG 2018
M. Reuter et al. (Eds.): ShapeMI 2018, LNCS 11167, pp. 268–276, 2018.
https://doi.org/10.1007/978-3-030-04747-4_25

1   Introduction

Quality control (QC) has become one of the main practical bottlenecks in big-data neuroimaging. Reducing human rater time via predictive modeling and automated quality control is bound to play an increasingly important role in maintaining and hastening the pace of scientific discovery in this field. Recently, the UK Biobank publicly released over 10,000 brain MRIs (and planning to release 90,000 more); as other biobanking initiatives scale up and follow suit, automated QC becomes crucial.

In this paper, we investigate the viability of deep convolutional neural nets for automatically labeling deep brain regional geometry models of failing quality after their extraction from brain MR images. We compare the performance of VGGNet, ResNet and Inception architectures, investigate the robustness of probability thresholds, and visualize decisions made by the trained neural nets. Our data consists of neuroimaging cohorts from the ENIGMA Schizophrenia and Major Depressive Disorder working groups participating in the ENIGMA-Shape project [1]. Using ENIGMAs shape analysis protocol and rater-labeled shapes, we train a discriminative model to separate FAIL(F) and PASS(P) cases. Features are derived from standard vertex-wise measures.

For all seven deep brain structures considered, we are able to reduce human rater time by 46 to 70 percent in out-of-sample validation, while maintaining FAIL recall rates similar to human inter-rater reliability. Our models generalize across datasets and disease samples. Our models' decision visualization, particularly ResNet, appears to capture structural abnormalities of the poor quality data that correspond to human raters' intuition.

2   Methods

Our goal in using deep learning (DL) for automated QC differs somewhat from most predictive modeling problems. Typical two-class discriminative solutions seek to balance misclassification rates of each class. In the case of QC, we focus primarily on correctly identifying FAIL cases, by far the smaller of the two classes (Table 1). In this first effort to automate shape QC, we do not attempt to eliminate human involvement, but simply to reduce it by focusing human rater time on a smaller subsample of the data containing nearly all the failing cases.

2.1   MRI Processing and Shape Features

Our deep brain structure shape measures are computed using a previously described pipeline [2,3], available via the ENIGMA Shape package. Briefly, structural MR images are parcellated into cortical and subcortical regions using FreeSurfer. Among the 19 cohorts participating in this study, FreeSurfer versions 5.1 and 5.3 were used. The binary region of interest (ROI) images are then surfaced with triangle meshes and spherically registered to a common region-specific template [4]. This leads to a one-to-one surface correspondence across the dataset at roughly 2,500 vertices per ROI. Our ROIs include the left and right thalamus, caudate, putamen, pallidum, hippocampus, amygdala, and nucleus accumbens. Each vertex p of mesh model $\mathcal{M}$ is endowed with two shape descriptors:

Medial Thickness, $D(p) = \|c_p - p\|$, where c_p is the point on the medial curve c closest to p.

LogJac(p), Log of the Jacobian determinant J arising from the template mapping, $J : T_{\phi(p)}\mathcal{M}_t \rightarrow T_p\mathcal{M}$.

Since the ENIGMA surface atlas is in symmetric correspondence, i.e., the left and right shapes are vertex-wise symmetrically registered, we can combine the two hemispheres for each region for the purposes of predictive modeling. Though we assume no hemispheric bias in QC failure, we effectively double our sample.

Our vertex-wise features are volume-normalized as follows: $\{D, J\}_{normed}(p) = \frac{\{D, J\}(p)}{V^{\{\frac{1}{3}, \frac{2}{3}\}}}$. Given discrete area elements of the template at vertex p, $A_t(p)$, we estimate volume as $V = \sum\limits_{p \in vrts(\mathcal{M})} 3A_t(p)J(p)D(p)$. We normalize our features subject-wise by this volume estimate to control for subcortical structure size.

2.2 Human Quality Rating

Human-rated quality control of shape models is performed following the ENIGMA-Shape QC protocol[1]. Briefly, raters are provided with several snapshots of each region model as well as its placement in several anatomical MR slices. A guide with examples of FAIL (QC = 1) and PASS (QC = 3) cases is provided to raters, with an additional category of MODERATE PASS (QC = 2) suggested for inexperienced raters. With sufficient experience, the rater typically switches to the binary FAIL/PASS rating. In this work, all QC = 2 cases are treated as PASS cases, consistent with ENIGMA shape studies.

2.3 Feature Mapping to 2D Images

Because our data resides on irregular mesh vertices, we first interpolate the features from an irregular spherical mesh onto an equiangular grid. The interpolated feature maps are then treated as regular 2D images by Mercator projection. Our map is based on the medial curve-based global orientation function (see [5]), which defines the latitude (θ) coordinate, as well as a rotational standardization of the thickness profile $D(p)$ to normalize the longitudinal (ϕ) coordinate. The resulting map normalizes the 2D appearance of $D(p)$, setting the poles to lie at the ends of the medial curve. In practice, the re-sampling is realized as matrix multiplication based on trilinear mesh interpolation, resulting in a 128 × 128 image for each measure.

---

[1] enigma.usc.edu/ongoing/enigma-shape-analysis.

2.4 Data Augmentation

Although our raw sample of roughly 13,500 examples is exceptionally large by the standards of neuroimaging, this dataset may not be large enough to train generalizable CNNs. Standard image augmentation techniques, e.g. cropping and rotations, are inapplicable to our data. To augment our sample of spherically mapped shape features, we sample from a distribution of spherical deformations, i.e. changes in the spherical coordinates of the thickness and Jacobian features. To do this, we first sample from a uniform distribution of vector spherical harmonic coefficients B_{lm}, C_{lm}, and apply a heat kernel operator [4] to the generated field on $T\mathbb{S}^2$. Change in spherical coordinates is then defined based on the tangential projection of the vector field, as in [4]. The width σ of the heat kernel defines the level of smoothness of the resulting deformation, and the maximum point norm M defines the magnitude. In practice, each random sampling is a composition of a large magnitude, smooth deformation ($\sigma = 10^{-1}$, $M = 3 \times 10^{-1}$) and a smaller noisier deformation ($\sigma = 10^{-2}$, $M = 3 \times 10^{-2}$). Once the deformation is generated, it is applied to the spherical coordinates of the irregular mesh, and a new sampling matrix is generated, as above.

2.5 Deep Learning Models

We train VGGNet [6], ResNet [7] and Inception [8] architectures on our data. We chose these architectures as they perform well in traditional image classification problems and are well-studied.

2.6 Model Decision Visualization

Deep learning models tend to learn superficial statistical patterns rather than high-level global or abstract concepts [9]. As we plan to provide a tool that both (1) classifies morphometric shapes, and (2) allows a user to visualize what the machine perceives as a 'FAIL', model decision visualization is an important part of our work. Here, we use Prediction Difference Analysis [10], and Grad-CAM [11] to visualize 'bad' and 'good' areas for each particular shape in question.

2.7 Predictive Model Assessment

We use two sets of measures to evaluate the performance of our models. To assess the validity of the models' estimated 'FAIL' probabilities, we calculate the area under the ROC curve (ROC AUC). We also use two supplementary measures: FAIL-recall and FAIL-share. In describing them below, we use the following definitions. TF stands for TRUE FAIL, FF stands for FALSE FAIL, TP stands for TRUE PASS, and FP stands for FALSE PASS. Our first measure, **F-recall** $= \frac{TF}{TF+FP}$, shows the proportion of FAILS that are correctly labeled by the predictive model with given probability threshold. The second measure, **F-share** $= \frac{TF+FF}{\text{Number of observations}}$, shows the proportion of the test sample labeled as FAIL by the model. Ideal models produce minimal **F-share**, and an **F-recall** of 1 for a given set of parameters.

3   Experiments

For each of the seven ROIs, we performed three experiments defined by three
DL models (VGGNet-, ResNet- and Inception-like architecture).

3.1   Datasets

Our experimental data from the ENIGMA working groups is described in
Table 1. Our predictive models were trained using 15 cohorts totaling 5218 sub-
jects' subcortical shape models from the ENIGMA-Schizophrenia working group.
For a complete overview of ENIGMA-SCZ projects and cohort details, see [12].

Table 1. Overview of FAIL percentage mean, standard deviation and maximum for
each site. Minimum is equal to 0 for all regions and sites except for hippocampus on
train (FAIL percentage 5%). Sample sizes for each ROI vary slightly due to FreeSurfer
segmentation failure.

	FAIL %	Accumbens	Caudate	Hippocampus	Thalamus	Putamen	Pallidum	Amygdala
Train	mean ± std	3.4 ± 4.7	0.9 ± 0.7	2.0 ± 1.1	0.8 ± 1.0	0.6 ± 0.6	2.3 ± 3.6	0.9 ± 0.9
	max	16.4	2.1	4.2	3.4	1.5	13.8	2.6
	size	10431	10433	10436	10436	10436	10435	10436
Test	mean ± std	4.7 ± 4.5	1.4 ± 1.5	4.9 ± 4.8	1.4 ± 1.5	0.4 ± 0.8	1.9 ± 2.0	0.8 ± 0.9
	max	10.5	3.5	11.4	3.5	1.6	3.8	2.1
	size	3017	3018	3018	3018	3017	3018	3018

To test our final models, we used data from 4 cohorts in the Major Depressive disorder working group (ENIGMA-MDD), totaling 1509 subjects, for final
out-of-fold testing. A detailed description of the ENIGMA-MDD sites and its
research objectives may be found here [13].

3.2   Model Validation

All experiments were performed separately for each ROI. The training dataset
was split into two parts referred to as 'TRAIN GRID' (90% of train data) and
'TRAIN EVAL.' (10% of the data). The two parts contained data from each
ENIGMA-SCZ cohort, stratified by the cohort-specific portion of FAIL cases.

Each model was trained on 'TRAIN GRID' using the original sampling
matrix and 30 augmentation matrices resulting in 31x augmented train dataset.
We also generated 31 instances of each mesh validation set using each sampling
matrix and validated models' ROC AUC on this big validation set during the
training.

As models produce probability estimates of FAIL (P_{FAIL}), we studied the
robustness of the probability thresholds for each model. To do so, we selected
P_{FAIL} values corresponding to regularly spaced percentiles values of **F-share**,

from 0.1 to 0.9 in 0.1 increments. For each such value, we examined **F-recall** the evaluation set.

Final thresholds were selected based on the lowest **F-share** on the TRAIN EVAL set, requiring that **F-recall** ≥ 0.8, a minimal estimate of inter-rater reliability. It is important to stress that while we used sample distribution information in selecting a threshold, the final out-of-sample prediction is made on an individual basis for each mesh.

4   Results

Trained models were deliberately set to use a loose threshold for FAIL detection, predicting 0.2–0.5 of observations as FAILs in the 'TRAIN EVAL' sample. These predicted FAIL observations contained 0.85–0.9 of all true FAILs, promising to reduce the human rater QC time by 50–80%. These results largely generalized to the test samples: Table 2 shows our best model and the threshold performance for each ROI. When applied to the test dataset, the models indicated modest over-fitting, with the amount of human effort reduced by 46–70%, while capturing 76–94% of poor quality meshes. The inverse relationship between FAIL percentage and F-share (Fig. 1) may indicate model failure to learn generalizable features on smaller number of FAIL examples. ROC AUC and F-recall performance generalize across the test sites. Since 68% of our test dataset is comprised of the Münster cohort, it is important that overall test performance is not skewed by it.

Our experiments with decision visualization (see Fig. 2) indicate that in most FAIL cases, the attention heat map generated by Grad-CAM corresponds to human raters' intuition while Prediction Difference Analysis tend to concentrate on local 'bumps' on shapes.

5   Discussion and Conclusion

We have presented potential deep learning solutions for semi-automated quality control of deep brain structure shape data. We believe this is the first DL approach for detecting end-of-the-pipeline feature failures in deep brain structure geometry. We showed that DL can robustly reduce human visual QC time by 46–70% for large-scale analyses, for all seven regions in question, across diverse MRI datasets and populations. Qualitative analysis of models decisions shows promise as a potential training and heuristic validation tool for human raters.

There are several limitations of our work. Our planar projection of vertex-wise features introduces space-varying distortions and boundary effects that can affect training, performance and visualization. Recently proposed spherical convolutional neural nets [14] may be useful to fix this issue. Second, our models' decision visualization only partly matches with human raters' intuition. In some cases, our models do not consider primary "failure" areas, as assessed by a human rater. Finally, our models are trained on purely geometrical features and do not include information on shape boundaries inside the brain. In rare cases, human

Table 2. Test performance of the best models for each region. ResNet performs the best in all cases. Overall models' performance generalizes to out-of-sample test data.

ROI	Augmented	Eval AUC	Test AUC	Eval F-share	Test F-share	Eval F-recall	Test F-recall
Accumbens	No	0.86	0.80	0.3	0.32	0.83	0.74
Accumbens	Yes	0.86	0.80	0.3	0.35	0.83	0.78
Amygdala	No	0.75	0.77	0.8	0.81	0.92	0.93
Amygdala	Yes	0.80	0.75	0.5	0.54	0.92	0.80
Caudate	No	0.91	0.78	0.1	0.16	0.82	0.58
Caudate	Yes	0.90	0.84	0.2	0.30	0.82	0.78
Hippocampus	No	0.86	0.92	0.4	0.41	0.90	0.94
Hippocampus	Yes	0.85	0.93	0.3	0.36	0.81	0.92
Pallidum	No	0.88	0.88	0.3	0.29	0.83	0.85
Pallidum	Yes	0.86	0.91	0.3	0.32	0.81	0.91
Putamen	No	0.82	0.69	0.5	0.54	0.86	0.76
Putamen	Yes	0.88	0.70	0.3	0.52	0.93	0.76
Thalamus	No	0.82	0.89	0.4	0.42	0.82	0.97
Thalamus	Yes	0.8	0.87	0.4	0.47	0.82	0.94

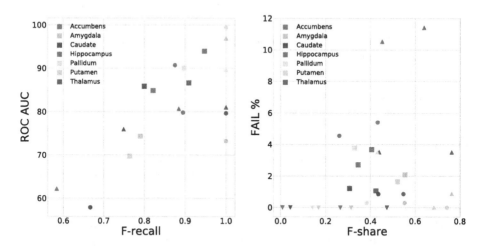

Fig. 1. Scatter plots of F-recall vs. ROC AUC on test datasets and F-share vs. proportion of predicted FAIL cases on test datasets (F-share). Left: F-recall vs ROC AUC. Right: Fail F-share vs FAIL percentage. F-share was calculated based on thresholds from Table 2. Mark size shows the dataset size. Mark shape represents dataset (site): ○ - CODE-Berlin (N = 176); □ - Münster (N = 1033); △ - Stanford (N = 105); ▽ - Houston (N = 195)

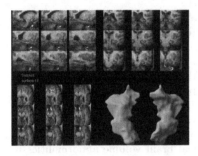

Fig. 2. QC report for human raters (left) and decision visualization example based on Grad-CAM for the ResNet model (right). Red colors correspond to points maximizing the model's FAIL decision in the last layer. Decision visualization corresponds to the observable deviations from underlying anatomical boundaries indicative of a "FAIL" rating according to an experienced rater. (Color figure online)

raters pass shapes with atypical geometry because their boundaries look reasonable, and conversely mark normal-appearing geometry as failing due to poor a fit with the MR image. Incorporating intensity as well as geometry features will be the focus of our future work.

Acknowledgements. This work was funded in part by NIH BD2K grant U54 EB020403 and Russian Science Foundation grant 17-11-01390.

References

1. Gutman, B., et al.: Harmonized large-scale anatomical shape analysis: mapping subcortical differences across the ENIGMA Bipolar, Schizophrenia, and Major Depression working groups. Biol. Psychiatry **81**(10), S308 (2017)
2. Gutman, B.A., et al.: Medial demons registration localizes the degree of genetic influence over subcortical shape variability: An n = 1480 meta-analysis. In: 2015 IEEE 12th International Symposium on Biomedical Imaging (ISBI), pp. 1402–1406. IEEE (2015)
3. Roshchupkin, G.V., Gutman, B.A., et al.: Heritability of the shape of subcortical brain structures in the general population. Nat. Commun. **7**, 13738 (2016)
4. Gutman, B.A., Madsen, S.K., Toga, A.W., Thompson, P.M.: A family of fast spherical registration algorithms for cortical shapes. In: Shen, L., Liu, T., Yap, P.-T., Huang, H., Shen, D., Westin, C.-F. (eds.) MBIA 2013. LNCS, vol. 8159, pp. 246–257. Springer, Cham (2013). https://doi.org/10.1007/978-3-319-02126-3_24
5. Gutman, B.A., Yalin, W., Rajagopalan, P., Toga, A.W., Thompson, P.M.: Shape matching with medial curves and 1-D group-wise registration. In: 2012 9th IEEE International Symposium on Biomedical Imaging (ISBI), pp.716–719 (2012)
6. Simonyan, K., Zisserman, A.: Very deep convolutional networks for large-scale image recognition. arXiv preprint arXiv:1409.1556 (2014)
7. He, K., Zhang, X., Ren, S., Sun, J.: Deep residual learning for image recognition. In: Proceedings of the IEEE Conference on Computer Vision and Pattern Recognition, pp. 770–778 (2016)

8. Szegedy, C., Ioffe, S., Vanhoucke, V., Alemi, A.A.: Inception-v4, inception-ResNet and the impact of residual connections on learning. In: AAAI, vol. 4, p. 12 (2017)

9. Jo, J., Bengio, Y.: Measuring the tendency of CNNs to learn surface statistical regularities. arXiv preprint arXiv:1711.11561 (2017)

10. Zintgraf, L.M., Cohen, T.S., Adel, T., Welling, M.: Visualizing deep neural network decisions: prediction difference analysis. arXiv preprint arXiv:1702.04595 (2017)

11. Selvaraju, R.R., Cogswell, M., Das, A., Vedantam, R., Parikh, D., Batra, D.: Grad-CAM: visual explanations from deep networks via gradient-based localization. See https://arxiv.org/abs/1610.02391 v3 **7**(8) (2016)

12. van Erp, T.G.M., Hibar, D.P., et al.: Subcortical brain volume abnormalities in 2028 individuals with Schizophrenia and 2540 healthy controls via the ENIGMA consortium. Mol. Psychiatry **21**, 547 (2016)

13. Schmaal, L., Hibar, D.P., et al.: Cortical abnormalities in adults and adolescents with major depression based on brain scans from 20 cohorts worldwide in the ENIGMA Major Depressive Disorder working group. Mol. Psychiatry **22**(6), 900–909 (2017)

14. Cohen, T.S., Geiger, M., Koehler, J., Welling, M.: Spherical CNNs. arXiv preprint arXiv:1801.10130 (2018)

Discrimination of Volumetric Shapes Using Orthogonal Tensor Decomposition

Hayato Itoh[1] and Atsushi Imiya[2(✉)]

[1] Graduate School of Informatics, Nagoya University,
Furo-cho, Chikusa-ku, Nagoya 464-8601, Japan
[2] Institute of Management and Information Technologies, Chiba University,
Yayoi-cho 1-33, Inage-ku, Chiba 263-8522, Japan
imiya@faculty.chiba-u.jp

Abstract. Organs, cells and microstructures in cells dealt with in medical image analysis are volumetric data. Sampled values of volumetric data are expressed as three-way array data. For the quantitative discrimination of multiway forms from the viewpoint of principal component analysis (PCA)-based pattern recognition, distance metrics for subspaces of multiway data arrays are desired. The paper aims to extend pattern recognition methodologies based on PCA for vector spaces to those for multilinear data. First, we extend the canonical angle between linear subspaces for vector-based pattern recognition to the canonical angle between multilinear subspaces for tensor-based pattern recognition. Furthermore, using transportation between the Stiefel manifolds, we introduce a new metric for a collection of linear subspaces. Then, we extend the transportation of between Stiefel manifolds in vector space to the transportation of the Stiefel manifolds in multilinear spaces for the discrimination analysis of multiway array data.

1 Introduction

We introduce distance metrics for discrimination and compression of multilinear forms which express multiway data arrays using the canonical angle between the Grassmann manifolds [1–4] and transportation [5] between the Stiefel manifolds [6] in the multilinear space. We deal with an extension of singular value decomposition (SVD) of two-dimensional arrays [7–9] to three-way arrays.

Principal component analysis (PCA) is a fundamental methodology for data processing in pattern recognition, computer vision, physiology and many natural and social sciences [10–14]. Sampled values of volumetric data [14] are expressed as three-way array data as elements in multilinear space. For the quantitative discrimination of multiway forms from the viewpoint of PCA-based pattern recognition, a distance metric for subspaces in multilinear space [15–22] is desired.

Object-oriented data analysis (OODA) [23–25] in bioinformatics is required for classification and retrieval structures discrete objects such as trees [25, 26]. A pattern is assumed to be a square integrable function in a linear space and to be defined on a finite support in n-dimensional Euclidean space [10, 13, 14].

© Springer Nature Switzerland AG 2018
M. Reuter et al. (Eds.): ShapeMI 2018, LNCS 11167, pp. 277–290, 2018.
https://doi.org/10.1007/978-3-030-04747-4_26

In pattern recognition by numerical computation, sampled patterns are dealt with. In traditional pattern recognition, these sampled patterns are embedded in an appropriate-dimensional Euclidean space as vectors. The other way is to deal with sampled patterns as three-way array data [15,23,24]. These three-way array data are expressed as tensors [16–19] in a multilinear space to preserve the linearity of the original pattern space. Since multiway array data are structured data in a square grid from the viewpoint of digital geometry, we introduce PCA for three-way array data from the viewpoint of the OODA using multilinear algebra [15,23]. The principal components in multilinear space derive distance metrics for discrimination and compression of multilinear forms.

Deformation of shapes induces the geodesic paths on the shape manifold [27]. Along these geodesic paths [28–30], local orthogonal bases are defined using PCA [31,32] for analysis of shape deformations and discrimination of shapes. These local orthogonal bases along the geodesic paths are effectively used for longitudinal analysis of shape deformation. We introduce a metric between shapes using a pair of these orthogonal bases along the trajectory path of deformation.

2   Distances Between Linear Subspaces

In this section, we summarize mathematical aspects of the subspace method in vector space [10,11,13] to extend the methodologies to the subspace method for tensors. Furthermore, we define the Stiefel distance as a metric between a pair of linear manifolds. The Stiefel distance is the transportation between a pair of collections of orthonormal bases [6], although the Grassmann distance is defined as the canonical angles between a pair of linear subspaces [1–3].

For $x \in \mathbf{R}^n$ and an orthogonal projection $P_{k,\alpha}$, we define the collection of linear subspaces

$$G_{k,n}^\alpha = \{x_\perp \mid x = x_\perp + x_\parallel, \ P_{k,\alpha} x_\perp = x_\perp, \ P_{k,\alpha} x_\parallel = 0\}. \tag{1}$$

For a pair of linear subspaces

$$L_{k,n}^\alpha = \mathcal{L}(\{\varphi_i^\alpha\}_{i=1}^k), \ L_{k,n}^\beta = \mathcal{L}(\{\varphi_i^\beta\}_{i=1}^{k'}) \tag{2}$$

and vectors $x, y \in \mathbf{R}^n$ which generate the Grassmann manifolds as

$$G_{k,n}^\alpha = x + L_{k,n}^\alpha, \ G_{k,n}^\beta = y + L_{k,n}^\beta, \tag{3}$$

we define a metric between $L_{k,n}^\alpha$ and $L_{k,n}^\beta$. We call the linear subspace $L_{k,n}^\alpha$ the generator linear manifold of the manifold $G_{k,n}^\alpha$.

The angle $\theta = \angle(a, b)$ between two vectors a and b is defined as $\cos\theta = \frac{a^\top b}{|a||b|}$. The angle between two linear spaces spanned by column vectors of U and V is the extremal of the criterion

$$\cos^2\theta = (Ua)^\top Vb \tag{4}$$

with respect to the conditions $|\boldsymbol{a}| = 1$ and $|\boldsymbol{b}| = 1$. The minimiser of Eq. (4) is the solution of the Euler-Lagrange equation

$$T_1 = \cos^2 \theta + \lambda(1 - |\boldsymbol{a}|^2) + \mu(1 - |\boldsymbol{b}|^2). \tag{5}$$

The extremals of Eq. (5) are computed from the solutions of the system equations

$$\boldsymbol{Ua} = \mu \boldsymbol{b}, \quad \boldsymbol{Vb} = \lambda \boldsymbol{a}. \tag{6}$$

Therefore, for the singular value problems

$$\boldsymbol{Pa} = \lambda \mu \boldsymbol{a}, \quad \boldsymbol{Qb} = \lambda \mu \boldsymbol{b}, \tag{7}$$

where $\boldsymbol{P} = \boldsymbol{UVU}$ and $\boldsymbol{Q} = \boldsymbol{VUV}$, the maximiser of Eq. (4) is $T_{\max} = \lambda_{\max}\mu_{\max}$ with the condition $\lambda = \mu$. This mathematical property implies the following proposition.

Proposition 1 [1–4]. *The canonical angle between the pair of linear subspaces spanned by column vectors of orthogonal matrices $\boldsymbol{U}$ and $\boldsymbol{V}$ is $\cos^{-1} \sigma$, where σ is the maximum eigenvalue of matrix $\boldsymbol{P} = \boldsymbol{UVU}$.*

The Stiefel manifold [6]

$$V_k^\alpha(\mathbf{R}^n) = \{\varphi_i^\alpha\}_{i=1}^k \tag{8}$$

defines the collection of orthogonal matrices which satisfy the condition

$$\boldsymbol{U}_{k,\alpha}^\top \boldsymbol{U}_{k,\alpha} = \boldsymbol{I}_k, \tag{9}$$

where $\boldsymbol{I}_k$ is the $k \times k$ identity matrix.

Definition 1. *Using the column vectors $\{\varphi_i^\alpha\}_{i=1}^k$ and $\{\varphi_i^\beta\}_{i=1}^k$ of $\boldsymbol{U}_{k,\alpha}$ and $\boldsymbol{U}_{k,\beta}$, respectively, we define the distances between a pair of linear subspaces spanned by the column vectors of $\boldsymbol{U}_{k,\alpha}$ and $\boldsymbol{U}_{k,\beta}$ as*

$$d_S(\{\varphi_i^1\}_{i=1}^k, \{\varphi_j^2\}_{j=1}^k)^p = \min_{w_{ij}} \sum_{i=1}^k \sum_{j=1}^k |\cos^{-1}(\varphi_i^{1\top} \varphi_j^2)|^p c_{ij}, \tag{10}$$

with respect to the constraints

$$c_{ij} \geq 0, \quad \sum_{i=1}^k c_{ij} = \frac{\lambda_{2,j}^p}{\sum_{i=1}^n \lambda_{2,i}^p}, \quad \sum_{j=1}^k c_{ij} = \frac{\lambda_{1,i}^p}{\sum_{j=1}^n \lambda_{1,j}^p}, \tag{11}$$

where $\lambda_{\alpha,i}$ $\alpha \geq 1$ is the eigenvalue associated with φ_i^α.

If the vector space of data $\mathfrak{D} \subset \mathbf{R}^n$ is the logical OR of categories $\{\mathfrak{C}_i\}_{i=1}^m$, that is, $\mathfrak{D} = \cup_{i=1}^m \mathfrak{C}_i$, elements in the common space $\mathfrak{C} = \cap_{i=1}^m \mathfrak{C}_i$ possess common properties of $\{f_{ij}\}_{j=1}^{m(i)} \in \mathfrak{C}_i$.

The orthogonal projection $\boldsymbol{Q}$ to the common linear space defined by $\{\boldsymbol{P}_i\}_{j=1}^m$ is the minimiser of the criterion

$$J_{\text{CMS1}} = \sum_{i=1}^m |\boldsymbol{Q}\boldsymbol{P}_i|_{\text{F}}^2 \tag{12}$$

with the condition $\boldsymbol{Q}^\top\boldsymbol{Q} = \boldsymbol{I}_k$ for $0 < k \le n$, where $|\boldsymbol{A}|_{\text{F}}^2 = \sum_{i=1}^m \sum_{j=1}^n |a_{ij}|^2$ for the $m \times n$ matrix $\boldsymbol{A} = ((a_{ij}))$. The Euler-Lagrange equation

$$J_{\text{CMS2}} = \sum_{i=1}^m |\boldsymbol{Q}\boldsymbol{P}_i|_{\text{F}}^2 + \langle(\boldsymbol{I}_k - \boldsymbol{Q}^\top\boldsymbol{Q}), \boldsymbol{\Lambda}\rangle. \tag{13}$$

for this constraint problem derives the eigenvalue problem

$$\left(\sum_{i=1}^m \boldsymbol{P}_i\right)\boldsymbol{Q} = \boldsymbol{Q}\boldsymbol{\Lambda}. \tag{14}$$

Equation (14) implies that the eigenvectors of $\boldsymbol{C} = \sum_{i=1}^m \boldsymbol{P}_i$ are the orthogonal basis of the linear subspace $\mathfrak{C} = \cap_{i=1}^m \mathfrak{C}_i$.

For an element $f_{kj} \in \mathfrak{C}_k$, $f_{ki}^C = (\boldsymbol{I}-\boldsymbol{Q})f_{kj}$ is the element in $\mathfrak{C}_k \setminus \mathfrak{C}$. Therefore, the categories $\mathfrak{C} \cap \mathfrak{C}_k f$ can be discriminated by f_{ki}^C and f_{kfi}^C using appropriate metrics for a pair of subspaces.

3   Linear Data Processing of Three-Way Array Data

3.1   Tensor PCA

For the triplet of positive integers I_1, I_2 and I_3, the third-order tensor $\mathbb{R}^{I_1 \times I_2 \times I_3}$ is expressed as $\mathcal{X} = ((x_{ijk}))$. Indices i, j and k are called the 1-mode, 2-mode and 3-mode of $\mathcal{X}$, respectively.

For a collection of 3-mode tensors $\{\mathcal{X}_i\}_{i=1}^N$, we define

$$\check{\mathcal{X}}_i = \mathcal{X}_i - \bar{\mathcal{X}}, \quad \bar{\mathcal{X}} = \frac{1}{N}\sum_{i=1}^N \mathcal{X}_i. \tag{15}$$

Then, the principal components of three-way multilinear form $\{\check{\mathcal{X}}_i\}_{i=1}^N$ are maximisers of the condition

$$J(\boldsymbol{U}^{(1)}, \boldsymbol{U}^{(2)}, \boldsymbol{U}^{(3)}) = \underset{i}{\text{E}}\left(|\check{\mathcal{X}}_i \times_1 \boldsymbol{U}^{(1)\top} \times_2 \boldsymbol{U}^{(2)\top} \times_3 \boldsymbol{U}^{(3)\top}|_{\text{F}}^2\right) \tag{16}$$

with respect to the conditions $\boldsymbol{U}^{(j)\top}\boldsymbol{U}^{(j)} = \boldsymbol{I}^{(j)}$ for $j = 1, 2, 3$. The column vectors of the collection of orthogonal matrices $\{\boldsymbol{U}^{(j)}\}_{j=1}^3$ are called the tensor principal components. Furthermore, computation of $\{\boldsymbol{U}^{(j)}\}_{j=1}^3$ called tensor principal component analysis (tensor PCA) based on the Tucker 3 decomposition of tensors.

The minimisers of Eq. (16) are the minimisers of the Euler-Lagrange equation

$$J_{33}(U^{(1)}, U^{(2)}, U^{(3)}) = E_k(|\mathcal{X}_k \times_1 U^{(1)} \times_2 U^{(2)} \times_3 U^{(3)}|_F^2)$$
$$+ \sum_{i=1}^{3} \langle (I - U^{(i)^\top} U^{(i)}), \Lambda^{(i)} \rangle, \tag{17}$$

where $\langle A, B \rangle = tr B^\top A$. This minimisation problem is solved by the iteration procedure in Algorithm 1.

Algorithm 1. Iterative method for tensor PCA

Data: $0 < \varepsilon \ll 1$
Data: $\alpha := 0$
Data: For $i = 1, 2, 3$, $U_{(0)}^i := Q^{(i)}$, where $Q^{(i)^\top} Q^{(i)} = I$
Result: Orthogonal matrices $U^{(i)}$ for $i = 1, 2, 3$
while $|U_{(\alpha+1)}^{(i)} - U_\alpha^{(i)}| \gg \varepsilon$ **do**

     maximise $E_i|U_{(\alpha+1)}^{(1)^\top} \mathcal{X}_{i1}^\top \mathcal{X}_{i1} U_{(\alpha+1)}^{(1)}|_F^2 + \langle (U_{(\alpha+1)}^{(1)^\top} U_{(\alpha+1)}^{(1)} - I), \Lambda_{(\alpha)}^{(1)} \rangle$;
     for $\mathcal{X}_{i1} = \mathcal{X}_i \times_2 U_{(\alpha)}^{(2)^\top} \times_3 U_{(\alpha)}^{(3)^\top}$;
     maximise $E_i|U_{(\alpha+1)}^{(2)^\top} \mathcal{X}_{i2}^\top \mathcal{X}_{i2} U_{(\alpha+1)}^{(2)}|_F^2 + \langle (U_{(\alpha+1)}^{(2)^\top} U_{(\alpha+1)}^{(2)} - I), \Lambda_{(\alpha)}^{(2)} \rangle$;
     for $\mathcal{X}_{i2} = \mathcal{X}_i \times_1 U_{(\alpha+1)}^{(1)^\top} \times_3 U_{(\alpha)}^{(3)^\top}$;
     maximise $E_i|U_{(\alpha+1)}^{(3)^\top} \mathcal{X}_{i3}^\top \mathcal{X}_{i3} U_{(\alpha+1)}^{(3)}|_F^2 + \langle (U_{(\alpha+1)}^{(3)^\top} U_{(\alpha+1)}^{(3)} - I), \Lambda_{(\alpha)}^{(3)} \rangle$;
     for $\mathcal{X}_{i3}$;
     $\alpha := \alpha + 1$

end

3.2 Distance Between Multilinear Grassmann Manifolds

The angle $\theta = \angle(A, B)$ between two tensors A and B is computed as $\cos \theta = \frac{\langle A, B \rangle}{|A|_F |B|_F}$. The angle between two multilinear spaces defined by $\{U^{(i)}, V^{(i)}\}_{i=1}^3$ is the extremal of the criterion

$$\cos^2 \theta = |\langle A \times_1 U^{(1)^\top} \times_2 U^{(2)^\top} \times_3 U^{(3)^\top}, B \times_1 V^{(1)^\top} \times_2 V^{(2)^\top} \times_3 V^{(3)^\top} \rangle|^2 \tag{18}$$

with respect to the conditions $|A|_F = 1$ and $|B|_F = 1$. Therefore, the minimiser of Eq. (18) is the solution of the Euler-Lagrange equation

$$T_1 = \cos^2 \theta + \lambda(1 - |A|_F^2) + \mu(1 - |B|_F^2). \tag{19}$$

The minimiser of Eq. (19) is the solution of the system of equations,

$$A \times_1 U^{(1)^\top} \times_2 U^{(2)^\top} \times_3 U^{(3)^\top} = \mu B, \tag{20}$$
$$B \times_1 V^{(1)^\top} \times_2 V^{(2)^\top} \times_3 V^{(3)^\top} = \lambda A. \tag{21}$$

The tensor singular value problems

$$\mathcal{A} \times_1 \boldsymbol{P}_1^\top \times_2 \boldsymbol{P}_2^\top \times_3 \boldsymbol{P}_3^\top = \lambda\mu\mathcal{A}, \ \mathcal{B} \times_1 \boldsymbol{Q}_1^\top \times_2 \boldsymbol{Q}_2^\top \times_3 \boldsymbol{Q}_3^\top = \lambda\mu\mathcal{B}, \qquad (22)$$

where $\boldsymbol{P}_i = \boldsymbol{U}^{(i)}\boldsymbol{V}^{(i)}\boldsymbol{U}^{(i)}$ and $\boldsymbol{Q}_i = \boldsymbol{V}^{(i)}\boldsymbol{U}^{(i)}\boldsymbol{V}^{(i)}$, derive the maximiser of Eq. (18) as $T_{\max} = \lambda_{\max}\mu_{\max}$ with the condition $\lambda = \mu$. This mathematical property implies the following theorem.

Theorem 1. *The canonical angle between a pair of linear subspaces spanned by triples of matrices $\{\boldsymbol{U}^{(i)}\}_{i=1}^3$ and $\{\boldsymbol{V}^{(i)}\}_{i=1}^3$ in a multilinear space is $\cos^{-1}\sigma$, where σ is the maximum eigenvalue of tensor $\boldsymbol{P}_1 \times_2 \boldsymbol{P}_2 \times_3 \boldsymbol{P}_3$.*

Setting $\boldsymbol{P}_\alpha^{(k)}$ to be the orthogonal projection to the linear subspace $\Pi_\alpha^{(k)}$, where $\alpha = 1, 2$ and $k = 1, 2, 3$, for the tensor subspace, the Grassmann distance is extended as

$$d_G(\Pi_1^{(1)} \otimes \Pi_1^{(2)} \otimes \Pi_1^{(3)}, \Pi_2^{(1)} \otimes \Pi_2^{(2)} \otimes \Pi_2^{(3)})^2$$
$$= \sum_{i=1}^k (\cos^{-1}\sqrt{\lambda_i^{(1)}\mu_i^{(1)}})^2 + \sum_{i=1}^k (\cos^{-1}\sqrt{\lambda_i^{(2)}\mu_i^{(2)}})^2 + \sum_{i=1}^k (\cos^{-1}\sqrt{\lambda_i^{(3)}\mu_i^{(3)}})^2, \qquad (23)$$

where $\boldsymbol{P}_1^{(k)}\boldsymbol{P}_2^{(k)}\boldsymbol{u}_i^{(k)} = \lambda_i^{(k)}\boldsymbol{v}_i^{(k)}$ and $\boldsymbol{P}_2^{(k)}\boldsymbol{P}_1^{(k)}\boldsymbol{v}_i^{(k)} = \mu_i^{(k)}\boldsymbol{u}_i^{(k)}$, for $\lambda_i^{(k)} = \mu_i^{(k)}$.

3.3 Distance Between Multilinear Stiefel Manifolds

For a tensor subspace, the distance between a pair of the Stiefel manifolds based on the Wasserstein distance based on transportation between a pair of manifolds is extended as

$$d_S(\boldsymbol{V}_1^{(1)} \otimes \boldsymbol{V}_1^{(2)} \otimes \boldsymbol{V}_1^{(3)}, \boldsymbol{V}_2^{(1)} \otimes \boldsymbol{V}_2^{(2)} \otimes \boldsymbol{V}_2^{(3)},)^p$$
$$= \min_{c_{ij}^{(1)}} \sum_{i=1}^k \sum_{j=1}^k |\cos^{-1}(\varphi_i^{1(1)\top}\varphi_j^{2(1)})|^p c_{ij}^{(1)} + \min_{c_{ij}^{(2)}} \sum_{i=1}^k \sum_{j=1}^k |\cos^{-1}(\varphi_i^{1(2)\top}\varphi_j^{2(2)})|^p c_{ij}^{(2)}$$
$$+ \min_{c_{ij}^{(3)}} \sum_{i=1}^k \sum_{j=1}^k |\cos^{-1}(\varphi_i^{1(3)\top}\varphi_j^{2(3)})|^p c_{ij}^{(3)}. \qquad (24)$$

We use the following three systems of inequalities for constraints:

$$\sum_j c_{ij}^{(n)} = \sqrt{\lambda_i^{(n)}}/\sum_{i=1}^{I_n} \sqrt{\lambda_i^{(n)}}, \quad \sum_i c_{ij}^{(n)} = \sqrt{\lambda_j^{(n)}}/\sum_{j=1}^{I_n} \sqrt{\lambda_j^{(n)}}, \qquad (25)$$

$$\sum_j c_{ij}^{(n)} = \lambda_i^{(n)}/\sum_{i=1}^{I_n} \lambda_i^{(n)}, \quad \sum_i c_{ij}^{(n)} = \lambda_j^{(n)}/\sum_{j=1}^{I_n} \lambda_j^{(n)}, \qquad (26)$$

and

$$\sum_j c_{ij}^{(n)} = \left(\lambda_i^{(n)}\right)^2 / \sum_{i=1}^{I_n} \left(\lambda_i^{(n)}\right)^2, \quad \sum_i c_{ij}^{(n)} = \left(\lambda_j^{(n)}\right)^2 / \sum_{j=1}^{I_n} \left(\lambda_j^{(n)}\right)^2, \quad (27)$$

for $n = 1, 2, 3$. These three constraints defined by Eqs. (25), (26) and (27) are the sum of singular values, the sum of eigenvalues and the energy, respectively.

3.4   Common Subspace in Multilinear Space

For the construction of the common space spanned by $\{P_1^{(j)} \otimes P_2^{(j)} \otimes P_2^{(j)}\}_{j=1}^m$, the orthogonal projection $Q = Q^{(1)} \otimes Q^{(2)} \otimes Q^{(3)}$ which minimises the criterion

$$J_{\text{CMS1}} = \sum_{i=1}^m |QP_i|_F^2 \qquad (28)$$

with the conditions

$$P_i = P_i^{(1)} \otimes P_i^{(2)} \qquad (29)$$

and

$$Q_i^{(j)\top} Q_i^{(j)} = I_{m_i}, \quad j = 1, 2, 3, \qquad (30)$$

derives the projection to the common space as the extension to tensor PCA. The minimiser of the Euler-Lagrange equation

$$J_{\text{CMS2}} = \sum_{i=1}^m |Q^{(j)} P_i|_F^2 + \sum_{j=1}^3 \langle (I_{m_j} - Q^{(j)\top} Q^{(j)}), \Lambda^{(j)} \rangle \qquad (31)$$

is the solution of the problem.

In each mode, the orthogonal projection $Q^{(j)}$ which maximises the criterion

$$J_{\text{CMSM}} = \sum_{i=1}^{N_j} |Q^{(j)} U_i^{(j)}|_F^2 \qquad (32)$$

for the collection of orthogonal projections $\{U_i^{(j)}\}_{i=1}^{N_j}$ approximates the common spaces spanned by $\{U_i^{(j)}\}_{i=1}^{N_j}$.

The projection $Q^{(j)}$ is the solution of the variational problem

$$J_{\text{CMSM-EL}} = \sum_{i=1}^N |Q^{(j)} U_i^{(j)}|_F^2 + \langle (I_{m_j} - Q^{(j)\top} Q^{(j)}), \Sigma^{(j)} \rangle. \qquad (33)$$

Therefore, the matrix $Q^{(j)}$ is the eigenmatrix of

$$\sum_{i=1}^{N_j} U_i^{(j)} Q^{(j)} = Q^{(j)} \Sigma^{(j)}. \qquad (34)$$

3.5   Dimension Reduction and Discrimination in Multilinear Space

We derive three-dimensional analogous of image singular value decomposition (imageSVD) [7–9] for tensors. Using this decomposition, we develop methods for dimension reduction and discrimination of sampled shapes embedded in multilinear space.

Let $\mathcal{X}$ be the $n_1 \times n_2 \times n_3$ tensor. Using a triplet of orthogonal matrices $\boldsymbol{U}^{(1)}$, $\boldsymbol{U}^{(2)}$ and $\boldsymbol{U}^{(3)}$ which minimise the criterion

$$J = |\mathcal{X} - \mathcal{X} \times_1 \boldsymbol{U}^{(1)\top} \times_2 \boldsymbol{U}^{(2)\top} \times_3 \boldsymbol{U}^{(3)\top}|, \tag{35}$$

the tensor $\mathcal{X}$ is approximated as

$$\mathcal{X} = \mathcal{X} \times_1 \boldsymbol{U}^{(1)\top} \times_2 \boldsymbol{U}^{(2)\top} \times_3 \boldsymbol{U}^{(3)\top} + \mathcal{E}, \tag{36}$$

where $\mathcal{E}$ is the residual error.

Uisng $\boldsymbol{U}^{(1)}$, $\boldsymbol{U}^{(2)}$ and $\boldsymbol{U}^{(3)}$, $\mathcal{X}$ is compressed as

$$\bar{\mathcal{X}} = \mathcal{X} \times_1 (\boldsymbol{U}^{(1)} \boldsymbol{P}_1)^\top \times_2 (\boldsymbol{U}^{(2)} \boldsymbol{P}_2)^\top \times_3 (\boldsymbol{U}^{(3)} \boldsymbol{P}_3)^\top, \tag{37}$$

where

$$\boldsymbol{P}_i = \begin{pmatrix} \boldsymbol{I}_{k_i}, \boldsymbol{O} \\ \boldsymbol{O}, \boldsymbol{O} \end{pmatrix}, \quad k_i \leq n_i, \tag{38}$$

for $i = 1, 2, 3$. We accept the $k_1 \times k_2 \times k_3$ leading sub-tensor of $\bar{\mathcal{X}}$ as the compressed approximation of $\mathcal{X}$.

Using PCA-based distances, we measure distances among a collection of sampled volumetric shapes. Here after, we assume that shapes are aligned using centroid, that is, the centroid is the origin of the geometrical expression of each shape. We embed sampled volumetric shapes $\{\mathcal{S}_i\}_{i=1}^m$ in the three-way multilinear space $\mathbf{R}^{n_1 \times n_2 \times n_3}$. Setting $\boldsymbol{U}_i^{(1)}$, $\boldsymbol{U}_i^{(2)}$ and $\boldsymbol{U}_i^{(3)}$ for $i = 1, 2, \cdots, m$ to be a triplet of orthogonal matrices computed from each shape $mathcalS_i$, these triplet of orthogonal matrices allow us to compute the Grassmann distance and the Wasserstein distance between shapes in the collection of shapes $\{\mathcal{S}_i\}_{i=1}^m$.

4   Numerical Evaluations

Using the volumetric image sequence in Fig. 1 from a cardiac dataset [33], we evaluate the mathematical properties of the Wasserstein distance for Stiefel manifolds. Performances for shape discrimination Euclidean distance for multilinear forms (See Apendix.) based on Frobenius norm of the multiway array, the Grassmann distance of multilinear forms and the distance of Stiefel manifolds in multilinear spaces are comparatively evaluated. Hereafter, we call the Wasserstein distance for multilinear Stiefel manifolds and the Grassmann distance of multilinear forms the Wasserstein distance and Grassmann distance, respectively.

First, we compared performances of the Euclidean, Wasserstein and Grassmann distances. Figure 2 illustrates comparisons on $D(i)$ between Wasserstein

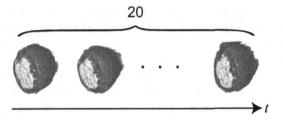

Fig. 1. Sequence of volumetric images. Each volumetric image in this sequence is extracted using landmarks of the endocardium of the left ventricle in cardiac MRI data [33]. The cardiac MRI dataset provides 17 volumetric sequences of the left ventricle for 17 patients. Each sequence contains 20 valumetric images. The resolution of each volumetric image is $81 \times 81 \times 63$ voxels.

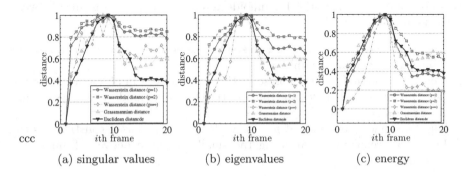

| (a) singular values | (b) eigenvalues | (c) energy |

Fig. 2. Comparison of three constraints between the first and jth frames. We use the Wasserstein, Grassmann and Euclidean distances. For the Wasserstein distance, we set $p = 1, 2, \infty$. The horizontal axis represents the number j of the target frame. The vertical axis represents the distance between frames. The left, middle and right column show the comparison among three distances for the constraints based on the sum of singular value, the sum of eigenvalues and the energy, respectively.

distance and Grassmann distance. From Fig. 2, comparison on $D(i)$ among the Euclidean, Wasserstein and Grassmann distances indicates that the Wasserstein distance can most accurately measure small deformations of the frames in a sequence. The outline shape of the beating heart shrinks from the first frame to the ninth frame. Then, the volume of the outline shape is smallest at the ninth frame. In the frames around the minimum volume, the beating motion of the heart rapidly deforms the volumes and outline shapes. The Wasserstein distance measures this biomechanical properties of the shape deformation of the beating heart.

Next, we compared the numerical properties of the Wasserstein distance of $p = 1, 2, \infty$, for the three conditions defined by Eqs. (25), (26) and (27). Setting $D(i)$ to be the distances between the first and ith frames for distance measures, Fig. 3 shows the curves of $D(i)$ for three distances.

The results for $p = 1, 2, \infty$ with the distances defined by Eqs. (25), (26) and (27) are shown in Fig. 3(a)-(c), (d)-(f) and (g)-(i), respectively. The performances for the discrimination of shapes are compared in each mode. The results indicate that the Wasserstein distance for $p = \infty$ represents small changes in the frames of a sequence more clearly than the Wasserstein distance for $p = 1, 2$. Comparisons of $D(i)$ in the left, middle and right columns in Fig. 3 indicate that the Wasserstein distance with the energy-based constraint measures small deformations the most clearly, since the curves $D(i)$ of the Wasserstein distance with the energy-based constraint preserves smooth profiles on the curves. These experimental results and comparisons on $D(i)$ indicate the validity of the Wasserstein distance with the energy-based constraint measuring small perturbations of deformation of the shape outlines in sequences of volumetric images.

From these numerical examples, we observe the following properties for the Wasserstein distance for Stiefel manifolds and the Grassmann distance between linear manifolds.

1. The Wasserstein distance measures small deformatoins between frames for sequences of volumetric images.
2. The Wasserstein distance represents the deformations in all modes while the Grassmann distance failed to represent the changes in mode 3 for the sequence of voxel images.
3. The Wasserstein distance of $p = \infty$ with the energy-based constraint is the best measurement for capturing the small difference between frames in a sequence.

5   Conclusions

We have reviewed several fundamental and well-established methodologies in pattern recognition to unify data processing for higher-dimensional spaces using tensor expressions and tensor PCA. Since organs, cells and microstructures in cells dealt with in biomedical image analysis are volumetric data, for the quantitative discrimination of such volumetric data, we have developed distance metrics using tensor principal component analysis for multiway array data, which express sampled data of volumetric data.

This research was supported by the "Multidisciplinary Computational Anatomy and Its Application to Highly Intelligent Diagnosis and Therapy" project funded by a Grant-in-Aid for Scientific Research on Innovative Areas from MEXT, Japan, and by Grants-in-Aid for Scientific Research funded by the Japan Society for the Promotion of Science.

Appendix

Image SVD (imageSVD) [8,9] for the image array $\boldsymbol{X} \in \mathbf{R}^{m \times n}$ establishes the decomposition

$$\boldsymbol{X} = \boldsymbol{U}\boldsymbol{X}\boldsymbol{V}^\top + \boldsymbol{E},$$

where $\boldsymbol{U}\boldsymbol{X}\boldsymbol{V}^\top$ has low-rank and $\boldsymbol{E}$ is the residual error. This decomposition is performed by minimising $|\boldsymbol{E}|_F^2$ with respect to the conditions

$$\boldsymbol{U}^\top\boldsymbol{U} = \begin{pmatrix} \boldsymbol{I}_k, \boldsymbol{O} \\ \boldsymbol{O}, \boldsymbol{O} \end{pmatrix}, \quad \boldsymbol{V}^\top\boldsymbol{V} = \begin{pmatrix} \boldsymbol{I}_l, \boldsymbol{O} \\ \boldsymbol{O}, \boldsymbol{O} \end{pmatrix}$$

for $k \le m$ and $l \le n$. Eigenmatrices of $\boldsymbol{X}\boldsymbol{X}^\top$ and $\boldsymbol{X}^\top\boldsymbol{X}$ derive matrices $\boldsymbol{U}$ and $\boldsymbol{V}$, respectively.

For a collection of $m \times n$ matrices $\{\boldsymbol{X}_i\}_{i=1}^N$, where $N \gg \max(m, n)$, we assume that

$$\frac{1}{N} \sum_{i=N} \boldsymbol{X}_i = \boldsymbol{O}.$$

The matrix PCA derives a pair of matrices $\boldsymbol{U}$ and $\boldsymbol{V}$ by minimising the criterion

$$J(\boldsymbol{U}, \boldsymbol{V}) = \frac{1}{N} \sum_{i=1}^N |\boldsymbol{X}_i - \boldsymbol{U}\boldsymbol{X}\boldsymbol{V}^\top|_F^2$$

with the constraints $\boldsymbol{U}^\top\boldsymbol{U} = \boldsymbol{I}_m$ and $\boldsymbol{V}^\top\boldsymbol{V} = \boldsymbol{I}_n$. A pair of orthogonal matrices $\boldsymbol{U}$ and $\boldsymbol{V}$ are eigenmatrices of

$$\boldsymbol{M} = \sum_{i=1}^N \boldsymbol{X}_i\boldsymbol{X}_i^\top, \quad \boldsymbol{N} = \sum_{i=1}^N \boldsymbol{X}_i^\top\boldsymbol{X}_i.$$

For a pair of $k \times m \times n$ three-ways $\boldsymbol{F} = ((f_{\alpha\beta\gamma}))$ and $\boldsymbol{G} = ((g_{\alpha\beta\gamma}))$, Euclidean distance d_E and the transportation d_T of intensities are

$$d_E(\boldsymbol{F}, \boldsymbol{G})^2 = \sum_{\alpha=1}^k \sum_{\beta=1}^m \sum_{\gamma=1}^n |f_{\alpha\beta\gamma} - g_{\alpha\beta\gamma}|^2$$

$$d_T(\boldsymbol{F}, \boldsymbol{G})^2 = \min_{c_{\alpha\alpha'\beta\beta'\gamma\gamma'}} \sum_{\alpha\,\alpha'=1}^k \sum_{\beta\,\beta'=1}^m \sum_{\gamma\,\gamma'=1}^n k_{\alpha\beta\gamma}^{\alpha'\beta'\gamma'} c_{\alpha\alpha'\beta\beta'\gamma\gamma'}$$

with respect to

$$g_{\alpha'\beta'\gamma'} \ge \sum_{\alpha=1}^k \sum_{\beta=1}^m \sum_{\gamma=1}^n c_{\alpha\alpha'\beta\beta'\gamma\gamma'}, \quad f_{\alpha\beta\gamma} \ge \sum_{\alpha'=1}^k \sum_{\beta'=1}^m \sum_{\gamma'=1}^n c_{\alpha\alpha'\beta\beta'\gamma\gamma'}, \quad c_{\alpha\alpha'\beta\beta'\gamma\gamma'} \ge 0$$

for $k_{\alpha\beta\gamma}^{\alpha'\beta'\gamma'} = |f_{\alpha\beta\gamma} - g_{\alpha'\beta'\gamma'}|^2$.

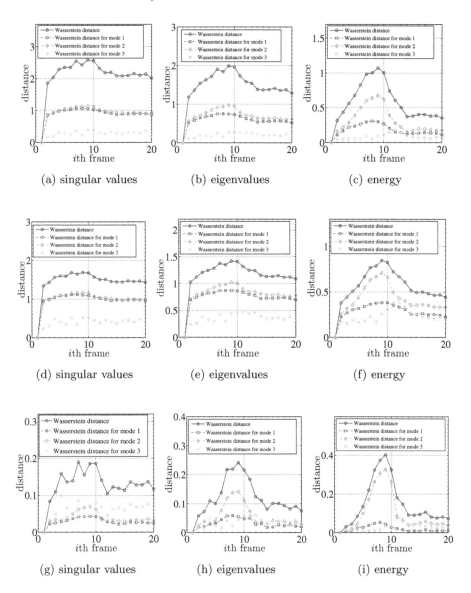

Fig. 3. Wasserstein distances between the first and jth frames in sequence of volumetric images. We use the sum of the singular values, the sum of the eigenvalues and the energy for constraints. The left, middle and right columns show the distances for the case of using sum of the singular values, sum of the eigenvalues and the energy, respectively, for constraints. The top, middle and bottom rows show the distances for $p = 1, 2, \infty$, respectively. The vertical axis represents the distance between frames. The horizontal axis represents the number j of the target frame.

References

1. Jordan, C.: Essai sur la géométrie àn n dimensions. Bull. Soc. Math. France **3**, 103–174 (1875)
2. Afriat, S.N.: Orthogonal and oblique projectors and the characterisation of pairs of vector spaces. Math. Proc. Cambridge Philos. Soc. **53**, 800–816 (1957)
3. Knyazev, A.V., Argentati, M.E.: Principal angles between subspaces in an a-based scalar product: algorithms and perturbation estimates. SIAM J. Sci. Comput. **23**, 2009–2041 (2002)
4. Cock, K.D., Moor, B.D.: Subspace angles between ARMA models. Syst. Control Lett. **46**, 265–270 (2002)
5. Villani, C.: Optimal Transport: Old and New. Grundlehren der mathematischen Wissenschaften. Springer, Heidelberg (2009). https://doi.org/10.1007/978-3-540-71050-9
6. Stiefel, E.: Richtungsfelder und Fernparallelismus in n-dimensionalen Mannigfaltigkeiten. Comment. Math. Helv. **8**, 305–353 (1935)
7. Hansen, P.-C.: Discrete Inverse Problems: Insight and Algorithms. SIAM, Philadelphia (2010)
8. Hansen, P.-C., Nagy, J.G., O'Leary, D.P.: Deblurring Images: Matrices, Spectra, and Filtering. SIAM, Philadelphia (2006)
9. Chung, J., Knepper, S., Nagy, J.: Large-scale inverse problems in imaging. In: Scherzer, O. (ed.) Handbook of Mathematical Methods in Imaging, pp. 43–86. Springer, New York (2011). https://doi.org/10.1007/978-0-387-92920-0_2
10. Iijima, T.: Pattern Recognition, Corona-sha (1974). (in Japanese)
11. Watanabe, S.: Pattern Recognition: Human and Mechanical. Wiley, Hoboken (1985)
12. Oja, E.: Subspace Methods of Pattern Recognition. Research Studies Press, Baldock (1983)
13. Otsu, N.: Mathematical Studies on Feature Extraction in Pattern Recognition, Researches of The Electrotechnical Laboratory, 818 (1981). (in Japanese)
14. Grenander, U., Miller, M.: Pattern Theory: From Representation to Inference. OUP, Oxford (2007)
15. Malcev, A.: Foundations of Linear Algebra. In: Russian, Gostekhizdat, 1948. English translation, W. H. Freeman and Company, New York (1963)
16. Cichocki, A., Zdunek, R., Phan, A.-H., Amari, S.: Nonnegative Matrix and Tensor Factorizations: Applications to Exploratory Multi-way Data Analysis and Blind Source Separation. Wiley, Hoboken (2009)
17. Itskov, M.: Tensor Algebra and Tensor Analysis for Engineers. ME. Springer, Cham (2015). https://doi.org/10.1007/978-3-319-16342-0
18. Mørup, M.: Applications of tensor (multiway array) factorizations and decompositions in data mining. Wiley Interdisc. Rev.: Data Min. Knowl. Disc. **1**, 24–40 (2011)
19. Kolda, T.G., Bader, B.W.: Tensor decompositions and applications. SIAM Review **51**, 455–500 (2009)
20. Itoh, H., Imiya, A., Sakai, T.: Approximation of N-way principal component analysis for organ data. In: Chen, C.-S., Lu, J., Ma, K.-K. (eds.) ACCV 2016. LNCS, vol. 10118, pp. 16–31. Springer, Cham (2017). https://doi.org/10.1007/978-3-319-54526-4_2
21. Edelman, A., Arias, T.A., Smith, S.T.: The geometry of algorithms with orthogonality constraints. SIAM J. Matrix Anal. Appl. **20**, 303–353 (1998)

22. Turaga, P., Veeraraghavan, A., Chellappa, R.: Statistical analysis on Stiefel and Grassmann manifolds with applications in computer vision. In: IEEE CVPR, pp. 1–8 (2008)

23. Kroonenberg, P.M.: Applied Multiway Data Analysis. Wiley, Hoboken (2008)

24. Marron, J.M., Alonso, A.M.: Overview of object oriented data analysis. Biometrical J. **56**, 732–753 (2014)

25. Ferrer, M., Valveny, E., Serratosa, F., Riesen, K., Bunke, H.: Generalized median graph computation by means of graph embedding in vector spaces. Pattern Recognit. **43**, 1642–1655 (2010)

26. Nye, T.M.W.: Principal component analysis in the space of phylogenetic trees. Ann. Stat. **39**, 2716–2739 (2011)

27. Fletcher, P., Lu, C., Pizer, S.M., Joshi, S.: Principal geodesic analysis for the study of nonlinear statistics of shape. IEEE TMD **23**, 995–1005 (2004)

28. Wong, Y.-C.: Differential geometry of Grassmann manifolds. Proc. Nat. Acad. Sci. **57**, 589–594 (1967)

29. Absil, P.-A., Mahony, R., Sepulchre, R.: Riemannian geometry of Grassmann manifolds with a view on algorithmic computation. Acta Applicandae Math. **80**, 199–220 (2004)

30. Hamm, J., Lee, D.D.: Grassmann discriminant analysis: a unifying view on subspace-based learning. In: Proceedings of the International Conference on Machine Learning, pp. 376–383 (2008)

31. Zhang, Z., Zha, H.: Principal manifolds and nonlinear dimension reduction via local tangent space alignment. SIAM J. Sci. Comput. **26**, 313–338 (2005)

32. Roweis, S.T., Saul, K.: Nonlinear dimensionality reduction by locally linear embedding. Science **290**, 2323–2326 (2000)

33. Andreopoulos, A., Tsotsos, J.K.: Efficient and generalizable statistical models of shape and appearance for analysis of cardiac MRI. Med. Image Anal. **12**, 335–357 (2008)

Organ-At-Risk Segmentation in Brain MRI Using Model-Based Segmentation: Benefits of Deep Learning-Based Boundary Detectors

Eliza Orasanu[1]([✉]), Tom Brosch[1], Carri Glide-Hurst[2], and Steffen Renisch[1]

[1] Philips Research, Hamburg, Germany
eliza.orasanu@philips.com
[2] Henry Ford Cancer Institute, Detroit, MI, USA

Abstract. Organ-at-risk (OAR) segmentation is a key step for radiotherapy treatment planning. Model-based segmentation (MBS) has been successfully used for the fully automatic segmentation of anatomical structures and it has proven to be robust to noise due to its incorporated shape prior knowledge. In this work, we investigate the advantages of combining neural networks with the prior anatomical shape knowledge of the model-based segmentation of organs-at-risk for brain radiotherapy (RT) on Magnetic Resonance Imaging (MRI). We train our boundary detectors using two different approaches: classic strong gradients as described in [4] and as a locally adaptive regression task, where for each triangle a convolutional neural network (CNN) was trained to estimate the distances between the mesh triangles and organ boundary, which were then combined into a single network, as described by [1]. We evaluate both methods using a 5-fold cross-validation on both T1w and T2w brain MRI data from sixteen primary and metastatic brain cancer patients (some post-surgical). Using CNN-based boundary detectors improved the results for all structures in both T1w and T2w data. The improvements were statistically significant ($p < 0.05$) for all segmented structures in the T1w images and only for the auditory system in the T2w images.

Keywords: Organ-at-risk brain segmentation
Model-based segmentation · Deep learning

1 Introduction

Organ-at-risk (OAR) segmentation is a key step for radiotherapy treatment planning. However, efficient and automated segmentation is still an unmet need. Manual delineation of these organs is a tedious process, time consuming, and prone to errors due to intra- and inter-observer variations.

Many automatic organ segmentation approaches work on a voxel-by-voxel basis by inspecting the local neighborhood of a voxel (e.g. region growing, front

© Springer Nature Switzerland AG 2018
M. Reuter et al. (Eds.): ShapeMI 2018, LNCS 11167, pp. 291–299, 2018.
https://doi.org/10.1007/978-3-030-04747-4_27

propagation, level sets etc., but also classification methods like decision forests or neural networks). However, those approaches are often prone to segmentation errors due to imaging artifacts. Another popular segmentation technique is model-based segmentation (MBS) [2]. With this technique a triangulated mesh representing the organ boundary is adapted to the medical image in a controlled way so that the general organ shape is preserved, thus regularizing the segmentation with prior anatomical knowledge. This makes the technique quite robust against many imaging artifacts. MBS usually uses simple features to detect organ boundaries, such as strong intensity gradients and a set of additional intensity-based constraints [4] or scale invariant feature transforms [5]. These features were proven to be reliable when used to segment well-defined grey values. Recent developments in deep learning have allowed the use of neural networks for boundary detection feature learning [1].

In this work, we propose to use an automatic model-based OAR segmentation to support MR-based treatment planning. We train our model features using two different boundary detection approaches: classic strong gradients as described in [4] and as a locally adaptive regression task, where for each triangle a convolutional neural network is trained to estimate the distance between the mesh and organ boundary, which are then combined into a single network, as described by [1]. We evaluate both methods using a 5-fold cross-validation on both T1-weighted (T1w) and T2-weighted (T2w) brain MRI data from sixteen primary and metastatic brain cancer patients (some post-surgical). CNN-based boundary detectors improve the results for all structures in both T1w and T2w data. The improvements were statistically significant ($p < 0.05$) for all segmented structures in the T1w images results and for the auditory system in the T2w images. Combining the strength and robustness of neural networks with the prior anatomical shape knowledge and shape regularisation of the model-based segmentation is a promising and powerful tool for organ segmentation.

2   Methods

In this section, we describe the basics of model-based segmentation and model development, as well as the data used and the two different trainings we performed.

2.1   Model-Based Segmentation

Model-based segmentation (MBS) is a popular segmentation framework. MBS was originally developed as a generic algorithm, but firstly applied mainly to cardiac applications [2], but has been widely used for a variety of other applications and modalities. The main idea of MBS is to adapt a triangulated surface mesh with a fixed number of vertices V and triangles T to an image.

This adaption is commonly performed in three steps: *Step 1: Shapefinder.* The first step places the surface mesh within the image to be segmented, using for example a Generalised Hough Transform. *Step 2: Parametric adaptation.* In the second step, global or local parametric transformations (rigid or affine) are applied to improve the alignment of the mesh to the image. *Step 3: Deformable adaption.* In the last step, the alignment of the mesh to the image is further improved by applying local mesh deformations.

The latter two steps are both based on triangle-specific features trained on reference populations. During segmentation, each mesh triangle detects an image boundary point along a search profile which is perpendicular to the triangle surface. Image segmentation is then achieved by aligning the mesh with the detected points. The adaptation of the image to the mesh is thus achieved by minimising the objective function E defined as:

$$E = E_{ext} + \alpha \cdot E_{int},\tag{1}$$

where E_{int} is the internal energy which attempts to minimise large deformations with respect to the mean mesh shape, E_{ext} is the external energy that attracts the mesh to the image boundary points and α is a parameter that balances the contribution of both E_{int} and E_{ext} [2].

2.2   Segmentation Model

The direct segmentation of the organs-at-risk is challenging due to variations in image orientation and due to image quality issues. Hence, we first segment the skull and hemispheres to provide an estimate of the initial location of OARs with respect to the other organs. The proposed head segmentation model is composed of triangle-based meshes for each individual structure to be segmented: skull; hemispheres; brainstem; optic nerves, globes, lenses, chiasm (optic system) and auditory system. To improve segmentation accuracy, we apply a hierarchical segmentation strategy, by segmenting larger-to-smaller structures. Hence, the skull is first segmented, providing a robust localisation of the head, after which the hemispheres are activated and segmented inside of the skull. Finally, the brainstem, and the remaining OARs are segmented.

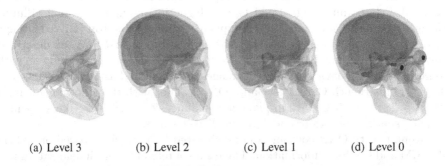

    (a) Level 3   (b) Level 2   (c) Level 1   (d) Level 0

Fig. 1. Head segmentation model with 4 different segmentation levels. Structures segmented include the skull, hemispheres and organs-at-risk

Image segmentation starts by adapting the model from the initial coarsest level to the image. This level is represented by a coarse mesh topology, i.e. only a few triangles are forming the mesh as shown in Fig. 1a. Then segmentation is refined by adapting the model of an intermediate level comprising more triangles (Fig. 1b). The next segmentation step includes an even finer representation of the skull being adapted, after which the hemispheres are also segmented (Fig. 1c). Lastly, the final and highest level of the segmentation is obtained of all structures present in the model: skull, hemispheres and organs-at-risk (Fig. 1d). The anatomical correspondence between the different level meshes is ensured by vertex correspondence look-up tables.

2.3 Boundary Detection

For each triangle, a boundary point is defined by searching along the triangle normal line. In the classical MBS, candidate points on the search line are evaluated using triangle-specific feature functions [4]. The candidate point with the strongest feature response is then selected as the boundary point [4].

Brosch et al. recently proposed that, instead of looking at discrete points along the search line, one can directly predict the signed distance of the centre of the triangle to the organ boundary using convolutional neural networks (CNN) [1]. This method was used in [1] for the segmentation of the prostate on T2w MRI data.

3 Experiments

3.1 Data and Ground Truth Generation

Sixteen primary and metastatic brain cancer patients (some post-surgical) underwent both CT-SIM and 1.0T MR-SIM (usual clinical protocol including T1-w and T2-w scans with resolutions of $0.9 \times 0.9 \times 1.25 \, \text{mm}^3$ and $0.7 \times 0.7 \times 2.5 \, \text{mm}^3$ respectively) within 1 week.

Patients were consented to an IRB-approved prospective protocol for imaging on a 1.0 T Panorama High Field Open Magnetic Resonance System (Philips Medical Systems, Cleveland, OH) equipped with flat table top (Civco, Orange City, IA) and external laser system (MR-simulation, or MR-SIM) as described previously. All brain MRI scans were acquired using an 8-channel head coil with no immobilization devices. Brain CT images were acquired using a Brilliance Big Bore (Philips Health Care, Cleveland, OH) scanner with the following settings: 120 kVp, 284 mAs, 512 × 512 in-plane image dimension, $0.8 - 0.9 \times 0.8 - 0.9 \, \text{mm}^2$ in-plane spatial resolution, and 1–3 mm slice thickness.

Ground truth OAR contours were delineated by physicians based on hybrid MR-SIM and CT-SIM information. The frame of reference for all delineation was the CT-SIM dataset, thus we resampled both MR T1w and T2w images into the CT space after elastic registration [3]. The references meshes were generated by adapting triangle-based model meshes to the physician-delineated contours. The reference meshes were further checked to assure consistency, especially for the optic lenses, which exhibit different locations between scans due to eye movement.

3.2 Model Training

We trained our model on both the T1-weighted and T2-weighted MRIs of the 16 subjects using a 5-fold cross-validation, and using two different trainings for the boundary detectors: classic gradient-based features ("classic" MBS) as described by [4] and the MBS with deep learning-based boundary detection (DL-MBS) as described by [1]. Both trainings of the boundary detectors are based on the method described in [4] used for selecting optimal boundary detectors from a large set of candidates, called Simulated Search. This method was further adapted for the CNN boundary detectors as described by [1]. Specifically, for each training iteration, mesh triangles were randomly and independently transformed using random translations along the triangle normal, small translations orthogonal to the triangle normal and small random rotations. Subvolumes were then extracted for each newly transformed triangle and the distance to the original reference mesh was computed. The network parameters in this case were optimised using stochastic gradient descent by minimising the root mean square error between the simulated distance and the predicted distance [1].

4 Results

We segmented the organs-at-risk in T1w and T2w brain MRI using the 2 different features on all 16 patients using a 5-fold cross validation. An example segmentation of both classic and DL-MBS on a T2w image is shown in Fig. 2.

Table 1. Mean and maximum distance (mm) per substructure over 16 subjects using 5-fold cross-validation on the T1w images using classic MBS and DL features. Note that 2 subjects presenting cataracts were excluded from both training and testing of the optic lenses.

Structure	Number of triangles	Mean distance (mm)		Maximum distance (mm)	
		Classic MBS	DL-MBS	Classic MBS	DL-MBS
Brainstem	6054	0.729	0.608	1.967	1.586
Optic globes	1002	0.853	0.563	2.133	1.447
Optic lenses	428	0.640	0.268	1.666	0.667
Chiasm and optic nerves	1263	0.729	0.410	1.990	1.089
Auditory system	2720	1.230	0.882	2.808	2.081

We computed the mean distance in mm between the segmentation and ground truth meshes as well as the maximum dista. Since the boundary between

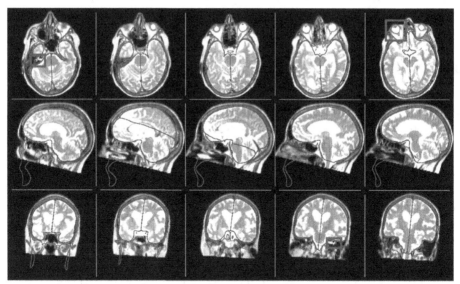

(a) classic MBS

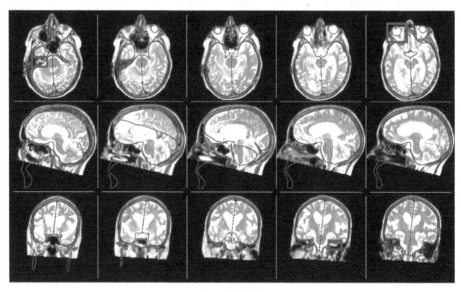

(b) DL-MBS

Fig. 2. Organs-at-risk segmentation of skull (red), hemispheres (blue), brainstem (orange), optic system (magenta) and auditory system (green). On T2w MR brain data using classic MBS and DL-MBS. It can be observed that DL-MBS provides a more robust segmentation, especially for smaller structures such as the optic lenses and auditory system, thus outperforming classic MBS. (Color figure online)

Table 2. Mean and maximum distance (mm) per substructure over 16 subjects using 5-fold cross-validation on the T2w images using classic MBS and DL features. Note that 2 subjects presenting cataracts were excluded from both training and testing of the optic lenses.

Structure	Number of triangles	Mean distance (mm)		Maximum distance (mm)	
		Classic MBS	DL-MBS	Classic MBS	DL-MBS
Brainstem	6054	0.564	0.557	1.542	1.507
Optic globes	1002	0.593	0.526	1.388	1.252
Optic lenses	428	0.752	0.674	1.554	1.568
Chiasm and optic nerves	1263	0.939	0.796	2.328	1.984
Auditory system	2720	1.163	0.639	2.764	1.640

the optic nerves and chiasm is not clearly defined in the MR images, we combined the two for the error analysis. The results are presented in Tables 1 and 2. The DL-MBS outperforms the classic MBS, giving smaller mean distances for both T1w and T2w over all structures of interest (organs-at-risk) investigated.

We performed a t-test to investigate if the differences between the classic MBS and DL-MBS are statistically significant. The difference T1w segmentation results between classic MBS and DL-MBS are statistically significant ($p < 0.05$) for all structures segmented, while for the T2w segmentation the results are statistically significant different ($p < 0.05$) only for the auditory system.

We plotted the maximum distance error for both feature training methods for th T1w (Fig. 3) and T2w (Fig. 4) on the organs-at-risk surfaces to investigate the regions were the segmentation presents the most differences. It can be observed that classic MBS is less consistent in segmenting the optical nerves and cochlea, especially in the T2w images with a lower resolution in the z-direction.

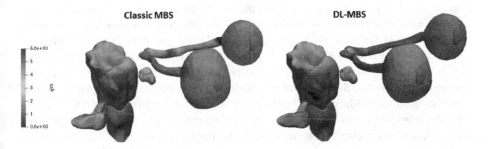

Fig. 3. Maximum segmentation error of the T1w MR images plotted on the organs-at-risk surfaces.

Classic MBS   **DL-MBS**

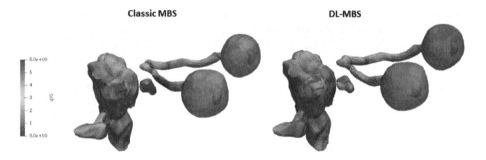

Fig. 4. Maximum segmentation error of the T2w MR images plotted on the organs-at-risk surfaces.

5   Discussion

In this paper, we investigated the advantages of combining neural networks with the prior anatomical shape knowledge of the model-based segmentation of organs-at-risk for brain RT on MRI. To that end, we trained and compared two boundary detectors for MBS using two different approaches: first using classic gradient-based features ("classic" MBS) [2] and then by using a convolutional neural network that predicts the organ boundary [1]. We validated the results on data from 16 brain cancer patients using a 5-fold cross-validation. The latter provided better segmentation results, with a smaller average distance between the ground truth and segmentation meshes for all organs-at-risk (brainstem, optic nerves, globes, lenses, chiasm, auditory system) on both T1w and T2w MR images, although statistically significant improvements were achieved only on the T1w data.

This work illustrates the strength of using neural networks for segmentation to support MR-based treatment planning in the brain. The CNN-based boundary detection was trained as it was done in [1], where the algorithm was developed and tested for prostate segmentation in T2-weighted images. Nonetheless, the method is also successful outside of the scope of the prostate segmentation, with its good results being translated also to brain segmentation, where it outperformed classic MBS segmentation. Results could be further improved in the future with small modifications to the training and/or network, in order to adapt it to the specific case of brain organs-at-risk segmentation, where the structures are small and their size is comparable to the image resolution.

We offer solutions to segment the skull, hemispheres and OARs (brainstem, optic nerves, globes, lenses, chiasm and auditory system). The skull segmentation currently has the main purpose of improving the robustness of the segmentation of the other structures, but it may also to be for the generation synthetic CT, the computed tomography substitute data set derived from MRI data and essential for treatment planning.

Furthermore, this study demonstrated the feasibility of developing automated OAR brain segmentation for MR-based treatment planning. Since the segmentation accuracy is below the voxel resolution, our results highlight the importance of acquiring data with high resolution to improve the accuracy of autosegmentation. One limitation of the current work might be the incompatibility of the immobilization masks with the MRI head coil, which may increase image registration uncertainty. Although in this work the images were acquired with dedicated MR-head coils, we hypothesis that the robustness of the CNN and regularising property of the model-based segmentation would provide an accurate segmentation even with an RT-compatible coil setup, with lower signal-to-noise ration. However, this hypothesis remains to be tested. Future work will also include using a broader database and to explore other body regions such as the head and neck.

References

1. Brosch, T., Peters, J., Groth, A., Stehle, T., Weese, J.: Deep learning-based boundary detection for model-based segmentation with application to MR prostate segmentation. In: Frangi, A.F., Schnabel, J.A., Davatzikos, C., Alberola-López, C., Fichtinger, G. (eds.) MICCAI 2018. LNCS, vol. 11073, pp. 515–522. Springer, Cham (2018). https://doi.org/10.1007/978-3-030-00937-3_59
2. Ecabert, O., et al.: Automatic model-based segmentation of the heart in CT images. IEEE Trans. Med. Imaging **27**(9), 1189–1201 (2008)
3. Kabus, S., Lorenz, C.: Fast elastic image registration. In: Proceedings of the Medical Image Analysis for the Clinic: A Grand Challenge, pp. 81–89 (2010)
4. Peters, J., Ecabert, O., Meyer, C., Kneser, R., Weese, J.: Optimizing boundary detection via simulated search with applications to multi-modal heart segmentation. Med. Image Anal. **14**(1), 70 (2010)
5. Yang, M., Yuan, Y., Li, X., Yan, P.: Medical image segmentation using descriptive image features. In: Proceedings of the British Machine Vision Conference, pp. 94.1–94.11 (2011)

Uncertainty Quantification in CNN-Based Surface Prediction Using Shape Priors

Katarína Tóthová[1][(✉)], Sarah Parisot[2], Matthew C. H. Lee[3],
Esther Puyol-Antón[4], Lisa M. Koch[1], Andrew P. King[4], Ender Konukoglu[1],
and Marc Pollefeys[1,5]

[1] ETH Zurich, Zürich, Switzerland
`katarina.tothova@inf.ethz.ch`
[2] Aimbrain Ltd., London, UK
[3] HeartFlow Inc., Redwood City, USA
[4] King's College London, London, UK
[5] Microsoft, Redmond, USA

Abstract. Surface reconstruction is a vital tool in a wide range of areas of medical image analysis and clinical research. Despite the fact that many methods have proposed solutions to the reconstruction problem, most, due to their deterministic nature, do not directly address the issue of quantifying uncertainty associated with their predictions. We remedy this by proposing a novel probabilistic deep learning approach capable of simultaneous surface reconstruction and associated uncertainty prediction. The method incorporates prior shape information in the form of a principal component analysis (PCA) model. Experiments using the UK Biobank data show that our probabilistic approach outperforms an analogous deterministic PCA-based method in the task of 2D organ delineation and quantifies uncertainty by formulating distributions over predicted surface vertex positions.

Keywords: Surface reconstruction · Uncertainty quantification
Deep learning · Shape prior

1 Introduction

Reconstruction of organ surfaces and segmentation of their bodies are amongst the most important tasks in medical image analysis. High-quality organ surface models are often sought after in disciplines such as cardiac or neuro-imaging, and provide a powerful tool in diagnosis, surgical planning, disease tracking, longitudinal studies and interpretation of functional data [1, 21, 22].

Traditional approaches to parametric surface modelling rely on evolving deformable shapes according to predefined forces [8, 11, 12, 23] or use atlas registration [2, 10, 21, 22]. Recent advances in machine learning have showed the possibility of training a deep neural network in an end-to-end manner: from images to parametrised shapes [19]. In their work, Milletari et al. [19] devised a convolutional neural network (CNN) to directly predict coordinates of the organ

© Springer Nature Switzerland AG 2018
M. Reuter et al. (Eds.): ShapeMI 2018, LNCS 11167, pp. 300–310, 2018.
https://doi.org/10.1007/978-3-030-04747-4_28

surface mesh from the imaging data. To build in prior shape knowledge, the network contains an explicit principal component analysis (PCA) layer and predictions are made as linear combinations of the modes of variation determined from the training data.

Despite the advances in organ surface modelling and associated segmentation, ways of estimating the precision of the prediction are still sparse. Yet, it is of vital importance for interpreting medical data to be able to not only measure the accuracy of the result as a deterministic sample but to quantify the uncertainty associated with it as well. We can distinguish between two types of uncertainty [14]: *aleatoric* uncertainty inherent to the data, modelled by probability distribution over model outputs, and *epistemic* uncertainty accounting for uncertainty in the model parameters, which typically decreases with increasing data size.

In the context of medical imaging, the need for addressing aleatoric uncertainty stems from the nature of the data. Medical imaging data often suffers from high levels of noise, coarse resolution and imaging artifacts - all the factors conspiring towards heightened need for quantification of uncertainty about the produced results. In image segmentation, this has been approached by means of segmentation sampling [6,17], where several plausible segmentations are gathered to estimate the variability of the output. While [6] uses MCMC to sample segmentations from an estimated posterior distribution where likelihood and prior functions are defined, [17] introduces Gaussian processes to sample from the posterior directly, knowing only its mean and covariance. On the other hand, uncertainties inherent to the prediction models can be captured by means of distributions over model parameters. Bayesian neural networks [7,9,18,20], where one puts priors over the model parameters instead of using deterministic values, have been employed to this end. Extensions combining both aleatoric and epistemic uncertainty into one model have been proposed in [14,16].

In our work, we build on a PCA-based method of surface reconstruction [19] and propose a probabilistic approach to integrate aleatoric uncertainty quantification within the model. We formulate the problem as a conditional probability estimation incorporating shape information in the form of a PCA model.

Hence, our approach addresses three main objectives:

- Direct probabilistic surface mesh prediction from imaging data. The proposed method improves upon a deterministic direct coordinate prediction by up to 12% on the UK BioBank dataset [25] as measured by DICE.
- Use of PCA-based shape priors to predict sensible shapes only. Here, our probabilistic approach improves upon the deterministic PCA-based method by up to 10.7% in terms of DICE score.
- Novel aleatoric uncertainty quantification formulation by means of assessing the posterior of the predicted surface.

2   Prediction Model

We formulate the surface prediction problem via a probabilistic model that utilises principles from probabilistic PCA [5]. Our goal is to build a model that goes beyond deterministic prediction and allows sampling 2D delineations of the organ surface based on the corresponding MRI data. To this end, we express the prediction as a probability conditioned on the image, $p(y|x)$, where x refers to the MRI image and y to the parametrised surface, i.e. set of surface vertices. We model the conditional probability $p(y|x)$ with a latent variable model

$$p(y|x) = \int p(y|z, x)p(z|x)dz, \tag{1}$$

where z is the set of latent variables.

The PCA aspect of the model lies within the definition of $p(y|z, x)$

$$p(y|z, x) = \mathcal{N}(y|US^{\frac{1}{2}}z + \mu + s(x), \sigma^2 I), \tag{2}$$

Here, U, μ and S are the principal component matrix (principal components are columns of the matrix), mean and diagonal covariance matrix respectively, all precomputed using the surfaces in the training set, and s is a global spatial shift that depends on the image x. In this formulation, the latent variable z can be interpreted as the PCA weights corresponding to the surface y. Variance σ^2 refers to the noise level in the data.

The conditioning to the image is modelled with $p(z|x)$ and we use a deep CNN architecture for this purpose. Specifically, we express

$$p(z|x) = \mathcal{N}(z|\mu(x), \Sigma(x)). \tag{3}$$

Here, a deep network takes the image x as input and predicts $\mu(x)$ and $\Sigma(x)$ simultaneously.

The last component of the proposed model is the prior for the latent variables $p(z)$. The probabilistic PCA model assumes a unit Gaussian distribution for the PCA weights, i.e. $p(z) \sim \mathcal{N}(0, I)$. In our model we assume the same, which becomes important when training the model.

Training. During training we optimise the parameters of $\mu(x)$, $\Sigma(x)$ and $s(x)$ using a training set. The optimisation objective consists of two terms: the first one aims to maximise the conditional probability $p(y|x)$ while the latter regularises the loss by minimising the Kullback-Leibler divergence (KLD) between the assumed prior distribution of z and the observed one in the training set, i.e. $\int p(z|x)p(x)dx \approx \sum_x p(z|x)$.

Direct maximisation of Eq. 1 requires marginalisation of the latent variable. The marginal distribution is also Gaussian with analytical mean and variance that allow direct computation and therefore, optimisation of $\ln p(y|x)$. However, this requires inverting a not-necessarily-diagonal covariance matrix of the size (num of vertices)^2 at each iteration, which can be infeasible due to the size and potential numerical instabilities, as we empirically observed. Therefore, instead of directly maximising $\ln p(y|x)$, we use Jensen's inequality to derive a lower bound as follows

$$\ln p(y|x) \geq \mathbb{E}_{z|x}\left[\ln p(y|z)\right] \cong \frac{1}{L}\sum_{l=1}^{L}\ln p(y|z_l), \tag{4}$$

where z_l is sampled from $p(z|x)$ defined in (3).

Maximisation of the lower bound in Eq. 4 will not necessarily satisfy the prior in the probabilistic PCA model. To address this, we use a regularisation term that aims to align the observed latent variable distribution with its prior. In order to satisfy the PCA model

$$p(z) \cong \sum p(z|x_n), \qquad x_n \sim p(x). \tag{5}$$

We use the KLD as a measure of deviation from this criteria and minimise

$$\mathrm{KLD}\left(\sum_{n=1}^{N} p(z|x_n), p(z) \right) \tag{6}$$

Using (4) and (6), our full model can then be trained by solving the following minimisation problem:

$$\min_{\theta} \left\{ \lambda\,\mathrm{KLD}\left(\sum_{n=1}^{N} p(z|x_n), p(z) \right) - \sum_{n=1}^{N} \frac{1}{L} \sum_{l=1}^{L} \ln p(y|z_l) \right\}, \tag{7}$$

where $z_l \sim \mathcal{N}(z|\mu(x_n), \Sigma(x_n))$ and λ is a regularisation parameter. For further details on the derivations please refer to Appendix A.

Inference. As we mentioned previously, in the proposed model $p(y|x)$ is a Gaussian distribution. For a given test image, we perform prediction by computing the mean and the covariance matrix of this distribution.

Given (2) and (3) we can write

$$\mathbb{E}(y|x) = U S^{\frac{1}{2}} \mu(x) + \mu + s, \tag{8}$$

$$\mathrm{var}(y|x) = \sigma^2 I + U S^{\frac{1}{2}} \Sigma(x) (U S^{\frac{1}{2}})^T. \tag{9}$$

Note that the first term of the predicted variance, i.e. $\sigma^2 I$, represents a fixed noise level in the data. Full derivation can be found in Appendix B.

3   Experiments and Results

We have tested the proposed method on a task of delineation of myocardium boundaries in cardiac MRI using imaging volumes from UK BioBank [25]. The 2D surface reconstruction consisting of the prediction of 50 vertices was evaluated on small (60×60 crops around the heart) and full (200×200 crops) field of view (FOV) images with the following characteristics:

- Small FOV: isotropic pixel of size 1.8 mm; 572 training, 160 testing and 195 validation examples
- Full FOV: isotropic pixel of size 1.8269 mm; 1532 training, 455 testing and 499 validation examples

Table 1. Vertex coordinate regression results. Comparison of direct vertex prediction (Direct Vertex), deterministic PCA (detPCA) and our proposed probabilistic PCA-based approach (probPCA) with varying number of principal components. Segmentations used for computation of DICE were obtained by flooding the corresponding delineations. RMSE directly compares the predicted vertex coordinates to the reference ones.

Small FOV	DICE	RMSE	Full FOV	DICE	RMSE
Direct Vertex	0.86 ± 0.06	2.21 ± 1.04	Direct Vertex	0.75 ± 0.14	4.20 ± 2.82
detPCA 12	0.87 ± 0.07	2.42 ± 1.27	detPCA 12	0.78 ± 0.13	4.20 ± 2.65
detPCA 8	0.84 ± 0.07	2.51 ± 1.26	detPCA 8	0.75 ± 0.14	4.48 ± 2.69
Ours:			*Ours:*		
probPCA 12	$\mathbf{0.88 \pm 0.09}$	1.91 ± 1.05	probPCA 12	$\mathbf{0.84 \pm 0.10}$	$\mathbf{2.59 \pm 2.37}$
probPCA 8	$\mathbf{0.88 \pm 0.09}$	$\mathbf{1.80 \pm 0.97}$	probPCA 8	0.84 ± 0.11	2.60 ± 2.38

We used one imaging slice per original MRI volume. Active contours [13] delineations consisting of 50 connected (corresponding throughout the subjects) vertices were obtained from reference segmentations extracted from the UK BioBank dataset. These were prepared automatically using expert-segmentations and combination of learning and registration methods described in [3,24].

The deep network architecture used in our model is analogous to the main branch described in [19] with 9 convolutional, 3 pooling and one dense layer (CL9P3DL1). Convolutional layers were followed by ReLU activations. Training was done by minimising loss (7) using RMS-Prop optimiser with a constant learning rate 10^{-6} for batches of size 5. Noise level in the data σ^2 and regularisation parameter λ were empirically set to $\sigma^2 = 5 \times 10^{-2}$ and $\lambda = 10^5$.

Table 1 shows evaluation of segmentations obtained from myocardium delineation in terms of DICE score measuring region overlap and Root Mean Square Error (RMSE) comparing distances between the corresponding predicted and reference vertices. We used two different methods as baselines for comparison. Firstly, a network with the same architecture as the one employed in our model (CL9P3DL1) was used to directly predict the coordinates of the surface vertices (Direct Vertex). Secondly, we utilised the deterministic PCA approach (detPCA) based on [19] again following the same architecture (without the spatial transformer refinement). For our method, the mean prediction $\mathbb{E}(y|x)$ served for computation of DICE scores and RMSE.

Working on the small FOV dataset, we exemplify the qualitative results of our probabilistic method in Fig. 1. Here, $p(y|x)$ distributions of predicted vertices are illustrated by plotting their variance as 30% confidence ellipses along the predicted mean delineation. We only plot the 30% confidence intervals and show results for small FOV for visualization purposes. Notice how direction and size of the ellipses vary along the perimeter of the shape - the larger the variance the bigger the uncertainty over the position of the vertex that can be sampled from this distribution.

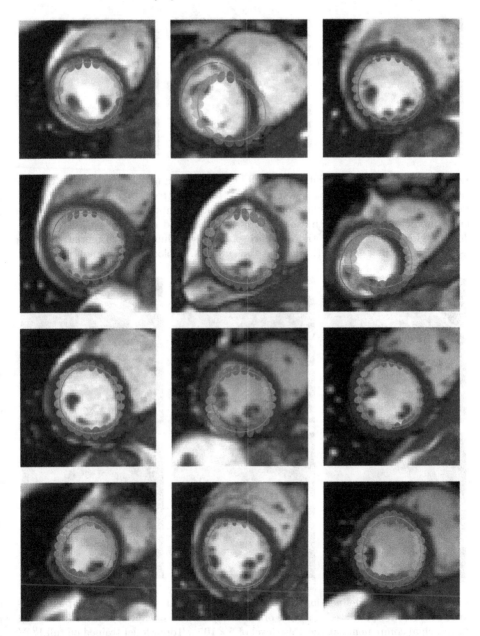

Fig. 1. Uncertainty quantification in small FOV myocardium delineations using 12 principal components at data noise level 5×10^{-2}: 30% confidence ellipses for points along the mean prediction. Colours correspond to the direction of the major axes. Only half of the points were plotted for clarity. (Color figure online)

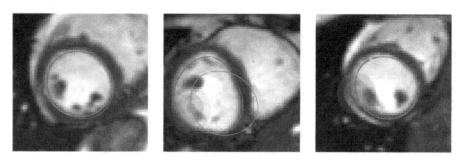

Fig. 2. Uncertainty quantification in small FOV myocardium delineation using 12 principal components at data noise level 5×10^{-2}: reference (red), predicted mean (cyan). Posterior distribution of specific points from predictions above (reference point and its mean prediction marked with a dot). Ellipses correspond to 30, 95 and 99.9% confidence regions. Observe how the reference point lies within the 99.9% area. Note we used corresponding vertices throughout the subjects. (Color figure online)

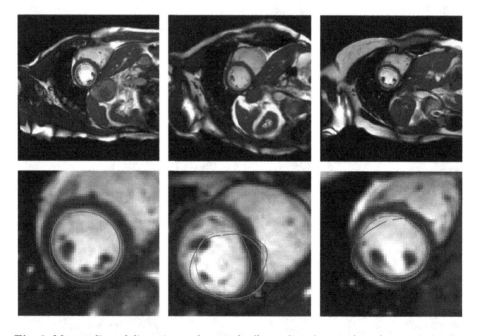

Fig. 3. Myocardium delineation: reference (red), predicted mean (cyan), sampled delineation (blue). We predicted positions of 50 vertices on the outline of myocardium using 12 principal components at the noise level of 5×10^{-2}. Top: Model trained on full FOV images. Bottom: Model trained on small FOV images. (Color figure online)

Figure 2 looks into the distribution of a specific vertex position in more detail. It essentially shows three types of results. On the left, we have high region overlap with high DICE (0.93) score, and relatively small variance; however large RMSE (3.23), which can lead to problems if one was to use the retrieved surface for e.g. registration purposes. The middle figure is a failure case with high variance, low DICE (0.66) and high RMSE (6.12). And finally on the right is a result with high DICE (0.92) and low RMSE (0.83), but higher uncertainty than in the first case. Several conclusions can be drawn from this. Firstly, failure to predict the correct delineation leads to heightened uncertainty about the prediction. Secondly, what may seem as a good solution in terms of overlap (and hence DICE) may not necessarily be ideal in terms of RMSE. While delineations may align, the corresponding vertices may not. Lastly, even if the corresponding points do not align, the uncertainty over their position may still be relatively low (compare images on the left and right in Fig. 2).

Finally, Fig. 3 illustrates results of the sampling process on full and small FOV images. Bottom row images here correspond to the cases outlined in Fig. 2. Observe how the samples become more variable as the uncertainty grows through subjects.

4   Conclusion

In this paper, we presented a novel probabilistic deep learning approach for simultaneous surface reconstruction and aleatoric uncertainty prediction. Inspired by the works on deterministic shape models [19] and probabilistic PCA [5], our surface reconstruction method incorporates prior shape knowledge via a linear PCA model. Experiments using the UK Biobank data have shown that our probabilistic approach outperforms an analogous deterministic PCA-based method. In contrast to deterministic approaches, which provide a single surface, our method yields a distribution of positions for every vertex on the surface. This way, we can not only sample numerous predictions from one model, but ascertain the vital uncertainty pertinent to each prediction.

Providing uncertainty estimations is essential in the medical domain, and in particular for surgery planning where precision and accuracy are of utmost importance. While the proposed method is capable of producing surface predictions of healthy 2D cardiac data, we intend to extend it to more challenging scenarios in the future. The aim is to generalise to 3D setting and other types of organs as well. Extensions to organs of more variable shapes may require adaptation of the shape model. Finally, transfer learning or domain adaptation techniques could be investigated to apply the proposed approach to datasets of substantially smaller size.

Acknowledgements. This research has been conducted using the UK Biobank Resource under Application Number 17806.

Appendix A

4.1   Posterior

From (2)

$$p(y|z, x) = \mathcal{N}(y| \underbrace{US^{\frac{1}{2}}z + \mu + s(x)}_{:=A}, \underbrace{\sigma^2 I}_{:=\Sigma}), \tag{10}$$

and Jensen's inequality we have

$$\ln p(y|x) \geq \int \ln[p(y|z)]p(z|x)dz = \mathbb{E}_{z|x}\left[\ln p(y|z)\right] \tag{11}$$

$$\cong \frac{1}{L}\sum_{l=1}^{L}\ln p(y|z_l), \tag{12}$$

where z_l is sampled from $p(z|x) = \mathcal{N}(z|\mu(x), \Sigma(x))$ and $\mu(x)$, $\Sigma(x)$ are provided by the network. In detail this translates to

$$\frac{1}{L}\sum_{l=1}^{L}\ln p(y|z_l) = \frac{1}{L}\sum_{l=1}^{L} -\frac{1}{2}\left\{r\ln(2\pi) + \ln|\Sigma| + (y - A)^T\Sigma^{-1}(y - A)\right\}, \tag{13}$$

r is the dimensionality of the vector y. In practice this value is summed over a batch of input vectors x_n. Note that to sample from $p(z|x)$ we employ the so-called "reparametrisation trick" [15], where we first sample $\epsilon \sim \mathcal{N}(0, I)$ and then compute $z_l = \mu(x) + \Sigma^{1/2}(x) * \epsilon$.

4.2   Regularisation

Considering

$$p(z) = \int p(z|x)p(x)dx \tag{14}$$

$$\cong \sum p(z|x_n), \qquad x_n \sim p(x), \tag{15}$$

the unitary Gaussian prior on z and the fact that

$$\mathrm{KLD}(p||q) = \mathbb{E}_p\left[\ln\frac{p(z)}{q(z)}\right] \tag{16}$$

$$\cong \sum_l (\ln p(z_l) - lnq(z_l)), \qquad z_l \sim p \tag{17}$$

we write

$$\mathrm{KLD}\left(\sum_{n=1}^{N} p(z|x_n), p(z)\right) \cong \frac{1}{L}\sum_l \left\{\underbrace{\ln\left[\sum_{n=1}^{N} p(z_l|x_n)\right]}_{:=LNP} \underbrace{-\ln[\mathcal{N}(0, I)]}_{:=LNQ}\right\} \tag{18}$$

where $\mu_n = \mu(x_n)$ and $\Sigma_n = \Sigma(x_n)$. Furthermore,

$$LNP = \ln\left[\sum_n \frac{1}{\sqrt{((2\pi)^s|\Sigma_n|)}}e^{-\frac{1}{2}(z_l-\mu_n)^T\Sigma_n^{-1}(z_l-\mu_n)}\right] \tag{19}$$

and

$$LNQ = -\left[-\frac{s}{2}\ln(2\pi) - \frac{z^Tz}{2}\right] = \frac{1}{2}\left[s\ln(2\pi) + z^Tz\right], \tag{20}$$

with s equal to the dimensionality of the latent space.

Appendix B

We obtain the posterior distribution of our vertex coordinates as follows. Given

$$p(y|z, x) = \mathcal{N}(y|US^{\frac{1}{2}}z + \mu + s(x), \sigma^2 I), \tag{21}$$

and

$$p(z|x) = p(z|\mu(x), \Sigma(x)), \tag{22}$$

we can write

$$
\begin{aligned}
\mathbb{E}(y|x) &= \mathbb{E}(\mathbb{E}(y|z)|x) \\
&= \mathbb{E}(US^{\frac{1}{2}}z + \mu + s|x) \\
&= \int (US^{\frac{1}{2}}z + \mu + s)p(z|x)dz \\
&= US^{\frac{1}{2}}\mathbb{E}(z|x) + \mu + s \\
&= US^{\frac{1}{2}}\mu(x) + \mu + s.
\end{aligned}
$$

As for the variance,

$$
\begin{aligned}
\text{var}(y|x) &= \mathbb{E}(\text{var}(y|z)|x) + \text{var}(\mathbb{E}(y|z)|x) \\
&= \sigma^2 I + \text{var}(US^{\frac{1}{2}}z + \mu + s|x) \\
&= \sigma^2 I + \text{var}(US^{\frac{1}{2}}z|x) \\
&= \sigma^2 I + US^{\frac{1}{2}}\text{var}(z|x)(US^{\frac{1}{2}})^T \\
&= \sigma^2 I + US^{\frac{1}{2}}\Sigma(x)(US^{\frac{1}{2}})^T.
\end{aligned}
$$

References

1. Bai, W., et al.: Automated cardiovascular magnetic resonance image analysis with fully convolutional networks. arXiv preprint, arXiv:1710.09289 (2017)
2. Bai, W., et al.: A probabilistic patch-based label fusion model for multi-atlas segmentation with registration refinement: application to cardiac MR images. IEEE Trans. Med. Imaging **32**(7), 1302–1315 (2013)
3. Bai, W., et al.: Semi-supervised learning for network-based cardiac MR image segmentation. In: Descoteaux, M., Maier-Hein, L., Franz, A., Jannin, P., Collins, D.L., Duchesne, S. (eds.) MICCAI 2017. LNCS, vol. 10434, pp. 253–260. Springer, Cham (2017). https://doi.org/10.1007/978-3-319-66185-8_29
4. Baumgartner, C.F., Koch, L.M., Pollefeys, M., Konukoglu, E.: An exploration of 2D and 3D deep learning techniques for cardiac MR image segmentation. In: Pop, M., et al. (eds.) STACOM 2017. LNCS, vol. 10663, pp. 111–119. Springer, Cham (2018). https://doi.org/10.1007/978-3-319-75541-0_12
5. Bishop, C.M.: Pattern Recognition and Machine Learning. Springer, Singapore (2006)

6. Chang, J., Fisher III, J.W.: Efficient MCMC sampling with implicit shape representations. In: 2011 IEEE Conference on Computer Vision and Pattern Recognition (CVPR), pp. 2081–2088. IEEE (2011)
7. Denker, J., LeCunn, Y.: Transforming neural-net output levels to probability distributions. In: Advances in Neural Information Processing Systems 3. Citeseer (1991)
8. Fischl, B.: Freesurfer. Neuroimage **62**, 774–781 (2012)
9. Gal, Y.: Uncertainty in Deep Learning. University of Cambridge, Cambridge (2016)
10. Garcia-Barnes, J., et al.: A normalized framework for the design of feature spaces assessing the left ventricular function. IEEE Trans. Med. Imaging **29**(3), 733–745 (2010)
11. Han, X., et al.: CRUISE: cortical reconstruction using implicit surface evolution. Neuroimage **23**, 997–1012 (2004)
12. Huo, Y., et al.: Consistent cortical reconstruction and multi-atlas brain segmentation. NeuroImage **138**, 197–210 (2016)
13. Kass, M., Witkin, A., Terzopoulos, D.: Snakes: active contour models. Int. J. Comput. Vis. **1**(4), 321–331 (1988)
14. Kendall, A., Gal, Y.: What uncertainties do we need in bayesian deep learning for computer vision. In: Advances in Neural Information Processing Systems 30 (NIPS 2017), pp. 5574–5584. Curran Associates (2017)
15. Kingma, D.P., Welling, M.: Auto-encoding variational bayes. In: ICLR (2014)
16. Kwon, Y., et al.: Uncertainty quantification using bayesian neural networks in classification: application to ischemic stroke lesion segmentation. In: Medical Imaging with Deep Learning (MIDL 2018) (2018, preprint)
17. Lê, M., Unkelbach, J., Ayache, N., Delingette, H.: Sampling image segmentations for uncertainty quantification. Med. Image Anal. **34**, 42–51 (2016)
18. MacKay, D.J.C.: A practical Bayesian framework for backpropagation networks. Neural Comput. **4**(3), 448–472 (1992)
19. Milletari, F., Rothberg, A., Jia, J., Sofka, M.: Integrating statistical prior knowledge into convolutional neural networks. In: Descoteaux, M., Maier-Hein, L., Franz, A., Jannin, P., Collins, D.L., Duchesne, S. (eds.) MICCAI 2017. LNCS, vol. 10433, pp. 161–168. Springer, Cham (2017). https://doi.org/10.1007/978-3-319-66182-7_19
20. Neal, R.M.: Bayesian Learning for Neural Networks. University of Toronto, Toronto (1995)
21. Peressutti, D., et al.: A framework for combining a motion atlas with non-motion information to learn clinically useful biomarkers: application to cardiac resynchronisation therapy response prediction. Med. Image Anal. **35**, 669–684 (2017)
22. Puyol-Antón, E., et al.: A multimodal spatiotemporal cardiac motion atlas from MR and ultrasound data. Med. Image Anal. **40**, 96–110 (2017)
23. Schuh, A., et al.: A deformable model for the reconstruction of the neaonatal cortex. In: IEEE 14th International Symposium on Biomedical Imaging (ISBI 2017). IEEE (2017)
24. Sinclair, M., Bai, W., Puyol-Antón, E., Oktay, O., Rueckert, D., King, A.P.: Fully automated segmentation-based respiratory motion correction of multiplanar cardiac magnetic resonance images for large-scale datasets. In: Descoteaux, M., et al. (eds.) MICCAI 2017. LNCS, vol. 10434, pp. 332–340. Springer, Cham (2017). https://doi.org/10.1007/978-3-319-66185-8_38
25. UK BioBank Homepage. https://www.ukbiobank.ac.uk/about-biobank-uk. Accessed 24 June 2018

Author Index

Printed in the United States
By Bookmasters